# A Practical Guide to
# Joint & Soft Tissue Injections

## Third Edition

**James W. McNabb, MD**
Private Practice—Family Medicine
Full Circle Family Medicine of Piedmont HealthCare
Mooresville, North Carolina

Wolters Kluwer
Philadelphia • Baltimore • New York • London
Buenos Aires • Hong Kong • Sydney • Tokyo

*Executive Editor*: Rebecca Gaertner
*Senior Product Development Editor*: Kristina Oberle
*Production Project Manager*: David Saltzberg
*Marketing Manager*: Stephanie Manzo
*Design Coordinator*: Doug Smock
*Senior Manufacturing Coordinator*: Beth Welsh
*Prepress Vendor*: SPi Global



9 8 7 6

Printed in China

---

**Library of Congress Cataloging-in-Publication Data**
McNabb, James W., author.
[Practical guide to joint & soft tissue injection & aspiration]
A practical guide to joint & soft tissue injections : an illustrated text for primary care providers / James W. McNabb. — Third edition.
p. ; cm.
Preceded by A practical guide to joint & soft tissue injection & aspiration / James W. McNabb. 2nd ed. 2010.
Includes bibliographical references and index.
ISBN 978-1-4511-8657-4 (alk. paper)
I. Title.
[DNLM: 1. Injections, Intra-Articular—methods. 2. Anesthesia, Local—methods. 3. Biopsy, Needle. 4. Injections—methods. 5. Joint Diseases—drug therapy. WB 354]
RC932
616.7'2—dc23

2014029297

---



LWW.com

CCS0719

This textbook is dedicated to my patients.

# Foreword

Medical delivery in the United States is rapidly changing. Multiple forces, including the implementation of the Affordable Care Act and the promotion of Patient Centered Medical Care, are calling on clinician's, in particular those who deliver primary care, to optimize treatment at the initial point of medical entry. Musculoskeletal disorders and complaints, in particular, are increasingly common with an aging population; many of whom remain active in recreational and competitive activities. In addition, new initiatives for improving patient-centered care regularly call on providers to confront pain as the "fifth vital sign," creating a need for office-specific and effective strategies to both diagnose and treat pain. Traditional systemic therapies addressing musculoskeletal disorders and pain, such as NSAIDs and narcotics, while effective in the short term, have inherent risks that are often compounded by individual patient comorbidities. Clinicians have the challenging task of balancing complications of these systemic therapies, such as gastric, renal, and cardiovascular morbidity, as well as potential addiction, with potential benefit. The need for targeted strategies, and alternative and integrative interventions, in the armamentarium and skill set for medical providers has never been greater.

The challenges identified in the preceding paragraph are a clear call for providers that have expertise in procedural training. Training programs, however, have in recent years faced their own challenges as there have been increasing demands for professional training, as well as limitations on time devoted to training with work hour restrictions. These limitations have created a "gap" in training with many providers seeking additional medical education programs outside of core professional training, including the utilization of professional CME courses, online training, and individual use of textbooks and DVDs. Dr. James McNabb has assisted in addressing this "gap" with his first two editions of *A Practical Guide to Joint & Soft Tissue Injection and Aspiration*. These texts have become landmark resources for both clinicians and training programs in their unparalleled ability to provide the student with what he or she needs to know to deliver care at the point of entry and improve the experience for both the patient and the provider. The second edition was a tremendous improvement over the first with the introduction of online high definition videos of the injection techniques as well as significant expansion of both injections and coding chapters.

The third edition builds on success of the first and second editions and provides the complete resource for the provider who administers injections. The third edition continues to build and expand on injection techniques and appropriate and current coding and covers new territory emerging in pain management. New chapters have been written on dry needling techniques, as well as local anesthesia. In his years of teaching for the AAFP, Dr. McNabb has been alerted to the deficits in training in the utilization of local anesthesia. The third edition has a detailed section that addresses the use of local anesthesia. Dr. McNabb's singular focus remains intact throughout the text as he is dedicated to assisting providers in delivering immediate relief of pain and dysfunction to patients in need.

In Medicine, many specialties identify core texts that are easily recognized and referred to by the original author's last name. Examples include **Harrison's** textbook of internal medicine, **Habif**'s textbook of dermatology, and **Sabiston's** textbook on surgery. In addition, few in the medical profession are unfamiliar with such classic's as **Cope's** approach to abdominal pain and **Sanford's** guide to antibiotic selection for infectious disease. In musculoskeletal medicine, there are many great textbooks that both primary care providers and orthopedic subspecialists reach to for readily available and current information, among those is Dr. McNabb's textbook. I have no doubt that this resource will emerge, if it has not already done so, as "the" resource on injection therapy for the MSK provider, and quite simply be referred to as **McNabb's**. I congratulate Dr. McNabb on yet again a wonderful contribution to our discipline, as I know this textbook will be an invaluable resource for providers and serve to improve care for thousands of patients.

Francis G. O'Connor, COL, MC, USA
Professor and Chair, Military and Emergency Medicine
Associate Director, Consortium for Health and Military Performance (CHAMP)
Uniformed Services University of the Health Sciences
"America's Medical School"

# Preface

"It was a dark and stormy night." I have always wanted to write a great melodramatic novel. However, I possess neither the time, talent, nor writing skill for that endeavor. Instead, I have borrowed this classic line from the Peanuts character, Snoopy, who was always going to write his great book. He in turn took this opening quote from the 1830 novel, *Paul Clifford* written by Edward Bulwer-Lytton.[1] When I was approached by the editors to write the third edition of this medical injection text, my only condition was that I begin with this phrase. I did not get their approval, but they also did not say no. I interpreted their response as an indication that I could take this project in a different direction from traditional musculoskeletal injection texts. I believe that the product of this work represents the spectrum of common, straightforward, effective, medical procedures that are performed with simple, inexpensive equipment in a variety of medical settings. Although written from the perspective of a practicing family physician in a busy private office, these procedures cross specialty lines. They may also be employed in settings as diverse as outpatient offices, urgent care centers, nursing homes, emergency rooms, and inpatient facilities. This text is also used in residency training programs and medical schools.

I am indeed fortunate to enjoy a professional career with a full-time practice of direct patient care at Full Circle Family Medicine. I truly am a simple country doctor, but also teach and write when I have time. While teaching musculoskeletal and dermatology courses, it has become evident that primary care providers' learning needs include procedures that extend beyond traditional musculoskeletal injections. For this reason, I have expanded the focus of this project to include more skin-related injections and to also include basic skin anesthesia techniques including facial nerve blocks. This text is meant to serve as an evidence-based, yet, practical guide for those providers who wish to learn the techniques and finer details of the most common needle-based procedures.

This edition is also an academically sound work. I have devoted a great deal of time and effort reviewing the peer-reviewed literature and citing references, where available. In recent years, there has been a significant expansion of basic science knowledge, discovery of additional medication toxicities, adoption of musculoskeletal ultrasound, and documentation of different techniques to access joint and soft tissue structures. I strongly advise that every provider using this text please read, study, and understand all of the information contained in the Foundation Concepts section BEFORE attempting to perform ANY of the procedures.

This third edition was infinitely more difficult to write and much more time consuming than even I anticipated. The challenge was to build on the success of the previous editions by expanding the content, while keeping the text truly relevant and accessible to practicing providers. This entire edition has been rewritten to incorporate recent information and add even more value. The first section titled Foundational Concepts updates and adds new information regarding medication toxicities, local anesthetics, injectable agents, musculoskeletal ultrasound, and others. A brand new section on Skin Anesthesia includes the administration of local anesthetics for direct local injection, field blocks, digital blocks, and facial nerve blocks. Skin and Skin Structures provides updated treatment of chalazions, keloids, and warts and presents corticosteroid intralesional treatment of both thin and thick benign, inflammatory dermatoses. The Head and Neck section updates existing chapters. The Upper Extremities section contains important updates of all injections, eliminates a carpal tunnel injection, includes a new preferred approach to treat CTS based on further understanding of the anatomy of the median nerve, and also adds a new section on digital mucous cysts. An important update has occurred in the Trunk section. The previous chapter on muscular trigger points has been replaced with a new, evidence-based chapter on myofascial trigger points documenting the preferred technique of "dry-needling." The Lower Extremities section has also been extensively rewritten with significant updates to the hip joint and knee joint chapters. A new chapter that provides a scientific overview of the different approaches and success rates for knee joint injections has also been added. The ancillary use of musculoskeletal ultrasound to guide these injections is emphasized.

Other features that add value include updated CPT, ICD-9 and ICD-10 codes. Examples of informed consent, aftercare instructions, and procedure documentation are found in the appendices. I am grateful to Wolters Kluwer Health for their commitment to improving the quality of this work by creating beautiful drawings that are consistent across all chapters.

High definition videos that demonstrate each procedure are included as part of this text. These are all case-based films that have been recorded in my office on real patients. Each gave their permission to use the images to advance medical education. A unique feature is that each of the videos is taken from the operator's viewpoint. This solidifies learning after the user reviews the background information, local anatomy, landmarks, and techniques for each procedure.

I would like to acknowledge the following people and organizations who taught, encouraged, and helped me write this text. This project is a culmination of 30 years of private practice and teaching. First, I must again thank my wife, Liz, for her support during my medical education, training, years of practice, teaching, and finally during the research and writing of this text. Without you I could never have done this. The leadership and faculty of family medicine residency training programs at the University of Wyoming – Casper, Scottsdale HealthCare, and Cabarrus Family Medicine were instrumental in allowing me to expand my knowledge base, develop sports medicine and procedural curricula, and build expertise in evidence-based medicine. My office staff has been great—putting up with my demands and politely getting out of my way when I rush down the hall with "another great idea" or carrying video camera equipment. Without the confidence of my patients, I would not have been able to achieve mastery of these techniques—for that I remain privileged to serve as your family physician. I must acknowledge the opportunity to teach the Joint Injections workshops for the American Academy and North Carolina Academy of Family Physicians and the Dermatologic Procedures workshops for National Procedures Institute over the last 15 years. Many thanks are directed to workshop participants for their involvement and honest feedback. Deserved recognition is extended to teaching faculty who have provided encouragement, support, and stimulated my thinking. These physicians include Drs. Richard Lord, Kevin Burroughs, Amrish Patel, Jack Pfenninger, Grant Fowler, Russ White, Gerald Admussen, Francis O'Connor, Joe Ruane, and A.J. Cianflocco. Special recognition is again extended to family physician, Dr. Roy "Chip" Watkins, who has served as my presentation partner for many of these workshops. Finally, a big thank you to those at Wolters Kluwer Health/Lippincott Williams & Wilkins. In particular, Kristina Oberle, Senior Product Development Editor, and Rebecca Gaertner, Executive Editor. They have treated me with the utmost professionalism, support and patience during the extremely long process of writing this third edition. To all involved, and so many more unintentionally left unnamed—Thank you!

Instead of a "dark and stormy night," let's make this a bright and sunny day!

---

[1] Lytton EB. *Paul Clifford*. New York: Cassell Pub. Co.; 1830:OCLC 19091989.

# Contents

## 7. TRUNK 161



## 8. LOWER EXTREMITIES 176



## APPENDIX 1: CONSENT FOR NEEDLE ASPIRATION AND/OR INJECTION 255

## APPENDIX 2: ASPIRATION AND INJECTION AFTERCARE HANDOUT 257

## APPENDIX 3: MEDICAL RECORD DOCUMENTATION 259

# Video Clips

Video clips of the following procedures can be found in the companion eBook edition.

## SKIN ANESTHESIA

Direct Local Injection
Field Block Local Injection
Digital Nerve Block
Supraorbital and Supratrochlear Nerve Blocks
Infraorbital Nerve Block
Mental Nerve Block
Mucosal Fold Block

## SKIN AND SKIN STRUCTURES

Chalazion
Keloid Scar
Common Warts
Granuloma Annulare and Other Thin, Benign, Inflammatory Dermatoses
Prurigo Nodularis and Other Thick, Benign, Inflammatory Dermatoses

## HEAD AND NECK

Temporomandibular Joint
Greater Occipital Neuralgia
Cervical Strain and Sprain

## UPPER EXTREMITIES

Subacromial Space Injection—Posterior Approach
Glenohumeral Joint—Posterior Approach
Glenohumeral Joint—Anterior Approach
Bicipital Tenosynovitis—Long Head
Cubital Tunnel Syndrome
Elbow Joint
Olecranon Bursitis
Lateral Epicondylitis
Medial Epicondylitis
Radial Nerve Entrapment
Carpal Tunnel Syndrome—Preferred Flexor Carpi Radialis Approach
Carpal Tunnel Syndrome—Traditional Approach
Wrist Joint
de Quervain Tenosynovitis
Dorsal Wrist Ganglion Cyst
Thumb Carpometacarpal Joint
Metacarpophalangeal Joint
Trigger Finger
Digital Mucous Cyst

## TRUNK

Myofascial Trigger Points
Suprascapular Neuropathy
Scapulothoracic Syndrome
Sacroiliac Joint

## LOWER EXTREMITIES

Hip Joint—Preferred Lateral Approach
Hip Joint—Anterior Approach
Piriformis Syndrome
Meralgia Paresthetica
Greater Trochanteric Pain Syndrome
Hip Adductor Tendonitis
Knee Joint—Preferred Lateral Suprapatellar Approach
Knee Joint—Lateral Midpatellar Approach
Knee Joint—Anteromedial and Anterolateral Approaches
Prepatellar Bursitis
Pes Anserine Syndrome
Iliotibial Band Friction Syndrome
Tibialis Posterior Tendonitis
Tarsal Tunnel Syndrome
Ankle Joint—Anterolateral Approach
Ankle Joint—Anteromedial Approach
Fibularis Brevis Tendonitis
Plantar Fasciitis
First Metatarsophalangeal Joint
Morton Interdigital Neuroma

# 1 Introduction

The performance of joint and soft tissue injections and aspirations is a valuable skill that can be mastered by primary care physicians and qualified medical providers. These procedures can help relieve pain and improve function for the patient, while at the same time, empowering the clinician, improving continuity of care, and decreasing health care costs. It is essential that these techniques be used thoughtfully and precisely—only after making the correct dermatologic or musculoskeletal diagnosis. This can be quite challenging at times but is no more difficult than diagnosing and treating any of the other many medical conditions that the primary care physician encounters on a daily basis. Learning how to confidently make an accurate diagnosis of these conditions is beyond the scope of this text.

Our primary consideration is the welfare of the patient. We must always endeavor to provide the best medical care at the least risk of harm. This can be achieved by developing a cognitive knowledge base along with an accompanying set of complementary procedural skills. In addition, our focus must remain on providing a positive patient experience. This involves the provision of a safe and supportive environment while ensuring a pain-free procedural experience. Patient satisfaction from a positive experience along with a good clinical outcome is the primary goal.

An important concept is that aspiration and injection therapy is not an end in itself. It is only one treatment option. The withdrawal of fluid or the precise deposition of a therapeutic agent is a temporary measure that is generally used as adjunctive therapy to other modalities. In many conditions, corticosteroid injection therapy used alone has been demonstrated to give short- to intermediate-term pain/functional relief, but no difference in long-term results. In these cases, initial injection treatment in combination with another treatment modality and activity modification gives patients optimal long-lasting results. Additional therapeutic options may include relative rest, compression, splinting/casting, ice, heat, ultrasound, stretching, physical therapy, and administration of other medications for pain control or even surgery. The performance of aspirations or injections alone, without correcting the underlying factors, is likely to result in recurrence if used without complementary treatment.

In this text, the following primary learning objectives are identified:

- Describe the indications and contraindications for each procedure.
- Review the current evidence-based medical literature.
- Select appropriate equipment/products for each injection or aspiration.
- Illustrate pertinent anatomic landmarks for each procedure.
- Demonstrate safe and effective technique.

2

# Foundation Concepts

*"The life so short, the craft so long to learn."*
—Hippocrates

## THOUGHTFUL CONSIDERATION

The evaluation and treatment of musculoskeletal conditions is a very important aspect of primary medical care. With improved understanding of anatomy, biomechanics, pathophysiology, and modern treatment options, the primary care provider is now in a position to make positive contributions to musculoskeletal patient care. Gone are the days when patients were treated with an oral nonsteroidal anti-inflammatory medication (NSAID) and ignored with the hope that the condition would heal itself. This text may be used to further understanding of techniques useful in the treatment of some of the most common musculoskeletal disorders as well as select skin conditions and anesthetic nerve blocks. As with any medical procedure, performing injections and aspirations places a great responsibility on the operator. These procedures should be done with a clear differential diagnosis and treatment plan in mind. They should never be performed indiscriminately. *Primum non nocere* or "first, do no harm" is one of the fundamental principles of medical care. Therefore, the physician is obligated to consider the indications, contraindications, weight of evidence in the medical literature, expected benefits, possible side effects, anticipated outcomes, diagnostic certainty, his or her personal experience with the procedure, clinical experience, the patient's response to previous interventions, and respect for the patient's values before making a decision on whether or not to perform any injection. This is a very complex process that requires thoughtful contemplation and a conversation with each patient. Furthermore, it is imperative that the clinician use common sense and know his or her limits before performing any medical procedure. In some cases, following a conversation with the patient, it may be preferable to use an alternative approach or request specialty consultation, rather than performing any invasive procedure.

## ALTERNATIVES TO MEDICATION MANAGEMENT

Musculoskeletal disorders are commonly encountered in practice by primary care providers. Traditionally, many of these have been treated using oral medications. However, the prescriber must be aware of their adverse reactions and potential toxicities.

Acetaminophen toxicity occurs on a frequent basis. From 1990 to 1998, there were 56,000 emergency room visits, 26,000 hospitalizations, and 458 deaths on average per year related to acetaminophen-associated overdoses.[1] In 2007, the Centers for Disease Control estimated 1,600 cases of acute liver failure each year, of which acetaminophen-related was the most common.[2] On January 13, 2011, the U.S. Food and Drug Administration (FDA) released a safety announcement requesting manufacturers to limit acetaminophen in prescription drug products to 325 mg/tablet/capsule. A boxed warning emphasizing the potential for severe liver injury and a warning highlighting the potential for allergic reactions (e.g., swelling of the face, mouth, and throat, difficulty breathing, itching, or rash) were added to the label of all acetaminophen prescription drug products.

Other reported side effects include anaphylaxis, acute renal tubular necrosis, anemia, thrombocytopenia, nausea, rash, and headache. On August 1, 2013, the FDA published a news release informing the public of the potential of rare but severe skin reactions reported in individuals following acetaminophen ingestion. These reactions include Stevens-Johnson syndrome, toxic epidermal necrolysis, and acute generalized exanthematous pustulosis. All of these skin conditions are potentially fatal and can occur with even first exposure.[3]

NSAIDs and coxibs are commonly employed classes of medications for use in the treatment of inflammatory conditions. However, many of the musculoskeletal conditions treated by primary care clinicians do not actually involve inflammation in their pathogenesis. Nevertheless, this class of medication is commonly employed. Unfortunately, NSAIDs and coxibs have side effects that extend beyond their well-recognized gastrointestinal (GI) side effects, hepatotoxicity, nephrotoxicity, edema, increase in blood pressure, and exacerbation of congestive heart failure. A meta-analysis of 754 trials in 353,809 patients with greater than 233,798 patient-years of follow-up was reported in 2013. Coxibs and diclofenac are found to increase major vascular events by a third—primarily due to an increase in coronary events. Ibuprofen significantly increases major coronary events. Naproxen, however, does not increase the incidence of major vascular events. All NSAIDs double the risk of heart failure and increase the risk of upper GI complications.[4] A nationwide cohort study determined that even short-term treatment with most NSAIDs is associated with an increase in the risk of death and recurrent myocardial infarction in patients with prior MI. Therefore, neither short- nor long-term treatment with NSAIDs is advised in this population. Any NSAID use should be limited from a cardiovascular safety point of view.[5] Most recently, two large European population-based studies show that traditional NSAIDs and COX-2 inhibitors increase the incidence of atrial fibrillation.[6,7] This is especially noted with recent use within 30 days of onset of atrial fibrillation. Since NSAIDs inhibit cyclooxygenase enzymes expressed in the kidneys, it is thought that this mechanism causes fluid retention, increases blood pressure, and leads to enlargement in both end-diastolic and end-systolic dimensions of the heart. Alternatively, because NSAIDs are used as anti-inflammatory drugs, the underlying inflammatory conditions and pain they treat may be associated with their cardiac effects.

Consequently, other treatment alternatives should be considered to avoid these potential toxicities. These include pharmacologic options including pain-modulating medications and injection management employing corticosteroids or intra-articular viscosupplement products/devices. Injections of botulinum toxin, platelet-rich plasma, and high concentrations of glucose (as utilized in prolotherapy) are used "off-label" by some practitioners. Finally, physical therapy techniques are available to use with great effect but are frequently underutilized.

## UNDERSTAND ANATOMY

It is critical that the clinician has a complete understanding of the three-dimensional anatomy and the structure's function in each area that is selected for injection or aspiration. A thorough knowledge of the target area brings a deeper understanding of the pathologic process causing the patient's symptoms. It also enables the provider to develop a list of alternative diagnostic possibilities. With this knowledge, the physician is able to take the next step. He or she can understand structural relationships beneath the surface of the skin. The physician is then able to think in three dimensions. While advancing the needle, it is important to "visualize" the location of the needle as it passes through the anatomic structures. Performing these thought processes enables the clinician to clinically determine the location of the needle tip in "real time." This results in improved clinical outcomes through the accurate placement of a therapeutic product or the insertion of a large-bore needle for fluid aspiration. Complications from needle trauma are also minimized by avoidance of critical structures.

## IDENTIFY LANDMARKS

For each injection or aspiration procedure, the physician must identify the pertinent local anatomic landmarks. These are areas that represent underlying bony prominences or easily identifiable soft tissues. The landmarks are specific to each injection site. After identification, the structures should be marked on overlying skin with ink by using either a ballpoint pen or a surgical marker. Next, the entry site for the needle is indicated with ink. Then an indentation in the skin is created by applying firm pressure over the ink mark using the retracted tip of a ballpoint pen. An indentation must be done since aseptic preparation of the area will remove the ink mark. This process gives the clinician a visual frame of reference and standardizes the procedure from one patient to the next. No matter how much experience a physician has with a procedure, the process of identifying and marking the landmarks and entry site should not be skipped. After committing the landmarks to a surface drawing, the patient is instructed not to move that area of the body. Repositioning will change the relationships between the skin markings and the underlying anatomy.

## WHEN TO REFER TO A SUBSPECIALIST

There will be situations where referral to subspecialist colleagues is desirable and necessary. This would be the case whenever the provider feels uncomfortable performing a procedure. Other indications include instances where there is uncertainty regarding the correct diagnosis; the expected response to treatment has not occurred; joints are not easily accessible (spine, hip, or sacroiliac joints); arthrocentesis attempts have been unsuccessful; and possible septic arthritis, suspected inflammatory polyarthritis, recurrent monoarthritis unresponsive to treatment, or undiagnosed chronic monoarthritis. In these instances, the patient may be referred to a sports medicine specialist, rheumatologist, orthopedic surgeon, interventional radiologist, or pain specialist. If an acute septic joint is suspected, the patient requires emergent inpatient hospitalization for joint drainage, debridement, irrigation, intravenous antibiotics, and possibly an infectious disease consultation in the case of an atypical infection.

## INDICATIONS FOR INJECTIONS AND ASPIRATIONS

There are many indications for performing injections and aspirations. From a diagnostic standpoint, the introduction of local anesthetic solution into a joint or soft tissue structure to temporarily decrease pain may allow the clinician to perform a more comprehensive examination. Pain limits the musculoskeletal exam through voluntary or involuntary guarding of the affected area. Muscle spasm commonly develops in response, further limiting the range of motion of the area examined.

Providing effective pain relief allows the clinician to adequately examine the area of interest. This is essential in order to determine the integrity of underlying structures including muscles, tendons, ligaments, and cartilage.

Important clinical management decisions may be made based on the results of a diagnostic injection. For example, a patient may present with acute shoulder pain. Upon examination, she complains of moderately severe pain, holds the shoulder at her side, and is unable to demonstrate shoulder abduction because of pain. The clinical question may be whether she has a complete tear of the shoulder rotator cuff complex or if impingement of the rotator cuff under the acromion is the cause of her pain. The clinician may elect to perform a subacromial space injection of 5 mL of 1% lidocaine. If after 1 min, the patient is able to demonstrate full range of motion including unrestricted abduction, then this "impingement test" indicates that pain was the limiting factor in her inability to abduct the shoulder. Consequently, there is not a complete tear of the rotator cuff structures. She may be able to continue to receive conservative care directed by the primary medical provider without specialty referral at that particular time.

Fluid may also be obtained upon aspiration of a joint or soft tissue space. If so, then it should be grossly examined for color, clarity, and the presence of blood. Normal synovial fluid is clear and transparent. The fluid may contain blood that indicates a hemorrhagic cause—most commonly acute trauma. It may also be yellow due to xanthochromia from the breakdown of hemoglobin leaking from inflamed synovium. The clarity of the fluid may be altered by the presence of white blood cells. Crystals and cellular debris can also decrease clarity. The information obtained from the microscopic examination of the fluid in order to assess it for cells, crystals, bacteria, and blood is critically important and is discussed in the Complications section.

Therapeutically, there are many reasons to perform injections and aspirations. Removal of fluid itself from a joint can result in significant pain relief and restore joint range of motion. With relatively small joints such as the elbow, this can occur with the removal of as little as 3 to 5 mL of fluid. In a large knee joint, it is not uncommon to remove as much as 100 to 150 mL of fluid in chronic conditions!

Indications for therapeutic injections include crystal arthropathies, synovitis, rheumatoid arthritis, other nonseptic inflammatory arthritides, osteoarthritis, and osteoarthrosis. Soft tissue indications include bursitis, tendonitis, tendinosis, epicondylitis, trigger points, ganglion cysts, neuromas, nerve entrapment syndromes, and fasciitis. With inflammatory joint and soft tissue conditions, therapeutic effect is achieved by the precise placement of a corticosteroid/local anesthetic mixture.

Injections of corticosteroids may also be given directly into lesions in patients with skin diseases as diverse as hypertrophic scars, keloids, lichen planus, lichen simplex chronicus, psoriasis, prurigo nodularis, alopecia areata, and discoid lupus.

Injection of local anesthetics into skin structures, and around nerves, temporarily eliminates pain. This is clinically important in order to allow the performance of otherwise-painful surgical procedures.

## CONTRAINDICATIONS TO INJECTIONS AND ASPIRATIONS

While understanding the indications of aspirations and injections is important, it is perhaps even more valuable to recognize the situations in which these procedures should not be performed. Absolute contraindications include performance of a procedure on an uncooperative patient, history of true allergy to the proposed injected medication, injection through infected tissues, and injection of corticosteroid into critical weight-bearing tendons. In particular, the injection of steroid into and around the Achilles, patellar, and quadriceps tendons may result in catastrophic rupture of these vital structures. Recovery from such rupture is often difficult, prolonged, and incomplete.

Many relative contraindications exist. These are variable and may apply only to certain patients or situations. Some of these include procedures near critical structures such as arteries, veins, nerves, or pleural surfaces. Also, caution must be exercised in patients with coagulation disorders, allergy to the preservative in the injected solution, immunocompromised states, brittle diabetes, history of avascular necrosis, previous joint replacement at the injection site, excessive anxiety concerning the procedure, and in patients who may not follow postprocedure instructions.

Patients receiving corticosteroids may experience activation of latent disease or an exacerbation of infections caused by ameba, *Borrelia burgdorferi* (Lyme disease), *Candida, Cryptococcus, Mycobacterium, Nocardia, Pneumocystis, Strongyloides* (threadworm), *Toxoplasma, or* others.

Patients taking the oral anticoagulant medication, warfarin, do not represent an absolute contraindication to injection or aspiration. In the journal *Arthritis and Rheumatism* in 1998, Thumboo[8] reported the results of a prospective cohort study of 32 joint and soft tissue injections and aspirations involving patients attending a rheumatology clinic taking warfarin with an INR less than 4.5. Patients followed up for 4 weeks after the procedure showed no significant hemorrhages.[8]

No studies concerning injection procedures have been reported to date on patients receiving antiplatelet drugs, thrombolytics, fibrinolytics, low molecular weight heparin, or the newer oral anticoagulant medications, including direct thrombin inhibitors (dabigatran and others) and factor Xa inhibitors (rivaroxaban, apixaban, and others). Data on the safety of the performance of injection procedures in patients taking warfarin should not be extended to these anticoagulation agents.

## SAFETY

In order to ensure patient and operator safety, the following procedures should be followed. First, the local anatomic landmarks must be defined. This assures the provider that the needle is being advanced with knowledge of the underlying structures. Next, always use universal precautions to avoid inadvertent contact with blood and body fluids. Personal protective equipment must be used. For almost all injections and aspirations, the use of nonsterile exam gloves is sufficient. In almost all clinical outpatient situations, it is unnecessary to use sterile gloves, drapes, gowns, or masks while performing these procedures—as long as medical antiseptic technique is strictly followed.

In order to decrease the chance of needle stick injury, there are a variety of safer sharps needle systems available for use. It is the practitioner's responsibility to utilize one of these safer designs to avoid injury and maintain compliance with OSHA regulations. After use, all sharps must be placed immediately in a puncture-resistant sharps container. Filled sharps containers are then disposed in accordance with state-regulated medical waste rules.

Medical antiseptic techniques are always used when performing invasive procedures. Common commercially available antiseptic products include 10% povidone–iodine–aqueous and 2% chlorhexidine–alcohol solutions. Both are broad-spectrum antiseptics with activity against gram-positive bacteria, gram-negative bacteria, fungi, and enveloped viruses. Chlorhexidine–alcohol has been shown to be significantly more effective than povidone–iodine in preventing postoperative superficial and deep incisional infections.[9] In patients undergoing neuraxial blockade procedures, chlorhexidine–alcohol significantly lowers the incidence of insertion-site colonization compared with the use of povidone–iodine.[10] These studies are consistent with others demonstrating superior clinical efficacy of chlorhexidine versus povidone–iodine in reducing the bacterial concentration in the operative field in foot-and-ankle surgery.[11,12] Further, chlorhexidine gluconate is not inactivated by blood or serum proteins, whereas this occurs with iodophors.[13,14] Lower postoperative infection rates with chlorhexidine–alcohol are thought to be related to chlorhexidine's more rapid action, persistent activity, and residual antimicrobial effect.[15] Antiseptics should be allowed to dry according to the manufacturer's recommendation.

Using a medical aseptic technique does not imply that the procedure needs to be done in a sterile operating room environment. However, it does require that the provider takes the necessary precautions to ensure a minimal chance that infectious organisms are carried into the tissues by the needle. When performing injections and aspirations, the operator must always follow the antiseptic, "no-touch" technique. This procedure does not allow for any contact of the injection site after sterile preparation of the skin. Following identification of the local landmarks, the injection site is marked with ink. Then, an impression in the skin is made at that site by applying firm pressure with the retracted tip of a ballpoint pen. Next, the injection site is cleansed with alcohol, followed by application of an antiseptic agent. After these steps are completed, there is no further contact or touching of the site with any nonsterile objects. The only object that comes into contact with this site is the tip of the sterile needle.

It is important to use needles and syringes for only a single patient. These must never be used on other patients. If, single-dose (single-use) medication vials are used, then they must only be used for one patient. Because these vials do not contain preservative, they can never be reused, even at a later time with the same patient. The rubber septum on a medication vial must be disinfected with alcohol prior to piercing. Medication vials are entered with a new needle and a new syringe, even when obtaining additional doses for the same patient.

Always attempt to aspirate before injecting any substance into tissues. This will confirm that the needle tip is not inside a blood vessel. Performing this simple maneuver ensures that inadvertent intravascular injection of the injection solution does not occur.

Place the injection *within* a joint or bursa and *around* a tendon. An injection into the substance of a tendon is likely to weaken that structure. Rupture may follow—especially if it is a weight-bearing tendon such as the Achilles, patellar, or quadriceps tendon. Also, avoid injecting directly into nerves. Such an injection is often evident since the patient usually reports pain, paresthesias, or numbness at the instant of needle contact with a nerve. In this case, simply withdraw the needle slightly and attempt to reposition it before proceeding with the injection.

After the injection has been completed, sterile gauze is used to wipe the site and, if necessary, apply direct pressure. Finally, a sterile adhesive dressing is applied. The needles are immediately disposed in a puncture-resistant sharps container. Following the procedure, the patient should remain in the office for a period of time in which the office staff observes the patient for any signs of systemic or local reactions.

## SYNOVIAL FLUID ANALYSIS

The acquisition of a sample of synovial fluid for microscopic analysis is the primary objective of arthrocentesis. Examination of the fluid can provide information critical to the diagnosis of the condition that has caused the joint effusion.[16,17] This is especially important in the case of acute monoarthritis in which either septic or crystal arthritis may be present. After arthrocentesis has been successfully performed, the appearance of the fluid is observed. Normal synovial fluid is clear and transparent. The gross appearance of the fluid should be noted. This provides a quick clinical estimation of the amount of inflammation present in the joint. Totally transparent fluid originates in normal joints and is observed with noninflammatory conditions such as osteoarthritis (Fig. 2.1). The degree of turbidity generally parallels the amount of inflammation. Most turbid to purulent synovial fluid usually occurs in septic joints, but exceptions are not uncommon (Fig. 2.2). Next, the fluid is either immediately examined under a microscope or transferred as quickly as possible to a laboratory capable of providing diagnostic testing. When the specimen is sent for synovial fluid analysis, it is placed in a glass tube anticoagulated with liquid ethylenediaminetetraacetate (EDTA). Do not use tubes that contain heparin, oxalate, or lithium since these anticoagulants confound crystal analysis. However, for best practices, contact the local laboratory to determine the preferred method for transportation of the fluid. Fluid submitted for culture is transferred from the syringe to appropriate culture media. A general bacterial culture medium is appropriate for most cases of septic arthritis. However, gonorrhea is a common cause of septic monoarthritis. If this is suspected, then transport it in the Thayer–Martin medium under carbon dioxide. Cultures from other sites including the pharynx, cervix, urethra, and rectum are necessary if gonococcal disease is suspected. Plate the specimen for growth in Sabouraud dextrose agar if a fungal infection is a consideration.

In the past, a number of tests for glucose, pH, and lactic acid were routinely performed, but evidence-based investigation has disproved their value. Traditionally, joint effusions have been classified as normal, noninflammatory, inflammatory, septic, and hemorrhagic. The absolute cell count is the major discriminating factor between an inflammatory fluid and a noninflammatory fluid. Fluids with cell counts less than 2,000 cells/$mm^3$ are likely to be noninflammatory, and inflammatory fluids generally have more than 2,000 cells/$mm^3$. The differential leukocyte count may add further information. Noninflammatory fluid generally contains less than 50% polymorphonuclear

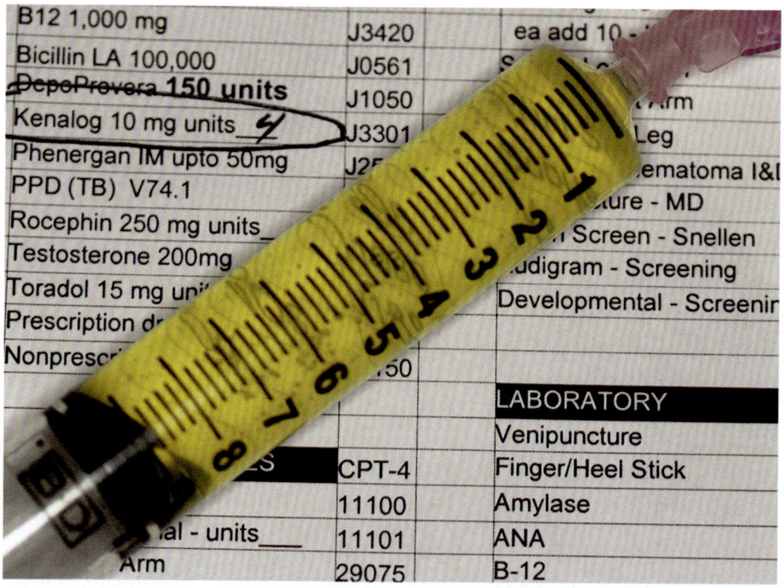


**FIGURE 2.1** ● Nonseptic, noninflammatory knee joint aspirate from a patient with advanced osteoarthritis.

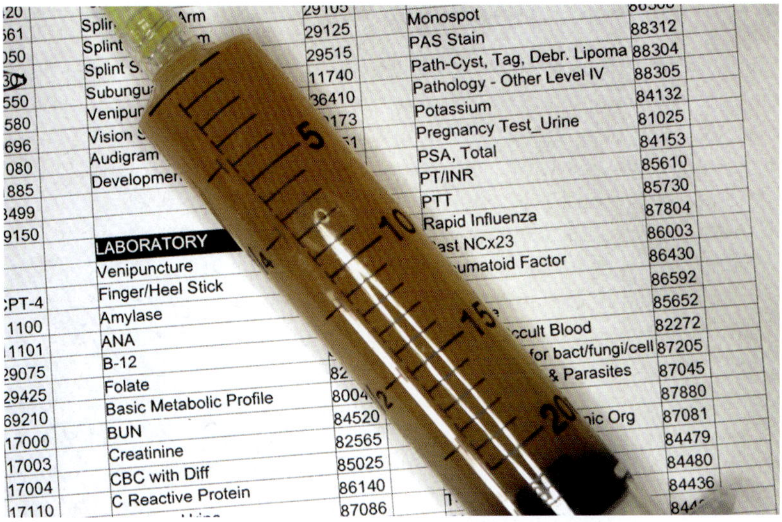


***FIGURE 2.2*** • Nonseptic, inflammatory knee joint aspirate with 20,365 WBCs from a patient with an acute flare of rheumatoid arthritis.

cells (PMNs) and an inflammatory fluid considerably more. Recent studies show that the only clinically useful synovial tests in the setting of septic arthritis are the WBC count, percentage of PMNs, Gram stain, and culture.

Crystal analysis can be performed in any office equipped with a microscope. A single drop of fluid is placed on a clean slide and is examined under a cover slip. Crystals can be observed with plain microscopy, and a preliminary identification made with regard to crystals, WBCs, and bacteria. A polarizing light microscope provides the gold standard for crystal identification. This is usually present only in a referral laboratory. Monosodium urate crystals found in gout appear needle shaped and are strongly negatively birefringent when examined under polarization. Calcium pyrophosphate dihydrate crystals are found in pseudogout. These are strongly refractile, short, rhomboid shaped, and weakly positively birefringent. The presence of intracellular crystals is an even more specific predictor for gout or pseudogout (Table 2.1).

## TABLE 2.1

### Synovial Fluid Properties

| | Appearance | Viscosity | Cells/mm$^3$ | % PMNs | Crystals |
|---|---|---|---|---|---|
| Normal | Transparent | High | <180 | <10% | None |
| Osteoarthritis | Transparent | High | 200–2,000 | <10% | None |
| Rheumatoid arthritis | Translucent | Low | 2,000–50,000 | Variable | None |
| Psoriatic arthritis | Translucent | Low | 2,000–50,000 | Variable | None |
| Reactive arthritis | Translucent | Low | 2,000–50,000 | Variable | None |
| Gout | Translucent to cloudy | Low | 2,000–50,000 | >90% | Needle-like – birefringence |
| Pseudogout | Translucent to cloudy | Low | 2,000–50,000 | >90% | Rhomboid-like + birefringence |
| Septic arthritis | Cloudy | Variable | 2,000–50,000+ | >90% | None |
| Hemarthrosis | Red | Low | 2,000–50,000 | <10% | None |

## SPECIAL MEDICAL CONDITIONS

Several medical conditions deserve special consideration. Diabetes is a common and increasingly prevalent medical condition in the primary care physician's patient population. Because of the frequent association with obesity, these patients place mechanical and metabolic stress on joint and soft tissues that may be amenable to treatment using therapeutic injections. Although there is concern that blood glucose levels may rise significantly, recent studies show that the transient elevation is not clinically significant. A single intra-articular steroid injection into the knee produces acute hyperglycemia for 2 to 3 days in patients with diabetes who otherwise have good glucose control.[18,19] Intra-articular steroid injections into the shoulder may briefly raise postprandial (but not mean) glucose levels with larger and repeated doses.[20] The rise in blood sugars can be well controlled with carbohydrate restriction, continuation of the usual diabetes treatment regimen, and close monitoring of blood sugars for a few days following injection. However, the presence of diabetes may make treatment using injected corticosteroids less effective.

Concern has been raised regarding the performance of injections in patients taking oral anticoagulants, including aspirin, NSAIDs, antiplatelet agents, warfarin, and other anticoagulant medications. There is only a single small investigation available for guidance. A prospective cohort study reported in 1998 demonstrated safe and effective joint and soft tissue injections and aspirations of 32 procedures on patients with therapeutic doses of warfarin. No episodes of hemarthrosis or abnormal bleeding were observed.[8] This has also been the author's experience in many more patients (unpublished). No studies concerning injection procedures have been conducted to date on patients receiving antiplatelet drugs, thrombolytics, fibrinolytics, low molecular weight heparin, or the newer oral anticoagulant medications, including direct thrombin inhibitors (dabigatran and others) and factor Xa inhibitors (rivaroxaban, apixaban, and others). Data on the safety of the performance of injection procedures in patients taking warfarin should not be extended to these anticoagulation agents.

Septic arthritis is a medical emergency. A joint infection is a very serious condition with dire consequences to the integrity of the joint and surrounding structures. All efforts must be made to diagnose septic arthritis as soon as possible and provide emergent hospitalization. The patient requires treatment including surgical drainage and irrigation of the affected joint, administration of intravenous antibiotics, and pain control. This is best done in a coordinated manner by the primary care physician with an orthopedic surgeon, and possibly an infectious disease subspecialist. Common organisms causing joint infections are *Streptococcus/Staphylococcus* species, *Neisseria gonorrhoeae* and, increasingly, methicillin-resistant *Staphylococcus aureus*.

Rheumatoid arthritis presents unique challenges to the primary care provider. This is a destructive, rapidly progressive inflammatory arthritis. Lytic enzymes rapidly degrade the joint surfaces, synovium, and supporting structures unless the process is interrupted and controlled. Joint and soft tissue injections play an important role in medical care because they can be used to deliver relatively small doses of corticosteroids locally in the affected joint(s) to augment the overall systemic management of this condition.

Management of pain involving joint replacement devices demands special consideration. Pain involving a joint replacement often occurs because the normal biomechanics are altered. Other causes of pain may include excessive postoperative scar tissue and poorly fitting or loose components of protheses. Simple injections of corticosteroids or other substances often do not lead to meaningful improvement in the patient's pain and certainly do not correct any underlying biomechanical abnormality.

There is also the possibility that an injection may be complicated by an infection of the prosthetic joint with catastrophic outcomes. In these patients, it is usually more prudent to not perform injections and to refer the patients back to their orthopedic surgeon for management of this challenging problem.

## TOPICAL ANESTHESIA

Providing the patient a pain-free experience is the responsibility of the primary care provider.[21] In select injections, such as the posterior approach to the subacromial space, techniques such as stretching/pinching the skin and other dermal stimulation may give adequate distraction to the patient so that pain from needle insertion is not experienced.

Painless local anesthesia via percutaneous needle introduction can be achieved by use of either skin cooling or application of a topical local anesthetic agent. A topical vapocoolant spray can be used to give rapid onset of brief, but effective, skin numbness. These skin refrigerants cause a brief period of noncytotoxic cooling of the epidermis. This provides up to 30 s of local anesthetic effect, which blocks the pain associated with needle injections. The mechanism of action for anesthesia is to decrease nerve conduction velocity of the A-delta fibers and C-fibers of the peripheral nervous system, thus interrupting nociceptive input to the spinal cord.

The classic vapocoolant agent, Gebauer's Ethyl Chloride, is available in glass bottle and metal can containers. Both vessels are held 3 to 9 in. away from the treatment area in a well-ventilated space. The bottle is held upside down, while the Accu-Stream 360 canister may be held in any position. The stream of Ethyl Chloride is sprayed continuously to the site for 3 to 7 s from the bottle and 4 to 10 s from the can, or until the skin just turns white—whichever occurs first. The needle is then immediately inserted into the skin. Extra caution must be exercised when using Ethyl Chloride as this product is flammable. It should never be used in the setting of open flames or sparks—including cautery units, hyfrecators, electrosurgical machines, radiofrequency devices, intense pulsed light generators, or lasers.

Alternatively, Gebauer's Pain Ease (a proprietary mixture of 1,1,1,3,3-pentafluoropropane and 1,1,1,2-tetrafluoroethane) is available both as a medium stream spray and as an aerosolized mist spray. These products are distributed in pressurized metal cans and are nonflammable products. Both Pain Ease products are administered at a distance of 3 to 7 in. from the target site by holding the can in an upright position. They are sprayed for 4 to 10 s until the skin begins to frost. Do not spray for longer than 10 s. The medium stream produces a pinpoint stream in a smaller target site. The fine droplets of mist are dispersed in a 3-cm-diameter circular pattern. Adequate local anesthesia for needle injection or minor surgical procedures lasts up to 30 s. Pain Ease is not carcinogenic or teratogenic and, thus, may be used safely in pregnancy when used as directed. Furthermore, this product offers advantages over Ethyl Chloride, including a larger field of anesthesia and lack of "running" of liquid down the skin (with use of the mist spray) and no fire hazard. In contrast to Ethyl Chloride, which is only approved for use on intact skin, Pain Ease may also be used on minor skin wounds and intact mucous membranes. With prolonged contact, both Ethyl Chloride and Pain Ease may damage polyvinylchloride coverings used to upholster examination tables. Barrier pads used during injections effectively keep the vapocoolant fluid from contact with the upholstery.

Ethyl Chloride and Pain Ease do not claim to be sterile, but the products have passed the Microbial Limit Test in accordance with the United States Pharmacopeia. These tests are designed to demonstrate that a substance is free from *S. aureus*, *Escherichia coli*, *Pseudomonas aeruginosa,* and *Salmonella* species. Those tests also measure total bacteria, mold, and yeast growth.[22] A 2012 study showed that Ethyl Chloride may be an effective disinfectant alone and may improve skin disinfection when used with povidone–iodine compared to povidone–iodine alone.[23] Thus, there does not appear to be a need to wipe the field with an antiseptic agent again following the application of a topical vapocoolant spray.

## LOCAL INFILTRATION ANESTHESIA

Local anesthetics are membrane-stabilizing drugs. They act by inhibiting sodium influx through sodium-specific ion channels in the neuronal cell membrane. They reversibly decrease the rate of depolarization and repolarization of excitable membranes in nociceptors—thus interrupting pain impulses.

Local anesthetics are commonly injected either alone or with another compound, such as a corticosteroid when treating painful conditions. The injection of local anesthetic into joints or soft tissues serves several purposes. Administration of the local anesthetic provides short-term pain relief. This allows for patient feedback. It may provide a more comprehensive examination of the affected area without the limitation of pain. Although mixing steroids with local anesthetics is not recommended by the manufacturers of injectable corticosteroids, it is common clinical practice to mix a local anesthetic in the same syringe as the corticosteroid solution prior to injection. By convention, the clear liquid (local anesthetic) is drawn up in the syringe first, followed by the cloudy fluid (steroid). The added volume of the local anesthetic helps dilute the corticosteroid. This enables dispersion of steroid in a large joint space or bursa. Pain relief following injection confirms the proper placement of corticosteroid both to the clinician and to the patient. Although pain may return after the effect of the anesthetic wears off, the patient can be assured that the injected corticosteroid is properly placed and should begin to exert its clinical effect within 24 to 48 h.

There are several choices of local anesthetics. Most commonly, the amino-amide class of local anesthetics is used. Lidocaine (ligocaine, Xylocaine) for local anesthetic injection is commercially available as 0.5%, 1%, and 2% concentrations with or without epinephrine. Duration of action for infiltration anesthesia is 60 to 120 min. For joint and soft tissue injections, the author exclusively uses 1% lidocaine without epinephrine. This is commonly available in multiuse bottles containing the preservative, methylparaben. Lidocaine is also available in 2-mL single-use preservative-free vials. The 2% solution of lidocaine confers no clinically important advantages and increases the risk of toxicity following administration of large amounts. The inclusion of epinephrine likewise offers no clinical advantages with musculoskeletal injections/aspirations and is not used in these procedures to dilute the corticosteroid. In fact, lidocaine with epinephrine is acidic and causes significant transient local burning pain upon injection.

Bupivacaine (Marcaine, Sensorcaine, Vivacaine, Exparel) is another commonly used local anesthetic. It has a longer onset of action but offers extended anesthetic effect. Duration of action for infiltration anesthesia is 240 to 480 min. Multidose vials also contain 1 mg of methylparaben as a preservative. Many physicians prefer to mix lidocaine with 0.25% bupivacaine in order to give the patient rapid onset of local anesthesia with an extended duration. However, there is no proven clinical benefit using this approach. Because of the additional steps required to draw up the separate anesthetics, preparation of this combination may increase the chance of contamination and needle stick injury. It may also give the patient a false sense of security since there is prolonged initial pain relief before the tissues have healed. Since the negative feedback from pain is absent for an extended period of time, the patient might suffer further injury such as tendon rupture through inadvertent use of the affected body area.

Ropivacaine (Naropin) is a newer agent that is the homolog of bupivacaine. It is available as a 0.5% solution for injection. Duration of action for infiltration anesthesia is 240 to 480 min. Levobupivacaine (Chirocaine) is the levo-enantiomer of bupivacaine. It is also a recently developed option for local anesthesia. Levobupivacaine is commercially available as 2.5, 5.0, and 7.5 mg/mL solutions. Both of these stereoisomers display less cardiovascular and central nervous system toxicity than racemic bupivacaine.[24]

The pH of local anesthetics can be buffered to decrease local pain. The pH of 1% lidocaine without epinephrine is 6.5 while the pH of 1% lidocaine with epinephrine is 4.5. Bupivacaine is isotonic. Adding sterile 8.4% sodium bicarbonate to lidocaine with epinephrine at a ratio of 1:10 neutralizes the mixture and has been shown to provide significant pain relief. However, this is not a clinically important issue with joint injections because plain lidocaine is used and not lidocaine with epinephrine.

A discussion of chondrocyte toxicity of amide local anesthetics is included in the "Complications" section of this chapter.

## INJECTABLE AGENTS

### Corticosteroids

Corticosteroids used for injection purposes are synthetic derivatives of hydrocortisone. The exact mechanism of action of corticosteroids is complex with various sites of action. They bind to glucocorticoid receptors regulating gene transcription. By altering the production of protein annexin-1, corticosteroids reduce cytokines and other inflammatory mediators.[25–27] They lead to down-regulation of immune function,[28] inhibition of cell-mediated immunity, and reduction in the number of macrophages and PMNs accumulating at inflammatory sites. There is also a vascular-stabilizing effect by the inhibition of endothelial expression of adhesion molecules for neutrophils. Capillary dilation and vascular permeability are therefore reduced.[25,26] The end effect is to reduce the amount of inflammation, thereby reducing swelling and pain.

Several corticosteroids are commercially available to use for joint and soft tissue injections (Table 2.2). These include triamcinolone acetonide (Kenalog), triamcinolone diacetate (Aristocort), triamcinolone hexacetonide (Aristospan), methylprednisolone acetate (Depo-Medrol), betamethasone acetate and sodium phosphate (Celestone Soluspan), and dexamethasone acetate (Decadron-LA). The agents differ with regard to their potency, solubility, and biologic half-life (Table 2.2). Potency is measured against hydrocortisone. Different products have varying effects and solubility in the tissues. The solubility is inversely proportional to the biologic duration of effect of the agent. Hydrocortisone is almost never used because of its high solubility and very short duration of action. It also has significant mineralocorticoid activity that is not shared by the other agents.

The common synthetic corticosteroids used in musculoskeletal procedures are derivatives of prednisolone. Corticosteroid preparations are either soluble or insoluble. Most corticosteroid preparations contain corticosteroid esters, which are highly insoluble in water and thus form microcrystalline suspensions.[29] The more insoluble, esterified corticosteroids remain at the injection sites far longer than the soluble forms.

Dexamethasone preparations, however, are not esters and are freely soluble in water; hence, the preparation is clear (i.e., nonparticulate). The potential advantage of corticosteroid ester preparations is that they require hydrolysis by cellular esterases to release the active moiety and consequently should last longer in the joint than do nonester preparations.[30] On the other hand, freely water-soluble preparations such as

## TABLE 2.2

### Properties of Injectable Corticosteroids

| Corticosteroid | Relative Anti-inflammatory Potency | Solubility (%Wt/Vol) | Biologic Half-life (h) |
|---|---|---|---|
| Hydrocortisone acetate (Hydrocortone) | 1 | High 0.002 | 8–12 |
| Triamcinolone acetonide (Kenalog) | 5 | Intermediate 0.004 | 12–36 |
| Triamcinolone hexacetonide (Aristospan) | 5 | Low 0.0002 | 12–36 |
| Methylprednisolone acetate (Depo-Medrol) | 5 | Intermediate 0.0014 | 12–36 |
| Betamethasone acetate and sodium phosphate (Celestone Soluspan) | 25 | Low/high | 26–54 |
| Dexamethasone acetate (Decadron-LA) | 25 | High | 26–54 |

dexamethasone sodium phosphate and betamethasone sodium phosphate are taken up rapidly by cells and thus have a quicker onset of effect but with a concomitant reduced duration of action.[27]

Notably, the betamethasone formulation, Celestone Soluspan, contains a combination of betamethasone salt and betamethasone ester and, therefore, may provide a dual action of quick onset and long duration of therapy. However, most clinical studies have not shown a significant difference between this product and other corticosteroid ester preparations in terms of onset or duration.[31,32]

Few studies have been conducted that directly compare the various agents in terms of their efficacy. A comparison of intra-articular administration of triamcinolone acetonide, triamcinolone hexacetonide, and a combination of betamethasone phosphate and acetate was conducted by Derendorf and colleagues.[33] They demonstrated complete absorption of all corticosteroids from the site of injection over a period of 2 to 3 weeks. Because of its lower solubility, triamcinolone hexacetonide was absorbed more slowly than triamcinolone acetonide, thus maintaining synovial levels for a longer time and creating lower systemic corticoid levels. Endogenous hydrocortisone suppression correlated with exogenous steroid levels.[33]

No studies have been done that conclusively determine which corticosteroid is preferred for injection of joints or soft tissues. Without good data, the selection of the particular corticosteroid agent is left to the preference of the individual clinician. Despite lack of literature support, some clinicians prefer to choose a relatively insoluble preparation for intra-articular use and a more soluble form for use in soft tissues and peritendinous injections. Considering medication availability, cost, and past experience, the author prefers to use triamcinolone acetonide (40 mg/mL) for all injections, regardless of site. If another corticosteroid is chosen, then the equivalent dosage and volume of administration may be calculated from the comparison table (Table 2.3).

The dose of corticosteroid to be used generally depends on the injection site, disease process, and degree of inflammation. Suggested doses of corticosteroid are listed in each individual chapter. Table 2.3 presents equivalent dosages of corticosteroids

## TABLE 2.3

### Equivalent Dosages of Injectable Corticosteroids

| Corticosteroid Preparation | Trade Name | Equivalent Dose/Volume (mg/mL) |
|---|---|---|
| Triamcinolone acetonide | Kenalog | 40 |
| Triamcinolone hexacetonide | Aristospan | 40 |
| Methylprednisolone acetate | Depo-Medrol | 40 |
| Dexamethasone acetate | Decadron-LA | 8 |
| Betamethasone acetate and sodium phosphate | Celestone Soluspan | 6 |

used for injection. For the purpose of this book, all doses are expressed in milligrams of triamcinolone acetonide suspension (Kenalog). If the physician chooses to use another steroid, then the comparative dosage can be simply calculated from the table. For instance, if the chapter in this text indicates that 20 mg of triamcinolone is to be used for injection into the wrist joint, then one could use 20 mg of Kenalog, 20 mg of Aristospan, 20 mg of Depo-Medrol, 4 mg of Decadron-LA, or 3 mg of Celestone Soluspan.

All published information concerning the frequency of intra-articular corticosteroid injection appears to be based upon professional opinion. A search of the peer-reviewed published medical literature failed to identify any studies that investigate how often corticosteroids can be injected into a joint. In general, most experts advocate that corticosteroid injections should be performed no more often than every 3 months. This non–evidence-based guide is an attempt to prevent potential steroid-related complications, including hypothalamic–pituitary–adrenal axis suppression, osteoporosis, and local articular degradation.

The author typically uses two syringe sizes when injecting corticosteroids. A 3-mL syringe is used for most injection sites of small joints, medium joints, and soft tissues. This accommodates 1 mL of 1% lidocaine without epinephrine and 1 mL of corticosteroid. A 5-mL syringe is used for large joints and bursa such as the subacromial space, sacroiliac joint, hip joint, knee joint, and trochanteric bursa. Each syringe is prepared at the time of the procedure. In the case of a large joint, 3 mL of 1% lidocaine is drawn up in the 5-mL syringe and then followed by drawing up 1 mL of the corticosteroid. Prior to injecting a patient with the local anesthetic/corticosteroid mixture, a common observation is that the insoluble corticosteroid often precipitates along the dependent aspect of the syringe. Immediately before the local anesthetic/corticosteroid mixture is injected, 1 mL of air is aspirated into the syringe creating a "mixing bubble" (Fig. 2.3). The syringe is then rapidly rotated in order to disperse the corticosteroid evenly within the volume of local anesthetic. The needle of the syringe is then pointed upward and the small volume of air expelled before the needle is inserted into the skin at the target site.

There is a common misconception that distributing the corticosteroid over a wide area enhances the effect from soft tissue injections. Practitioners frequently use a "fanning" or "peppering" technique to distribute the solution across the area of involvement. However, this practice is usually unnecessary. Solution injected as a bolus will passively move along tendon sheaths and local fascia planes. Consideration might be given to "fanning" when injecting trochanteric bursitis because the involved area is frequently quite large.

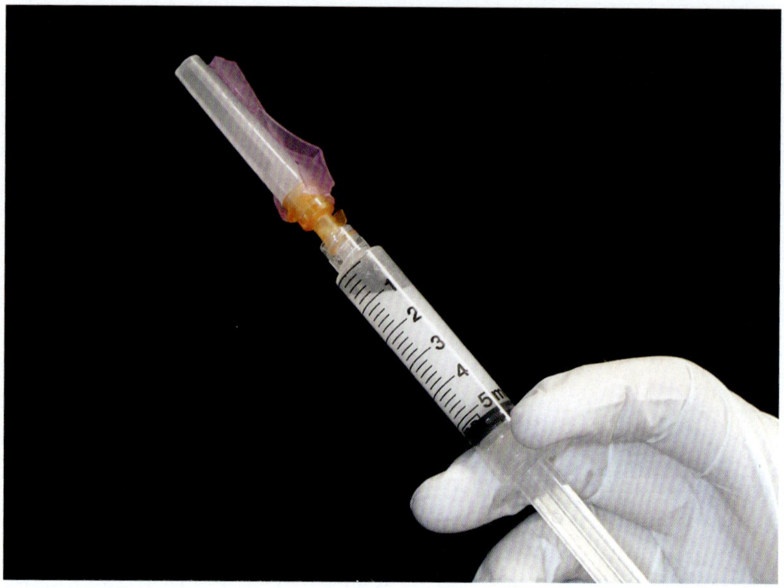

***FIGURE 2.3*** Mixing bubble.

## Viscosupplementation

Hyaluronan (sodium hyaluronate) is a natural complex sugar of the glycosaminoglycan family. The concentration and size of endogenous hyaluronan are reduced in the joint fluid of patients with osteoarthritis. Currently, there are several products available for injection that can be used to supplement this substance in joint fluid. These commercial agents are high molecular weight derivatives of hyaluronan, which are synthetically derived from rooster combs or produced by bacterial fermentation and extraction. The exact mechanism of action of viscosupplements is unknown but may involve physical cushioning of the knee joint, anti-inflammatory action, and/or the stimulation of production of endogenous hyaluronan by synoviocytes.

Viscosupplements serve an important role in the treatment of osteoarthritis of the knee. This condition is a chronic disease state that has a number of therapeutic options. Of these, weight reduction and physical therapy are the most effective measures. However, when pain persists, pharmacologic options may be utilized. Unfortunately, oral NSAIDs and acetaminophen are only modestly effective and possess significant toxicity. Narcotic medications should not be used on a chronic basis in this condition. Corticosteroid injections are effective for short- to medium-term use especially in patients experiencing an acute flare in pain and swelling. Viscosupplements occupy an important position in the mid- (3 months) to long-term (6 months) treatment of knee osteoarthritis. Their use may allow appropriate postponement of knee replacement surgery. They have an excellent record of effectiveness and long-term safety.

Injectable hyaluronan is commercially available in the United States as the products Synvisc (Genzyme), Synvisc-One (Genzyme), Gel-One (Zimmer), Orthovisc (Depuy Mitek), Hyalgan (Fidia Pharma), Supartz (Bioventus), and Euflexxa (Ferring) (Table 2.4). They are classified not as medications, but actually as medical devices by the FDA. These agents are approved only for the treatment of pain in osteoarthritis of the knee in patients who have failed to respond adequately to conservative nonpharmacologic therapy and simple analgesics such as acetaminophen. The safety and effectiveness of the use of these viscosupplements in other joints have not been established.

## TABLE 2.4

### Viscosupplementation Products

*Viscosupplementation products—synthetically derived from rooster combs*

Gel-One (Zimmer) http://www.zimmer.com/en-US/hcp/common/product/gel-one.jspx?cate=biologics#
30 mg/mL—3-mL syringe given as a single injection

Synvisc (Genzyme) www.synvisc.com
8 mg/mL—2-mL syringe given as three weekly injections

Synvisc-One (Genzyme) www.synviscone.com
8 mg/mL—6-mL syringe given as a single injection

Hyalgan (Fidia Pharma) www.hyalgan.com
10 mg/mL—2-mL syringe given as five weekly injections

Supartz (Bioventus) www.supartz.com
10 mg/mL—2.5-mL syringe given as five weekly injections

*Viscosupplementation products—produced by bacterial fermentation and extraction*

Euflexxa (Ferring) www.euflexxa.com
10 mg/mL—2-mL syringe given as three weekly injections

Durolane (Bioventus) www.durolane.com (European and Canadian approval only at this time.)
20 mg/mL—3-mL syringe given as a single injection

Orthovisc® (Depuy Mitek) www.orthovisc.com
15 mg/mL—2-mL syringe given as three weekly injections

*Non–animal-stabilized hyaluronic acid (NASHA)*

Neovisc (Tribute) www.tributepharma.com/products/NeoVisc (European and Canadian approval only at this time.)
10 mg/mL—2-mL syringe given as three to five weekly injections

Ostenil (TRB Chemedica) www.ostenil.ca (European and Canadian approval only at this time.)
10 mg/mL—2-mL syringe given as three weekly injections

Suplasyn (Bioniche) www.suplasyn.com (European and Canadian approval only at this time.)
10 mg/mL—2-mL syringe given as three weekly injections

Evidence-based support in the medical literature for the use of hyaluronan derivatives remains incomplete. However, there is an increasing body of literature that is supportive. An investigation of hylan G-F 20 (Synvisc-One), demonstrated a significant improvement in pain and function up to 26 weeks as compared to saline control. There were no serious adverse events and was no increased risk of adverse events with repeat exposure to hylan G-F 20.[34]

In addition to the mid- to long-term treatment of knee osteoarthritis, there may be specific advantages of viscosupplements in the treatment of patients who have brittle diabetes mellitus, those who have failed corticosteroid injections, patients who have received frequent corticosteroids and are in danger of the significant side effects from repeated administration, or those patients who have a rare allergy to corticosteroids.

Although these products are similar in many respects, there are significant differences in the physical properties of each product (Table 2.5). Some hyaluronate products are derived from processing of rooster combs. Others are extracted from bacteria that have been genetically engineered to produce exact copies of human hyaluronic acid. More importantly from a clinical standpoint are the molecular weight of the product and cross-linking of the molecules. A higher molecular weight and the presence of

**TABLE 2.5**

**FDA-Approved Viscosupplements: Physical Properties**

| Product | Molecular Weight | Elasticity | Viscosity | Cross-linked | Injections | Duration |
|---|---|---|---|---|---|---|
| Healthy young synovial fluid | 6 | 117 | 45 | | | N/A |
| Osteoarthritic synovial fluid | 1.1–1.9 | 1.9 | 1.4 | | | |
| Euflexa | 2.4–3.6 | 92 | 38 | No | 3 | 26 wk |
| Gel-One | Unknown | Unknown | Unknown | Yes | 1 | 13 wk |
| Hyalgan | 0.5–0.7 | 0.8 | 4 | No | 5 | 26 wk |
| Orthovisc | 1.0–2.9 | 60 | 46 | No | 3–4 | 22 wk |
| Supartz | 0.6–1.2 | 9 | 15 | No | 5 | 26 wk |
| Synvisc | 6 | 111 | 25 | Yes | 3 | 26 wk |
| Synvisc-One | 6 | 111 | 25 | Yes | 1 | 26 wk |

cross-linking increase the residence time in the joint and predict a longer-term response to treatment. Some products have demonstrated a duration of effect of 13 weeks, while others (Synvisc and Synvisc-One) have proven effectiveness up to 26 weeks. The products also differ very significantly in the frequency that the injections must be performed to complete a treatment cycle. Synvisc-One and Gel-One are injected intra-articularly as a single dose. Synvisc, Orthovisc, and Euflexxa are administered as a series of three weekly injections. Both Hyalgan and Supartz are given in a series of five injections at weekly intervals. All of these preparations are prepackaged in sterile syringes. They are expensive, and provider knowledge of the reimbursement process is recommended.

Administration is contraindicated in patients with known hypersensitivity to hyaluronan products or in patients with current infections in or around the target knee. It is extremely important to ensure that injection of the viscosupplement is accurately placed within the knee joint. Thus, when performing an intra-articular knee injection of any viscosupplement, the operator must aspirate synovial fluid in order to document successful entry through the knee joint capsule. Ultrasound guidance of the aspiration and injection procedure is quite helpful in ensuring a successful procedure. Inadvertent injection extra-articularly, into the synovial tissues, into the fat pad, or intravascularly greatly increases the risk of adverse reactions. The most commonly reported adverse effects of the viscosupplements injections are transient local pain, arthralgia, joint stiffness, joint swelling, joint warmth, and gait disturbance. Use caution when injecting the rooster comb–derived products in patients allergic to avian proteins, feathers, or egg products.

### Botulinum Toxin

Botulinum neurotoxin is a group of seven related proteins produced by *Clostridium botulinum*. Of these, only type A and type B neurotoxins are approved for use in the United States. Botulinum toxin irreversibly binds to the presynaptic nerve membrane and blocks formation and transmission of acetylcholine at the neuromuscular junction. The neuromuscular effect of botulinum causes a flaccid paralysis of the injected muscles. It effectively creates "medical splinting" of the target musculotendinous unit that prevents continued use. This functional-forced rest of the area for approximately 3 months allows the pathology to heal.

Injections are performed using anatomic landmarks or with electromyographic guidance. Those affected muscles with highest clinical and EMG activity are injected. Therapeutic effect from the injection usually occurs in the first 7 days, and the response lasts for an average of 12 weeks. Injections may be repeated every 3 to 4 months. Recovery occurs through proximal axonal sprouting and muscle reinnervation by formation of a new neuromuscular junction.

Effective treatment using botulinum toxin has been demonstrated in clinical studies to be effective in the treatment of various musculoskeletal disorders, including cervical dystonias, cervicogenic headache, migraine headache, temporomandibular joint disorders associated with increased muscle activity, myofascial pain disorder, piriformis syndrome, limb dystonia (writer's cramp), lateral epicondylitis, and plantar fasciitis. A list of the botulinum toxin products currently approved for use in the United States is displayed in Table 2.6. At this time of publication, the use of botulinum neurotoxin for the treatment of musculoskeletal pain is approved by the FDA only for cervical dystonia in adult patients, upper limb spasticity in adult patients, and for prophylaxis of headaches in adult patients with chronic migraine (≥15 days/month with headache lasting 4 h a day or longer).[35] Use of botulinum toxin for other pain is considered off-label use. An individual practitioner however may consider it appropriate for use in patients with a condition that does not respond to, or is judged inappropriate for, other treatment options.

### Other

Other investigational agents may earn a future role in the practice of medicine and be delivered via intra-articular injections. These include ketorolac (Toradol)[36,37] and biologic agents such as etanercept (Enbrel).[38] An exciting future treatment may involve injecting appropriate viral vectors into joints to transfer genes into synoviocytes for the treatment of rheumatoid arthritis, psoriatic arthritis, other inflammatory arthritis, and osteoarthritis.[39,40]

Autologous blood and platelet-rich plasma injections of tendinopathies and structural injuries have received considerable attention from the sports medicine community in recent years. However, there is insufficient evidence to support their use.[41] Sarapin, an extract of the *Sarracenia purpurea* (pitcher plant), has been injected primarily by practitioners treated spine disorders. There too is no quality, peer-reviewed literature that supports the use of this product.[42]

**TABLE 2.6**

**Botulinum Neurotoxin**

| |
|---|
| *Botulinum neurotoxin type A products* |
| Botox (Allergan) http://www.allergan.com/products/eye_care/botox.htm |
| 100 units/vial |
| Dysport (Ipsen) www.dysport.com |
| 500 units/vial |
| *Botulinum neurotoxin type B product* |
| MyoBloc (Solstice Neurosciences) http://www.myobloc.com |
| 5,000 units/mL |

## EQUIPMENT

It is highly recommended that medical providers organize all of the equipment and supplies needed to perform injections and aspirations. Organizing them presents the materials conveniently to the practitioner. This decreases the amount of time required to gather all of the necessary items. It also reduces the possibility of inadvertent medical errors. Organizing all equipment/supplies should be done well before the procedure is performed. Based on provider or organization preference, four options can be utilized.

1. A dedicated cabinet
2. An injection tray
3. An injection cart
4. Injection packs

A cabinet works well in a setting where the provider consistently works out of the same room. It keeps the supplies centralized and visible but requires collection of the various components at the time a procedure is performed. A large plastic tray or an injection cart provides a portable option for organizing materials. These may work well in a large clinic or teaching setting. Another option is to create "injection packs" that include all of the supplies used universally in these procedures.

After many years of performing these procedures, the author's preferred option in his private medical office is to store materials in a central location. Then, individual injection packs are organized by clinical staff assistants prior to patient visits. These are placed with associated medications and various syringe and needle options inside a secure cabinet in each examination room. When a patient presents with a condition that requires an injection or aspiration, a pack is simply retrieved from the cabinet and placed on the counter in the exam room. The author uses those materials but is also free to select other syringe sizes and/or needle lengths from the cabinet. At the time of the injection, the author or his staff fills the injection syringe with the appropriate medication(s) and secures the correct needle. This preprocedure organization enhances office efficiency and reduces the possibility of a medical mistake.

Items that should be collected and organized (Fig. 2.4):

- Gloves—nonsterile exam gloves
- Barrier "chucks" pads—nonsterile
- Alcohol pads
- 10% Povidone–iodine pads or 2% chlorhexidine–70% alcohol pads
- Gauze pads—nonsterile
- Adhesive bandages
- Hemostat surgical clamp (optional)
- Syringes
  - 3 mL
  - 5 mL
  - 10 mL
  - 20 mL
  - 60 mL
  - Insulin syringe for superficial dermatologic injections
- Needles
  - 20 gauge—1 in.—for drawing medications and aspiration of small joints
  - 18 gauge—1½ in.—for aspiration of large joints and bursa
  - 25 gauge—1/2, 1, 1½, and 2 in.—for injections
  - 25 gauge—3½ in. spinal needles—for deep injections (infrequently used)
- Pain Ease mist or medium stream vapocoolant spray

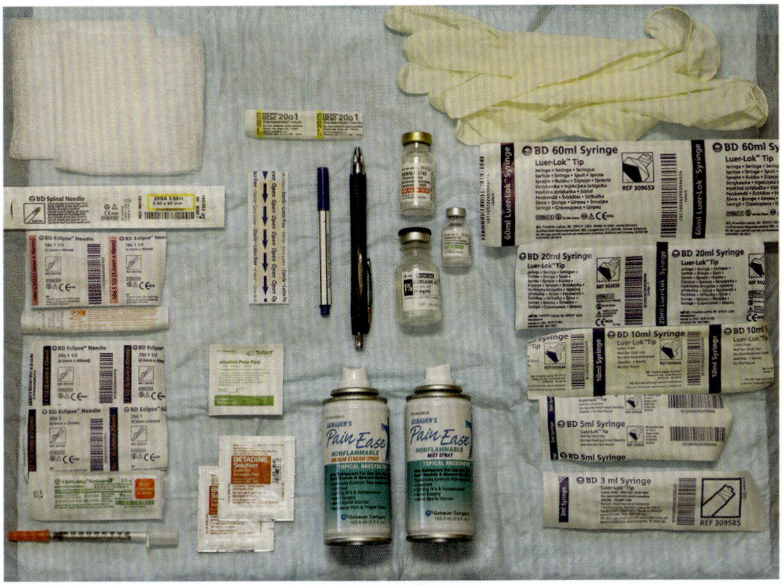


*FIGURE 2.4* • Equipment for injections and aspirations.

- Lidocaine: 1% plain
- Steroid of choice (generally triamcinolone 40 mg/mL for joint and soft tissue injections, 10 mg/ml for dermatologic injections)
- Viscosupplementation agent of choice (ordered as needed)

## TECHNIQUE

When performing injections and/or aspirations, it is important that the medical provider follows a standardized routine. This helps organize the clinician, prepares the patient, and reduces the possibility of procedural omissions. The following steps should be done in the order presented:

1. Determine the medical diagnosis and consider relevant differential diagnoses.
2. Consider all contraindications to the procedure.
3. Discuss the proposed procedure and alternatives with the patient and/or responsible party.
4. Obtain written informed consent from the patient and/or responsible party.
5. Collect and prepare the required materials.
6. Correctly position the patient for the procedure.
7. Identify and mark the anatomic landmarks and injection site with ink. (Do not allow the patient to move the affected area from the time that the marks are placed until after the procedure is completed.)
8. Press firmly on the skin with the retracted tip of a ballpoint pen to further identify the injection site.
9. Perform hand-hygiene procedures, by washing hands either with conventional soap and water or with alcohol-based hand rubs.
10. Put on clean exam gloves.
11. Prepare clean skin with an alcohol pad followed by either a 10% povidone–iodine pad or a 2% chlorhexidine–70% alcohol pad. Then allow this to dry according to the manufacturer's recommendations.
12. Provide local anesthesia as indicated through use of tactile distraction, vapocoolant spray (Pain Ease), and/or injected local anesthesia.

13. Using the no-touch technique, introduce the needle at the insertion site and advance it precisely into the treatment area.
14. If using ultrasound guidance, follow the instructions regarding technique in the following section. (Optional)
15. Aspirate synovial or bursa fluid (optional) and send it for laboratory examination if indicated. If injecting corticosteroid solution or viscosupplement immediately following aspiration, do not remove the needle from the joint or bursa. In this case, grasp the needle hub firmly (with a hemostat clamp if necessary), twist off the original syringe, and then immediately attach the second syringe that contains the corticosteroid.
16. Inject corticosteroid solution or viscosupplement into the target site. Always aspirate before injection to avoid intravascular administration. Do not inject the medication against resistance.
17. Withdraw the needle.
18. Apply direct pressure over the injection site with a sterile gauze pad.
19. Apply a sterile adhesive bandage.
20. Provide the patient with specific postinjection instructions.

## MUSCULOSKELETAL ULTRASOUND

Conventional palpation or "anatomic landmark-guided" injections frequently result in inaccurate needle placement into extra-articular tissue and adjacent structures.[43,44] There is a growing body of literature that demonstrates the efficacy of musculoskeletal ultrasound as a valuable adjunct for accurate needle placement. The goal of image-guided procedures is to maximize patient safety, improve procedural accuracy, and optimize clinical outcomes. In "expert" hands, the discrete placement of a needle tip into even a large joint may occur only half of the time. Without confirmation of needle placement by diagnostic imaging, the only way to ensure joint entry is by aspiration of synovial fluid.

A number of studies now demonstrate significantly increased accuracy rates of injections and improved clinical outcomes when using ultrasound-guided techniques. The use of ultrasound increases the success rate to nearly 100%—particularly when used to guide injections of the glenohumeral joint, subacromial space, and acromioclavicular joint and the knee.[45,46] In fact, a recent review of 13 studies of the knee and shoulder showed that imaging guidance with ultrasound improved the accuracy of intra-articular injections of the knee (95.8% vs. 77.8%, $P < 0.001$) and shoulder (97.3% vs. 65.4%, $P < 0.001$).[47] In addition, the use of image-guided techniques are particularly important in patients without joint effusion and when injecting intra-articular viscosupplements to treat osteoarthritis of the knee.[48]

There is statistically significant improvement in patient outcomes of pain and function with a reduction in adverse events when ultrasound-guided injections are compared to those guided by palpation of landmarks.[49,50] These image-guided techniques also cause significantly less procedural pain, take no additional time to perform, lead to greater provider confidence with the procedure, and improve cost-effectiveness.[47,51–53]

As imaging is done concurrently with the injection, the entire procedure may be performed within a sterile field using sterile gel and a sterile sheath for the ultrasound probe. Alternatively, the ultrasound imaging may utilize an acoustic window adjacent to, but not directly involving, the injection site. The advantage in this situation is that the ultrasound field does not require a sterile environment and the injection/aspiration is done as previously described. In both cases, the needle tip is guided to its target in a live image and recorded for documentation purposes.

Ultrasound-guided articular, bursa, or tendon injection is performed utilizing standard sterile precautions and appropriate preparation of the site. A high-frequency, 15- to 6-MHz linear ultrasound transducer provides good visualization of superficial structures. A low-frequency 5- to 2-MHz curvilinear probe may be needed to visualize deep joint articular surfaces such as the hip joint, especially in large patients. The area is scanned to inspect regional anatomy and identify any nearby neurovascular structures. In the case of tendon injections, the muscle and tendon should be scanned throughout their course to determine the safest and most optimal injection site. For articular injections, the joint space is scanned in all dimensions to determine the safest/optimal injection site. When the injection site is determined, the ultrasound probe may be placed either remote to the injection site or directly over that site. When positioned remotely, the procedure can be visualized and guided without the use of sterile ultrasound gel. Otherwise, the ultrasound probe is placed within a sterile cover. Ultrasound gel may then be placed within the cover or sterile gel placed directly over the intended site. The needle is inserted such that it is visible at all times and can be directly guided into the articular space, bursa, or tendon. Injection of the agent should be done under direct visualization to confirm placement into the intended target and to prevent inadvertent placement into periarticular or peritendinous structures.

## COMPLICATIONS

Complications from injections and aspirations fall into two categories—systemic and local. Systemic complications include vasovagal reactions, local anesthetic–related complications, and corticosteroid-related complications. Patients can develop allergic reactions including anaphylaxis. Other serious toxicities involving cardiac arrhythmias and seizures may occur—but usually with inadvertent administration of intravascular doses far in excess of the amounts used with soft tissue and joint injections. Systemic complications linked to corticosteroid injections include vascular flushing, elevated blood sugar levels in patients with diabetes, impaired immune response, psychological disturbances, hypothalamic–pituitary–adrenal axis suppression, irregular menses, abnormal vaginal bleeding, and osteoporosis.

Patients receiving corticosteroid therapy are at increased risk for infection or reactivation of an infection due to potentially decreased immune resistance with an inability to localize infections. The risk of infection exists with any pathogen (viral, bacterial, fungal, protozoan, or helminthic) at any location of the body. Infections may be mild or severe, and the risk for complications increases with corticosteroid dose. In addition, corticosteroid therapy may mask the signs and symptoms of an active infection.

Local complications may include subcutaneous fat atrophy, dermal atrophy, and skin depigmentation. These are most noticeable after injection of superficial structures but can also be seen after an intra-articular injection. This is presumably due to inadvertent superficial injection of corticosteroid or reflux of corticosteroid along the needle track back into the subcutaneous fat or dermis. It can take up to 2 months for skin effects to manifest. Skin depigmentation normalizes in most patients over a period of 1 year.[54] Although skin atrophy usually resolves, effects lasting longer than 5 years have been reported.[55] The extent and duration of such skin complications are likely related to the solubility and concentration of the corticosteroid preparation. Interestingly, normal saline infiltration has been shown to rapidly reverse local corticosteroid skin atrophy.[56] Other local complications may involve bleeding, infection, osteonecrosis of juxta-articular bone, ligament rupture, or tendon rupture. Intratendinous corticosteroid injection can lead to tendon rupture.[57–59] This is likely to occur through the inhibition of tenocyte proliferation[60] and the reduction in the strength of isolated collagen fascicles. Pneumothorax has been reported as a complication of trigger point injections of back muscles.[61] Injuries to the radial artery can occur with attempted aspiration of large volar wrist ganglion cysts.[62]

Postinjection flare is a local phenomenon commonly believed to be due to a reaction to steroid crystals in the soft tissue and/or synovial space. The reaction occurs 6 to 24 h following corticosteroid injection. Although the flare has been attributed in the past to crystalline corticosteroids, this is controversial and has no support in the medical literature. A clinically identical reaction occurs from chemical synovitis due to preservatives, including methylparaben.[63,64] Multidose vials of plain lidocaine, lidocaine with epinephrine, and bupivacaine all contain 1 mg of methylparaben. If a patient has a history of a "steroid flare" or "lidocaine allergy," single-use vials of 1% lidocaine that do not contain a preservative might be carefully used instead. In either case, an acute postinjection reaction can be managed by the use of NSAIDs, and ice application after a repeat aspiration confirms that there is no infection.

There has been increasing concern following recent reports of toxicity of amide local anesthetics on chondrocytes. This effect has been reported with lidocaine, bupivacaine, and ropivacaine in in vitro studies[65,66] and confirmed with in vivo trials.[67,68] Of these, bupivacaine and ropivacaine may be the least toxic agents.[66,69] The evidence suggests that there is a greater risk for chondrolysis with longer exposure to a high concentration of local anesthetic, such as with the use of a continuous infusion of anesthetic via a pain pump following orthopedic surgery.[69] However, toxic late cellular and metabolic changes are seen even after a single injection of local anesthetic in animal models.[66] Some studies suggest that the preservatives and the pH of the local anesthetic solution may also play a role in chondrotoxicity.[70]

Intra-articular injection of local anesthetics differs from that of continuous intra-articular infusion. Chondrocyte toxicity to the anesthetic directly correlates with the length of exposure to the product. The uptake and clearance of the anesthetic in the joint or soft tissues are dependent on several factors related to the physiochemical properties of the local anesthetic and local blood flow. Uptake tends to be delayed for local anesthetics with high lipophilicity and protein binding.[71] Of the amide local anesthetics, bupivacaine has the greatest values for these properties and probably has the longest residence time in tissues.[72] A single intra-articular injection of lidocaine most likely has no clinically significant deleterious effects. However, there are no studies that have quantified the length of time that local anesthetics actually persist in the joints following a single injection. Thus, the consequences of a single intra-articular injection of local anesthetics in humans remain unclear and require further investigation.

## AFTERCARE

Immediately following the aspiration and/or injection, apply pressure to the sterile bandage, covering the site. Once the provider is assured that the patient is stable and is not at risk of falling, the patient should be brought down from the exam/procedure table. Gentle massage and slow range of motion should be encouraged to enable distribution of the corticosteroid throughout the joint space or soft tissues. After discharge from the office, patients should be advised to look for and immediately report any adverse reactions. Of primary importance is recognizing the early signs of infection. Therefore, any swelling, redness, increased warmth, proximal red streaking, or fever greater than 100°F should be reported immediately.

Patients often experience complete resolution of pain following injection with a local anesthetic. Because of pain relief and absence of negative feedback, there is an increased risk of further injury to the treated area. They should be informed that the initial pain relief is provided by the injected local anesthetic and that its effect will only be temporary. In the case of plain 1% lidocaine, pain relief can be expected to last only about 1 h. The anti-inflammatory effect of the injected corticosteroid product usually has a 24- to 48-hour onset of action. Thus, patients should be informed that the pain is expected to return in about an hour and decrease again in 1 to 2 days.

Additional instructions may be given following aspiration and/or injection. The patient might be directed to apply ice to the affected area. However, there is no evidence that this is beneficial. NSAIDs may be prescribed depending on the clinical situation—but with full knowledge of the side effects and potential toxicities discussed earlier in this chapter. Studies have shown that immobilization of the affected area is not necessary,[73,74] but reduced usage and activity modification are often helpful. A compressive elastic wrap or splint may be desired, but again, there is no support for routinely splinting injected areas in the medical literature. An aftercare patient education handout that outlines the most common possible adverse reactions and specific instructions is a useful document (see Appendix 2).

## DOCUMENTATION OF THE PROCEDURE

A very important step in the provision of medical services is the full and accurate description of the events that occurred before, during, and after the procedure. This serves not only as the official medical record but also as a billing record and a legal document. The note should affirm that discussion of the proposed procedure and the alternative treatments occurred, possible complications were discussed, and all questions were answered. The note must include the fact that written informed consent was obtained. Then, it should document patient position, anesthesia, supplies used, and the physical steps involved in performing the procedure. The record should include any pertinent findings, complications encountered, and the patient's postprocedure condition. Finally, a list of patient instructions, treatment plan, and follow-up care should be documented and signed by the medical provider and any supervisors if necessary.

See the example of documentation for a knee joint aspiration and injection in Appendix 3. This may be modified as needed to meet the needs of the specific aspiration/injection procedure, patient, provider, and medical organization. A review of this document by legal counsel prior to implementation is recommended.

## BILLING AND CODING

In order to receive appropriate payment, it is essential that the clinician assigns the proper code(s) for the procedure(s) performed. This ensures fair payment for the work done at the visit and reimbursement for any eligible supplies. A complete description of the procedure(s) performed during the patient encounter must be documented in the medical record in order to support the level of coding. At the time of publication, the following Current Procedural Terminology (CPT) 2014 codes are employed to bill for injections and aspirations:

- 20526—Injection, therapeutic, carpal tunnel
- 20550—Injection(s), single tendon sheath, or ligament, aponeurosis (e.g., plantar "fascia")
- 20551—Injection, single tendon origin/insertion

- 20552—Injection(s), single or multiple trigger point(s), one or two muscles
- 20553—Injection(s), trigger point(s), three or more muscles
- 20600—Arthrocentesis, aspiration and/or injection, *small* joint or bursa
- 20605—Arthrocentesis, aspiration and/or injection, *intermediate* joint or bursa
- 20610—Arthrocentesis, aspiration and/or injection, *major* joint or bursa
- 20612—Aspiration and/or injection of ganglion cyst(s), any location
- 64400—Injection, anesthetic agent, trigeminal nerve, any division or branch.
- 64405—Injection, anesthetic agent, greater occipital nerve
- 64418—Injection, anesthetic agent, suprascapular nerve
- 64450—Injection, anesthetic agent, other peripheral nerve or branch
- 64455—Injection(s), anesthetic agent and/or steroid, plantar common digital nerve(s) (e.g., Morton neuroma)

CPT 2014 defines small joints as those in the fingers and toes. Temporomandibular, acromioclavicular, wrist, elbow, ankle, and olecranon bursae are defined as intermediate joints or bursa. Large structures are the glenohumeral joint, sacroiliac joint, hip joint, knee joint, and the subacromial bursa.

According to their definitions, the CPT codes 20550, 20551, 20600, 20605, and 20610 are used once for each tendon, joint, or bursa injected. If more than one tendon, joint, or bursa is injected at a visit, then the codes are listed multiple times for each separate structure that is injected. In addition, the modifiers –51 or –59 should be used to indicate when multiple procedures are performed. Usually –59 is used to code for multiple injections at different sites, but the specific modifier used is determined by the preference of each insurance carrier. Note that trigger point injection CPT codes 20552 and 20553 are used only once each session, regardless of the number of injections performed. CPT 2014 gives specific instructions when reporting multiple ganglion cyst aspirations/injections. In this case, the code 20612 is used and the modifier –59 appended.

CPT 2014 does not specifically define codes to be used for corticosteroid injections of either the ulnar nerve in cubital tunnel syndrome, or with the entrapment of the deep branch of the radial nerve (posterior interosseous nerve). The author feels that until CPT descriptors change, the code 64450 (injection, anesthetic agent, other peripheral nerve or branch) most accurately reflects the procedure performed in these conditions.

Medicare and most commercial insurance companies apply the multiple surgery rule when paying for multiple injections. They generally pay 100% for the first procedure, 50% for the second, and 25% for third and subsequent procedures.

Diagnostic codes must also be submitted in order for an insurance company to justify payment for the injection/aspiration procedure. These codes follow the standard International Classification of Diseases (ICD) system. In each of the injection chapters of this book, both the most commonly used ICD-9 (http://www.cdc.gov/nchs/icd/icd9cm.htm) and ICD-10 (http://www.cdc.gov/nchs/icd/icd10cm.htm) codes are listed.

J codes are utilized to charge for the injected medication/device used during the procedure. Therapeutic injectable products, such as corticosteroids and viscosupplementation agents, are billed in addition to the injection administration codes. The J codes are not used for local anesthetics since their use is considered a necessary part of the procedure much like the needle and syringe. The charge is reflected as the number of units used during the procedure. For instance, the J code for Kenalog is expressed in 10-mg units. If the injection is done with 40 mg of Kenalog, then the patient is charged 4 units of J3301. The most common current J codes used for injection are listed in Table 2.7.

**TABLE 2.7**

**2014 HCPCS J Codes for Injectables**

| J-Code | Material | Unit (mg) |
|---|---|---|
| J3301 | Kenalog | 10 |
| J3303 | Aristospan | 5 |
| J1020 | Depo-Medrol | 20 |
| J1030 | Depo-Medrol | 40 |
| J1040 | Depo-Medrol | 80 |
| J0704 | Celestone Soluspan | 6 |
| J1094 | Decadron-LA | 1 |
| J7322 | Synvisc | 16 |
| J7324 | Orthovisc | 30 |
| J7321 | Hyalgan | 20 |
| J7321 | Supartz | 25 |
| J7323 | Euflexxa | 20 |
| J0585 | Botulinum toxin type A | 1 |
| J0587 | Botulinum toxin type B | 1 |

An evaluation and management (E&M) code can be billed if the documentation of the visit supports the necessity and completeness of the evaluation. This requires the –25 modifier and may be used only if there is a "significant, separately identifiable evaluation and management service by the same physician or other qualified health care professional on the same day of the procedure or other service."[75] Otherwise, only the CPT code and associated J code can be used if the evaluation is not performed or does not meet those conditions.

## INFORMED CONSENT

As with any invasive procedure, informed consent must be obtained from the patient. For the purpose of documentation, this should be done in a written format. The patient must also have an adequate opportunity to ask questions, including a discussion of alternative methods of diagnosis and treatment. An example of an informed consent form is included in Appendix 1.

## EVIDENCE-BASED MEDICINE

Intra-articular and soft tissue corticosteroid injections are common procedures performed by primary care physicians. They are accepted interventions and are frequently used to treat various musculoskeletal conditions. Although significant therapeutic efficacy is claimed from over 50 years of published research, a closer examination of the literature yields less convincing evidence of significant long-term improvement of specific, measured outcomes. The available data support short-term benefit from injected corticosteroids. There are currently insufficient high-quality data to provide a definitive answer on the efficacy of corticosteroid injections. However, lack of discrete medical evidence does not necessarily mean that these procedures are ineffective. Even gold standard evidence-based medicine resources such as Cochrane Reviews suffer from performing meta-analysis on studies with data that are themselves flawed. New investigations that are methodologically sound are needed to measure outcomes of corticosteroid injections given for the treatment of specific conditions.

## REFERENCES


1. Nourjah P, et al. Estimates of acetaminophen (Paracetamol)-associated overdoses in the United States. *Pharmacoepidemiol Drug Saf.* 2006;15:398–405.
2. Bower WA, et al. Population-based surveillance for acute liver failure. *Am J Gastroenterol.* 2007;102: 2459–2463.
3. FDA Drug Safety Communication: FDA warns of rare but serious skin reactions with the pain reliever/fever reducer acetaminophen. Available at: http://www.fda.gov/Drugs/DrugSafety/ucm363041.htm. Accessed on December 29, 2013.
4. Coxib and Traditional NSAID Trialists' Collaboration. Vascular and upper gastrointestinal effects of non-steroidal anti-inflammatory drugs: Meta-analyses of individual participant data from randomised trials. *Lancet.* 2013;382(9894):769–779.
5. Olsen AS, Fosbøl EL, Lindhardsen J, et al. Duration of treatment with nonsteroidal anti-inflammatory drugs and impact on risk of death and recurrent myocardial infarction in patients with prior myocardial infarction. A nationwide cohort study. *Circulation.* 2011;123:2226–2235.
6. Schmidt M, Christiansen CF, Mehnert F, et al. Non-steroidal anti-inflammatory drug use and risk of atrial fibrillation or flutter: Population based case–control study. *BMJ.* 2011;343:d3450.
7. Krijthe BP, Heeringa J, Hofman A, et al. Non-steroidal anti-inflammatory drugs and the risk of atrial fibrillation: a population-based follow-up study. *BMJ Open.* 2014;4(4):e004059.
8. Thumboo J, O'Duffy JD. A prospective study of the safety of joint and soft tissue aspiration and injections in patients taking warfarin sodium. *Arthritis Rheum.* 1998;41(4):736–739.
9. Rabih O, Darouiche MD, et al. Chlorhexidine-alcohol versus povidone-iodine for surgical-site antisepsis. *New Engl J Med.* 2010;362:18–26.
10. Krobbuaban B, Diregpoke S, et al. Alcohol-based chlorhexidine vs. povidone iodine in reducing skin colonization prior to regional anesthesia procedures. *J Med Assoc Thai.* 2011;94(7):807–812.
11. Ostrander RV, Botte MJ, Brage ME. Efficacy of surgical preparation solutions in foot and ankle surgery. *J Bone Joint Surg Am.* 2005;87:980–985.
12. Bibbo C, Patel DV, Gehrmann RM, et al. Chlorhexidine provides superior skin decontamination in foot and ankle surgery: A prospective randomized study. *Clin Orthop Relat Res.* 2005;438:204–208.
13. Mangram AJ, et al. CDC: Guideline for prevention of surgical site infection, 1999. *Infect Control.* 1999;20(4):250–266. Available at: http://www.cdc.gov/hicpac/pdf/guidelines/SSI_1999.pdf
14. Brown TR, et al. A clinical evaluation of chlorhexidine gluconate spray as compared with iodophor scrub for preoperative skin preparation. *Surg Gynecol Obstet.* 1984;158:363–366.
15. Denton GW. Chlorhexidine. In: Block SS, ed. *Disinfection, Sterilization, and Preservation,* 5th Ed. Philadelphia, PA: Lippincott Williams & Wilkins, 2001:321–336.
16. Courtney P, Doherty M. Joint aspiration and injection and synovial fluid analysis. *Best Pract Res Clin Rheumatol.* 2013;27(2):137–169.
17. Pascual E, Sivera F, Andrés M. Synovial fluid analysis for crystals. *Curr Opin Rheumatol.* 2011;23(2): 161–169.
18. Habib GS, Bashir M, Jabbour A. Increased blood glucose levels following intra-articular injection of methylprednisolone acetate in patients with controlled diabetes and symptomatic osteoarthritis of the knee. *Ann Rheum Dis.* 2008;67:1790–1791.
19. Habib G, Safia A. The effect of intra-articular injection of betamethasone acetate/betamethasone sodium phosphate on blood glucose levels in controlled diabetic patients with symptomatic osteoarthritis of the knee. *Clin Rheumatol.* 2009;28:85–87.
20. Habib GS, Abu-Ahmad R. Lack of effect of corticosteroid injection at the shoulder joint on blood glucose levels in diabetic patients. *Clin Rheumatol.* 2007;26:566–568.
21. Berry PH, Dahl JD. The new JCAHO pain standards: Implications for pain management nurses. *Pain Manag Nurs.* 2000;1(1):3–12.
22. Gebauer's Pain Ease® Topical Anesthetic Skin Refrigerant Technical Data Document. Available at: http://www.gebauer.com/Portals/150313/docs/pe%20technical%20data%20document.pdf. Accessed on May 3, 2014.
23. Azar FM, Lake JE, Grace SP, et al. Ethyl chloride improves antiseptic effect of Betadine skin preparation for office procedures. *J Surg Orthop Adv.* 2012;21(2):84–87.
24. Miller RD, Pardo MC, Jr. *Basics of Anesthesia,* 6th Ed. Philadelphia, PA: Elsevier Saunders, 2011:140–141.
25. Schramm R, Thorlacius H. Neutrophil recruitment in mast cell-dependent inflammation: Inhibitory mechanisms of glucocorticoids. *Inflamm Res.* 2004;53:644–652.
26. Malemud CJ. Cytokines as therapeutic targets for osteoarthritis. *BioDrugs.* 2004;18:23–35.
27. Barnes PJ. Anti-inflammatory actions of glucocorticoids: Molecular mechanisms. *Clin Sci (Lond).* 1998;94:557–572.
28. Eymontt MJ, Gordon GV, Schumacher HR, et al. The effects on synovial permeability and synovial fluid leukocyte counts in symptomatic osteoarthritis after intraarticular corticosteroid administration. *J Rheumatol.* 1982;9:198–203.

29. MacMahon PJ, Eustace SJ, Kavanagh EC. Injectable corticosteroid and local anesthetic preparations: A review for radiologists. *Radiology*. 2009;252(3):647–661.
30. Wright JM, Cowper JJ, Page Thomas DP, et al. The hydrolysis of cortisol 21-esters by a homogenate of inflamed rabbit synovium and by rheumatoid synovial fluid. *Clin Exp Rheumatol*. 1983;1:137–141.
31. Blankenbaker DG, De Smet AA, Stanczak JD, et al. Lumbar radiculopathy: Treatment with selective lumbar nerve blocks—comparison of effectiveness of triamcinolone and betamethasone injectable suspensions. *Radiology*. 2005;237:738–741.
32. Stanczak J, Blankenbaker DG, De Smet AA, et al. Efficacy of epidural injections of Kenalog and Celestone in the treatment of lower back pain. *AJR Am J Roentgenol*. 2003;181:1255–1258.
33. Derendorf H, Möllmann H, Grüner A, et al. Pharmacokinetics and pharmacodynamics of glucocorticoid suspensions after intra-articular administration. *Clin Pharmacol Ther*. 1986;39(3):313–317.
34. Chevalier X, Jerosch J, Goupille P, et al. Single, intra-articular treatment with 6 ml hylan G-F 20 in patients with symptomatic primary osteoarthritis of the knee: A randomised, multicentre, double-blind, placebo controlled trial. *Ann Rheum Dis*. 2010;69(1):113–119.
35. Botox Prescribing Information. Available at: http://www.allergan.com/assets/pdf/botox_pi.pdf. Accessed on May 4, 2014.
36. Min KS, St Pierre P, Ryan PM, et al. A double-blind randomized controlled trial comparing the effects of subacromial injection with corticosteroid versus NSAID in patients with shoulder impingement syndrome. *J Shoulder Elbow Surg*. 2013;22(5):595–601.
37. Lee SC, Rha DW, Chang WH. Rapid analgesic onset of intra-articular hyaluronic acid with ketorolac in osteoarthritis of the knee. *J Back Musculoskelet Rehabil*. 2011;24(1):31–38.
38. Roux CH, Breuil V, Valerio L, et al. Etanercept compared to intraarticular corticosteroid injection in rheumatoid arthritis: Double-blind, randomized pilot study. *J Rheumatol*. 2011;38(6):1009–1011.
39. Evans CH, Ghivizzani SC, Robbins PD. Arthritis gene therapy and its tortuous path into the clinic. *Transl Res*. 2013;161(4):205–216.
40. Weber C, Armbruster N, Scheller C, et al. Foamy virus-adenovirus hybrid vectors for gene therapy of the arthritides. *J Gene Med*. 2013;15(3–4):155–167.
41. Moraes VY, Lenza M, Tamaoki MJ, et al. Platelet-rich therapies for musculoskeletal soft tissue injuries. *Cochrane Database Syst Rev*. 2014;4:CD010071.
42. Levin JH. Prospective, double-blind, randomized placebo-controlled trials in interventional spine: What the highest quality literature tells us. *Spine J*. 2009;9(8):690–703.
43. Jackson DW, Evans NA, Thomas BM. Accuracy of needle placement into the intra-articular space of the knee. *J Bone Joint Surg Am*. 2002;84-A(9):1522–1527.
44. Bum Park Y, Ah Choi W, Kim YK, et al. Accuracy of blind versus ultrasound-guided suprapatellar bursal injection. *J Clin Ultrasound*. 2012;40(1):20–25.
45. Curtiss HM, Finnoff JT, Peck E, et al. Accuracy of ultrasound-guided and palpation-guided knee injections by an experienced and less-experienced injector using a superolateral approach: A cadaveric study. *PM R*. 2011;3(6):507–515.
46. Daley EL, Bajaj S, Bisson LJ, et al. Improving injection accuracy of the elbow, knee, and shoulder: Does injection site and imaging make a difference? A systematic review. *Am J Sports Med*. 2011;39(3):656–662.
47. Berkoff DJ, Miller LE, Block JE. Clinical utility of ultrasound guidance for intra-articular knee injections: A review. *Clin Interv Aging*. 2012;7:89–95.
48. Punzi L, Oliviero F. Arthrocentesis and synovial fluid analysis in clinical practice: Value of sonography in difficult cases. *Ann N Y Acad Sci*. 2009;1154:152–158.
49. Naredo E, Cabero F, Beneyto P, et al. A randomized comparative study of short term response to blind injection versus sonographic-guided injection of local corticosteroids in patients with painful shoulder. *J Rheumatol*. 2004;31(2):308–314.
50. Ucuncu F, Capkin E, Karkucak M, et al. A comparison of the effectiveness of landmark-guided injections and ultrasonography guided injections for shoulder pain. *Clin J Pain*. 2009;25(9):786–789.
51. Sibbitt WL Jr, et al. Does sonographic needle guidance affect the clinical outcome of intraarticular injections? *J Rheumatol*. 2009;36(9):1892–1902.
52. Wiler JL, Costantino TG, et al. Comparison of ultrasound-guided and standard landmark techniques for knee arthrocentesis. *J Emerg Med*. 2010;39(1):76–82.
53. Sibbitt WL Jr, Kettwich LG, Band PA, et al. Does ultrasound guidance improve the outcomes of arthrocentesis and corticosteroid injection of the knee? *Scand J Rheumatol*. 2012;41(1):66–72.
54. Rogojan C, Hetland ML. Depigmentation: A rare side effect to intra-articular glucocorticoid treatment. *Clin Rheumatol*. 2004;23:373–375.
55. Lund IM, Donde R, Knudsen EA. Persistent local cutaneous atrophy following corticosteroid injection for tendinitis. *Rheumatol Rehabil*. 1979;18:91–93.
56. Shumaker PR, Rao J, Goldman MP. Treatment of local, persistent cutaneous atrophy following corticosteroid injection with normal saline infiltration. *Dermatol Surg*. 2005;31:1340–1343.
57. Clark SC, et al. Bilateral patellar tendon rupture secondary to repeated local steroid injections. *J Accid Emerg Med*. 1995;12:300–301.
58. Ford LT, DeBender J. Tendon rupture after local steroid injection. *South Med J*. 1979;72:827–830.
59. Chen SK, et al. Patellar tendon ruptures in weight lifters after local steroid injections. *Arch Orthop Trauma Surg*. 2009;129:369–372.
60. Scutt N, Rolf CG, Scutt A. Glucocorticoids inhibit tenocyte proliferation and tendon progenitor cell recruitment. *J Orthop Res*. 2006;24:173–182.
61. Paik NC, Seo JW. CT-guided needle aspiration of pneumothorax from a trigger point injection. *Pain Med*. 2011;12(5):837–841.

62. Jalul M, Humphrey AR. Radial artery injury caused by a sclerosant injected into a palmar wrist ganglion. *J Hand Surg Eur Vol*. 2009;34(5):698–699.
63. Fujita F, Moriyama T, Higashi T, et al. Methyl p-hydroxybenzoate causes pain sensation through activation of TRPA1 channels. *Br J Pharmacol*. 2007;151(1):153–160.
64. Epstein SP, Ahdoot M, Marcus E, et al. Comparative toxicity of preservatives on immortalized corneal and conjunctival epithelial cells. *J Ocul Pharmacol Ther*. 2009;25(2):113–119.
65. Dragoo JL, et al. The in vitro chondrotoxicity of single-dose local anesthetics. *Am J Sports Med*. 2012;40(4):794–799.
66. Jacobs TF, et al. The effect of Lidocaine on the viability of cultivated mature human cartilage cells: An in vitro study. *Knee Surg Sports Traumatol Arthrosc*. 2011;19(7):1206–1213.
67. Wiater BP, et al. Risk factors for chondrolysis of the glenohumeral joint: A study of three hundred and seventy-five shoulder arthroscopic procedures in the practice of an individual community surgeon. *J Bone Joint Surg Am*. 2011;93(7):615–625.
68. Scheffel PT, et al. Glenohumeral chondrolysis: A systematic review of 100 cases from the English language literature. *J Shoulder Elbow Surg*. 2010;19(6):944–949.
69. Grishko V, et al. Apoptosis and mitochondrial dysfunction in human chondrocytes following exposure to lidocaine, bupivacaine, and ropivacaine. *J Bone Joint Surg Am*. 2010;92(3):609–618.
70. Dragoo JL, et al. Chondrotoxicity of low pH, epinephrine, and preservatives found in local anesthetics containing epinephrine. *Am J Sports Med*. 2010;38(6):1154–1159.
71. Miller RD, Pardo MC Jr. *Basics of Anesthesia*, 6th Ed. Philadelphia, PA: Elsevier Saunders, 2011:136.
72. Becker DE, Reed KL. Essentials of local anesthetic pharmacology. *Anesth Prog*. 2006;53(3):98–109.
73. Charalambous C, Paschalides C, Sadiq S, et al. Weight bearing following intra-articular steroid injection of the knee: Survey of current practice and review of the available evidence. *Rheumatol Int*. 2002;22(5): 185–187.
74. Chatham W, et al. Intraarticular corticosteroid injections: Should we rest the joints? *Arthritis Care Res*. 1989;2(2):70–74.
75. American Medical Association. CPT® 2014 Professional Edition, 2014:976. ISBN#: 978-1-60359-844-6.

# 3 Direct Local Injection

Direct injection by infiltration of a local anesthetic into the skin is a valuable method to provide precise anesthesia. This injection is done in a discrete area so that a minor skin procedure may be performed painlessly. Generally, *1% lidocaine with epinephrine* at 1:100,000 (5 μg/mL) is the anesthetic choice for most skin procedures—whereas *1% lidocaine without epinephrine* is used for musculoskeletal injections. If anesthesia is required for more than 60 min, bupivacaine with or without epinephrine may be considered. The addition of epinephrine to lidocaine provides certain advantages, including prolongation of anesthetic duration of action and vasoconstriction to provide some hemostasis. Due to dermal vasoconstriction, there is blanching of the skin in the affected area. This affords the advantage of allowing visual estimation of the area of anesthesia—thus decreasing the possibility of cutting skin that is not anesthetized. The epinephrine-induced vasoconstriction delays absorption of lidocaine. The prolongation in the rate of absorption decreases the chance of toxicity and increases the maximum recommended dose of lidocaine from 4 to 7 mg/kg.[1] The addition of epinephrine permits the use of larger volumes of the local anesthetic, if needed. It is theoretically safer to avoid injecting epinephrine in areas that contain end arterioles such as fingers, toes, penis, tip of the nose, earlobes, or skin flaps with marginal viability. This may be particularly important in patients who have medical conditions that lead to vascular compromise, including Raynaud phenomenon, advanced diabetes, connective tissue disease, peripheral vascular disease, and Buerger disease (thromboangiitis obliterans). However, there is now extensive evidence that withholding epinephrine in these areas in patients with normal vascular flow is not necessary and is in fact a "medical myth." Historical reviews,[2] a prospective series in more than 3,000 patients[3] and a retrospective review of 1,100 cases,[4] have documented that it is safe to use lidocaine with epinephrine in the digits. In addition, a review of 4,953 cases involving surgery of the nose, ears, extensive flaps, and skin grafts using lidocaine with epinephrine did not result in any complications associated with the use of epinephrine.[5] If necessary, phentolamine, an alpha-adrenergic blocker, may be injected to reverse severe digital ischemia.[6]

Several methods may be used to reduce the pain of injection caused by insertion of the needle and infiltration of the anesthetic into the skin. Ideally, the smallest needle, usually 30 gauge, should be used. Adjunctive techniques include use of topical vapocoolant spray or physical skin distraction to decrease the pain associated with needle insertion. Quick insertion of the needle into the skin, warming the injection fluid,[7] and injecting the anesthetic solution slowly all decrease pain. If clinically indicated, injecting into the subcutaneous tissue is less painful than infiltrating directly into the dermis. However, placement subcutaneously increases the time to full-skin anesthesia to approximately 5 min.

The pH of lidocaine with epinephrine is 4.5. Thus, it is acidic and causes an intense burning pain upon injection. Buffering lidocaine/epinephrine with sodium bicarbonate to achieve a neutral pH above 6.8[8] significantly decreases the injection pain.[9,10] Buffering of the solution is particularly useful in circumstances where the pain of local anesthetic injection is not tolerated such as in large areas of infiltration, in sensitive areas such as the face or genitalia, and in children.[11] To buffer the anesthetic, mix 1 part sodium bicarbonate (8.4%) to 9 parts lidocaine (1% to 2%) immediately before the procedure. Mixing of the solutions may be done within the syringe that is to be used for the injection. Simply, draw up both solutions, add 0.5 mL of air, and rotate the syringe to mix. Then, invert the syringe and expel the air bubble before proceeding. Raising the pH reduces the pain of injection without affecting the onset or efficacy of local anesthesia.

## PATIENT POSITION

- Any, but generally recumbent on the examination/procedure table with the area of concern presented to the clinician.

## ANESTHESIA

- Usually, topical vapocoolant spray is used to decrease the pain associated with injection. Alternatively, skin distraction methods may be employed. Furthermore, the needle used for injection is the smallest possible—that is, 30 gauge if possible; thus, only minimal discomfort is experienced when it is inserted into the skin.

## EQUIPMENT

- 3-mL syringe
- 30-gauge, 1/2-in. needle
- 1.8 mL of 1% lidocaine with epinephrine (larger volume if multiple injections)
- 0.2 mL of 8.4% sodium bicarbonate (larger volume if multiple injections)
- One alcohol prep pad
- Topical vapocoolant spray
- Sterile gauze pads

## TECHNIQUE

1. Mix the volumes of 1% lidocaine/epinephrine with 8.4% sodium bicarbonate within the syringe.
2. Prep the insertion site with an alcohol pad.
3. Use topical vapocoolant spray to achieve transient local anesthesia.
4. Using the no-touch technique, insert the needle through the skin by a single, quick needle stick (Fig. 3.1).
5. Advance the needle at an angle below the center of the lesion in the deep dermis.
6. An intradermal injection produces a wheal directly underneath the lesion.
7. The lesion is thus "floated" upwards. This adds to procedure safety by increasing tissue depth and separating subcutaneous structures (vessels, nerves, tendons) from the surgical instrument (Fig. 3.2).
8. The injection can also be placed first in the subdermal tissues and then intradermal to decrease pain of the procedure.
9. Remove the needle and apply direct pressure with the gauze pad.
10. Perform the skin procedure only after complete anesthesia is achieved in the target area.

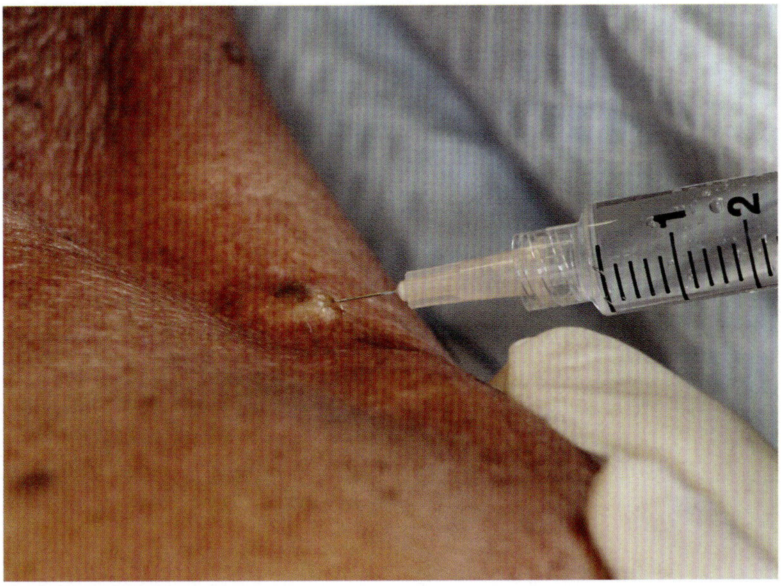


FIGURE 3.1 • Direct local injection.

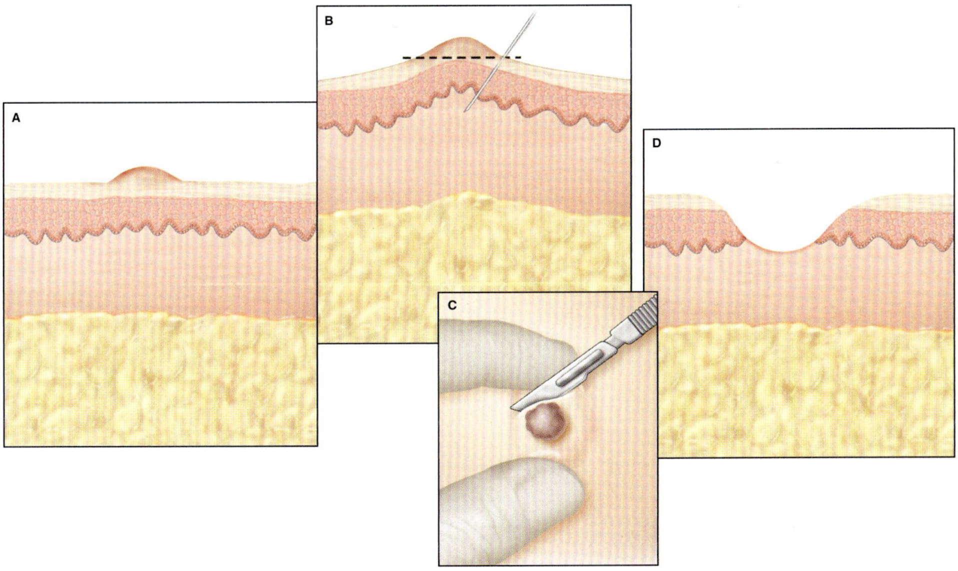


FIGURE 3.2 • Steps in direct local injection.

## AFTERCARE

- None needed.

**CPT code:** None (injected local anesthesia is included as part of the skin procedure CPT code.)

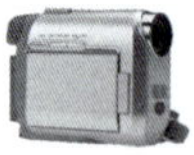

A video clip showing a direct local anesthetic injection can be found in the companion eBook.

## REFERENCES


1. Tetzlaff JE. The pharmacology of local anesthetics. *Anesthesiol Clin North Am.* 2000;18:217–233.
2. Denkler K. A comprehensive review of epinephrine in the finger: To do or not to do. *Plast Reconstr Surg.* 2001;108(1):114–124.
3. Lalonde D, Bell M, Benoit P, et al. A multicenter prospective study of 3,110 consecutive cases of elective epinephrine use in the fingers and hand: The Dalhousie Project clinical phase. *J Hand Surg Am.* 2005;30(5):1061–1067.
4. Chowdhry S, Seidenstricker L, Cooney DS, et al. Do not use epinephrine in digital blocks: Myth or truth? Part II. A retrospective review of 1111 cases. *Plast Reconstr Surg.* 2010;126(6):2031–2034.
5. Häfner HM, Röcken M, Breuninger H. Epinephrine-supplemented local anesthetics for ear and nose surgery: Clinical use without complications in more than 10,000 surgical procedures. *J Dtsch Dermatol Ges.* 2005;3(3):195–199.
6. Hardy SJ, Agostini DE. Accidental epinephrine auto-injector-induced digital ischemia reversed by phentolamine digital block. *J Am Osteopath Assoc.* 1995;95(6):377–378.
7. Hogan ME, vanderVaart S, Perampaladas K, et al. Systematic review and meta-analysis of the effect of warming local anesthetics on injection pain. *Emerg Med.* 2011;58(1):86–98.
8. Bancroft JW, et al. Neutralized lidocaine: Use in pain reduction in local anesthesia. *J Vasc Interv Radiol.* 1992;3(1):107–109.
9. Masters JE. Randomised control trial of pH buffered lignocaine with adrenaline in outpatient operations. *Br J Plast Surg.* 1998;51(5):385–387.
10. Hanna MN, et al. Efficacy of bicarbonate in decreasing pain on intradermal injection of local anesthetics: A meta-analysis. *Reg Anesth Pain Med.* 2009;34(2):122–125.
11. Davies RJ. Buffering the pain of local anaesthetics: A systematic review. *Emerg Med (Fremantle).* 2003;15(1):81–88.

# Field Block Local Injection

The injection of local anesthetic around the target area is a useful method to provide anesthesia to a larger area than that is achieved with direct local injection. This is termed a field block and is commonly used to provide anesthesia for surgical excision of a skin lesion. It is also used when direct injection into the surgical field or distortion of the surgical site is not desired. Use of a field block allows a smaller volume of anesthetic to affect a larger area. In this case, the local anesthetic is injected circumferentially in the dermis around the surgical site. This infiltration prevents the nerve impulses from leaving the area. For the reasons noted in "Direct Local Injection", 1% lidocaine with epinephrine (perhaps buffered with sodium bicarbonate) is the anesthetic choice for this skin procedure—with the previous exceptions considered.

Instead of inserting the needle in a vertical orientation, this procedure is performed in a horizontal plane. The operator identifies the area that requires anesthesia, which includes the lesion and surrounding margins for excision. Surgical excisions are usually performed with a fusiform shape. The insertion site of the needle is positioned just beyond the corners of the fusiform outline. A longer needle (usually a 1-in. 30-gauge needle for use on the face or a 1½-in. 27-gauge or 25-gauge needle for other areas) is inserted into the skin and advanced within the dermis outside of the margin of the excision to the midpoint of the lesion. The local anesthetic is injected into the dermis as the needle is slowly withdrawn. Before the needle is removed from the skin, the tip is redirected and advanced to the other side of the planned excision. After the local anesthetic is injected, the needle is withdrawn completely and the process repeated on the opposite side of the lesion.

## PATIENT POSITION

- Any, but generally recumbent on the examination/procedure table with the area of interest presented to the clinician.

## ANESTHESIA

- Usually, topical vapocoolant spray is used to decrease the pain associated with injection. Alternatively, skin distraction methods may be employed.

## EQUIPMENT

- 5-mL or 10-mL syringe
- 1-in. 30-gauge needle for face or a 1½-in. 27-gauge or 25-gauge needle
- 4.5 mL or 9 mL of 1% lidocaine with epinephrine
- 0.5 mL or 1 mL of 8.4% sodium bicarbonate

- One alcohol prep pad
- Topical vapocoolant spray
- Sterile gauze pads

## TECHNIQUE

1. Mix the volumes of 1% lidocaine/epinephrine with 8.4% sodium bicarbonate within the syringe.
2. Prep the insertion site with an alcohol pad.
3. Use topical vapocoolant spray to achieve transient local anesthesia.
4. Using the no-touch technique, insert the needle through the skin by a single, quick needle stick.
5. The insertion site of the needle is positioned just beyond the points of the fusiform shape (Fig. 3.3).
6. A long needle (usually a 1-in. 30-gauge needle for use on the face or a 1½-in. 27-gauge or 25-gauge needle for other areas) is inserted into the skin and advanced within the dermis outside of the margin of the excision to the midpoint of the lesion.
7. The local anesthetic is injected into the dermis as the needle is slowly withdrawn. The intradermal injection produces a wheal along the injection tract (Fig. 3.4).
8. Before the needle is removed from the skin, the tip is redirected and advanced to the other side of the width of the excision.
9. After the local anesthetic is injected, the needle is withdrawn completely and the process repeated on the opposite side of the lesion.
10. Remove the needle and apply direct pressure with the gauze pad.
11. Perform the skin procedure only after complete anesthesia is achieved in the target area.

## AFTERCARE

- None needed.

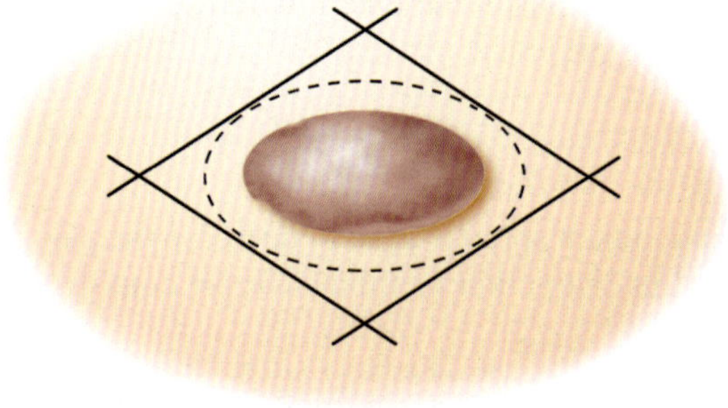

***FIGURE 3.3*** Location for field-block local anesthesia injection.

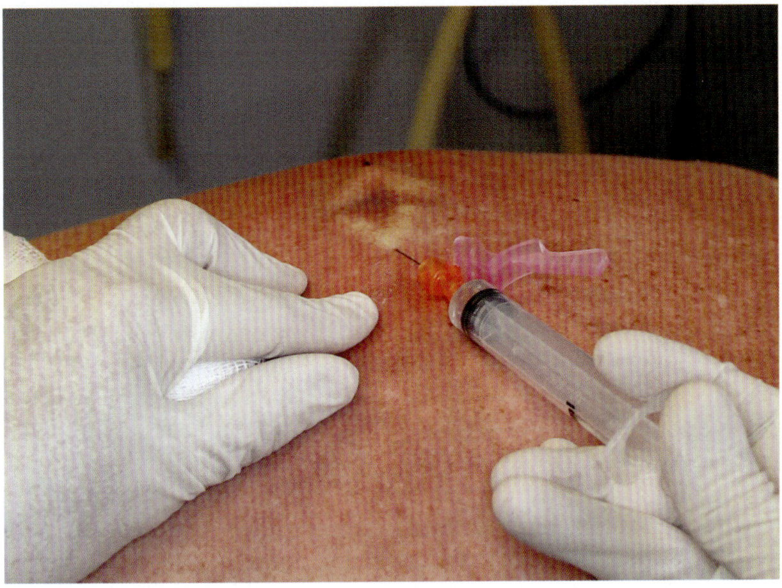

***FIGURE 3.4*** ● Field block.

**CPT code:** None (injected local anesthesia is included as part of the skin procedure CPT code.)

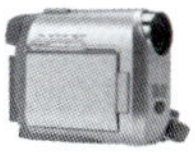

A video clip showing a field-block local anesthetic injection can be found in the companion eBook.

# Digital Nerve Block

Injection of local anesthetic around the digital nerves is a useful method to provide anesthesia of the fingers and toes so that surgical procedures may be conducted on those digits. The fingers and toes are innervated by two sets of nerves that course in the lateral aspect of each digit. There are a pair of dorsal and another pair of palmar/plantar nerves. Each nerve is associated with a corresponding artery. The objective of a digital nerve block is to bathe each of the four nerves with lidocaine to achieve total digital anesthesia while avoiding injury to the vascular structures. Traditionally, this procedure has been performed utilizing a two-injection dorsal technique. However, there is a large body of evidence that demonstrates superior efficacy and preference for a single-injection technique into the volar subcutaneous space at the proximal digit.[1–4]

As noted previously, there is now extensive evidence that withholding epinephrine in areas that contain end arterioles (including the digits) in patients with normal vascular flow is not necessary and is in fact a "medical myth." Historical reviews,[5] a prospective series in more than 3,000 patients[6] and a retrospective review of 1,100 cases,[7] have documented that it is safe to use lidocaine with epinephrine in the digits.

Lidocaine (1%) with epinephrine has a similar onset of action, but is significantly less painful and has a shorter duration of action than bupivacaine (0.5%).[8–10] Therefore, the preferred method to perform a digital nerve block is a single injection of 1% lidocaine with epinephrine (1:100,000) into the volar subcutaneous space at the proximal digit to create a firm, turgid feel to the tissue.

**Relevant Anatomy:** (Fig. 3.5)

## PATIENT POSITION

- Recumbent on the examination/procedure table with the hand or foot extended to the clinician.

## ANESTHESIA

- Topical vapocoolant spray is used to decrease the pain associated with injection.

## EQUIPMENT

- 5-mL syringe
- 25-gauge, 1-in. needle
- 5 mL of 1% lidocaine with epinephrine
- One alcohol prep pad
- Topical vapocoolant stream spray
- Sterile gauze pads

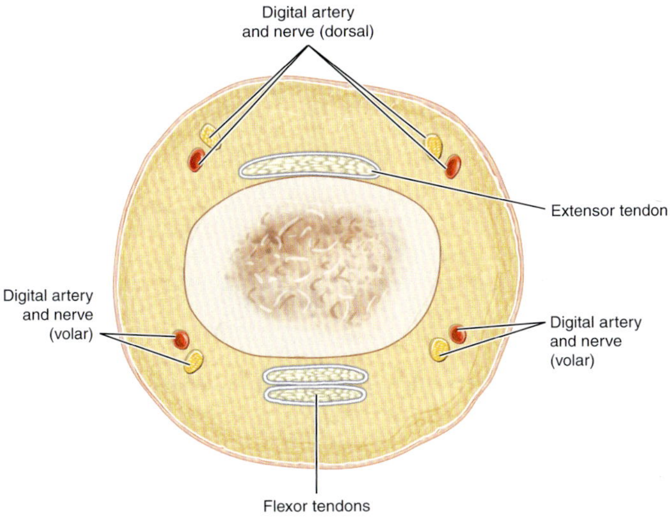


*FIGURE 3.5* • Digital anatomy.

## TECHNIQUE

1. Locate the needle insertion site over the palmar/plantar crease at the junction of the digit and the palm or foot.[4]
2. Prep the insertion site with an alcohol pad.
3. Use topical vapocoolant stream spray to achieve transient local anesthesia.[11]
4. Using the no-touch technique, insert the 25-gauge 1-in. needle through the skin by a single, quick needle stick. Advance the needle in a few millimeters through the skin into the subcutaneous tissue (Fig. 3.6).
5. Inject about 2.5 mL of lidocaine with epinephrine as a bolus in the subcutaneous tissue.
6. Remove the needle and apply direct pressure with the gauze pad—spreading the local anesthetic up to the digital nerves.

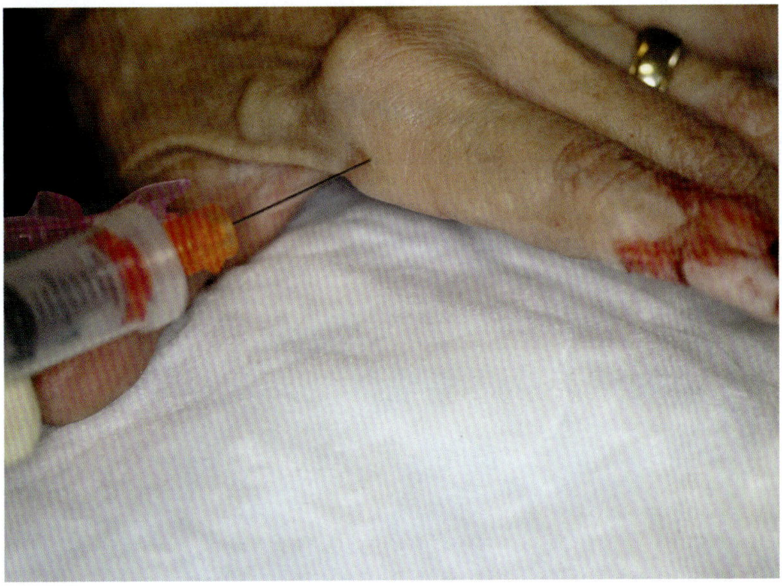

*FIGURE 3.6* • Digital nerve block.

7. Allow at least 5 to 10 min for the anesthesia to take effect.
8. Repeat the procedure if necessary.
9. Perform the digital procedure only after complete anesthesia is achieved.

## AFTERCARE

- None needed.

**CPT code:** 64450—Injection, nerve block, therapeutic, other peripheral nerve or branch

**CPT code:** None (injected local anesthesia is included as part of the skin procedure CPT code.)

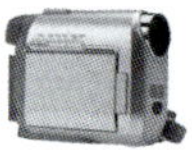

A video clip showing a digital nerve block can be found in the companion eBook.

## REFERENCES

1. Hung VS, Bodavula VK, Dubin NH. Digital anaesthesia: Comparison of the efficacy and pain associated with three digital nerve block techniques. *J Hand Surg Br*. 2005;30(6):581–584.
2. Williams JG, Lalonde DH. Randomized comparison of the single-injection volar subcutaneous block and the two-injection dorsal block for digital anesthesia. *Plast Reconstr Surg*. 2006;118(5):1195–1200.
3. Cannon B, Chan L, Rowlinson JS, et al. Digital anaesthesia: One injection or two? *Emerg Med J*. 2010;27(7):533–536.
4. Tzeng YS, Chen SG. Tumescent technique in digits: A subcutaneous single-injection digital block. *Am J Emerg Med*. 2012;30(4):592–596.
5. Denkler K. A comprehensive review of epinephrine in the finger: To do or not to do. *Plast Reconstr Surg*. 2001;108(1):114–124.
6. Lalonde D, Bell M, Benoit P, et al. A multicenter prospective study of 3,110 consecutive cases of elective epinephrine use in the fingers and hand: The Dalhousie Project clinical phase. *J Hand Surg Am*. 2005;30(5):1061–1067.
7. Chowdhry S, Seidenstricker L, Cooney DS, et al. Do not use epinephrine in digital blocks: Myth or truth? Part II. A retrospective review of 1111 cases. *Plast Reconstr Surg*. 2010;126(6):2031–2034.
8. Schnabl SM, Unglaub F, Leitz Z, et al. Skin perfusion and pain evaluation with different local anaesthetics in a double blind randomized study following digital nerve block anaesthesia. *Clin Hemorheol Microcirc*. 2013;55(2):241–253.
9. Alhelail M, Al-Salamah M, Al-Mulhim M, et al. Comparison of bupivacaine and lidocaine with epinephrine for digital nerve blocks. *Emerg Med J*. 2009;26(5):347–350.
10. Thomson CJ, Lalonde DH. Randomized double-blind comparison of duration of anesthesia among three commonly used agents in digital nerve block. *Plast Reconstr Surg*. 2006;118(2):429–432.
11. Kose O, Saylan S, Ediz N, et al. Effects of topical alkane vapocoolant spray on pain intensity prior to digital nerve block for ingrown nail surgery. *Foot Ankle Spec*. 2010;3(2):73–75.

# Facial Nerve Blocks

Facial nerve blocks are utilized to achieve anesthesia of different regions of the face. The technique is used when direct injection into the surgical field or distortion of the surgical site is not desired. In this case, a small volume of the local anesthetic is injected around the specific nerve that innervates a defined area of skin. Therefore, a small volume affects a much larger area than would otherwise be possible using local injections. This decreases excessive pain and bruising associated with multiple injections. It also reduces the total amount of local anesthetic required, thus minimizing the potential for medication toxicity.

There are three classic nerve blocks that are commonly performed to provide anesthesia of the face. These are the supraorbital/supratrochlear, infraorbital, and mental nerve blocks. Each of these nerves is a terminal sensory branch of the fifth cranial nerve, and each has its own discrete foramen to exit the bony structures. Once the foramen is located, a small amount of anesthetic (0.5 to 1 mL) can be injected at that site to provide the desired effect. As shown in Figure 3.7, all of the three facial foramen are located along a line drawn in a vertical (sagittal) orientation from the center of the patient's pupil. The supraorbital foramen is the easiest to identify. It is located superior to the center of the pupil and palpated as a subtle depression in the supraorbital ridge underneath the eyebrow. The supratrochlear nerve is commonly injected along with the supraorbital nerve to extend the anesthetic effect to the midline of the forehead. The nerve is located at the supraorbital ridge immediately vertical (sagittal) to the inner canthus of the eye. In most people, this is usually located at the medial aspect of the eyebrow. The infraorbital foramen may be found in the maxilla about 1.5 cm inferior to the infraorbital rim—and in line with the pupil. A depression in the maxilla cannot be palpated. Finally, the mental nerve is located along the same line drawn in a vertical (sagittal) orientation from the center of the patient's pupil. It is positioned at the midpoint of the height of the mandible. A discrete depression is also not possible to palpate. To confirm the correct location, firm palpation directly over each of the foramen elicits a sensation of intense, dull pain, not found in adjacent areas.

From a coding standpoint, all injections to establish local anesthesia for a surgical procedure are considered part of that procedure. As such, they are included in the CPT procedural code and not billed separately.

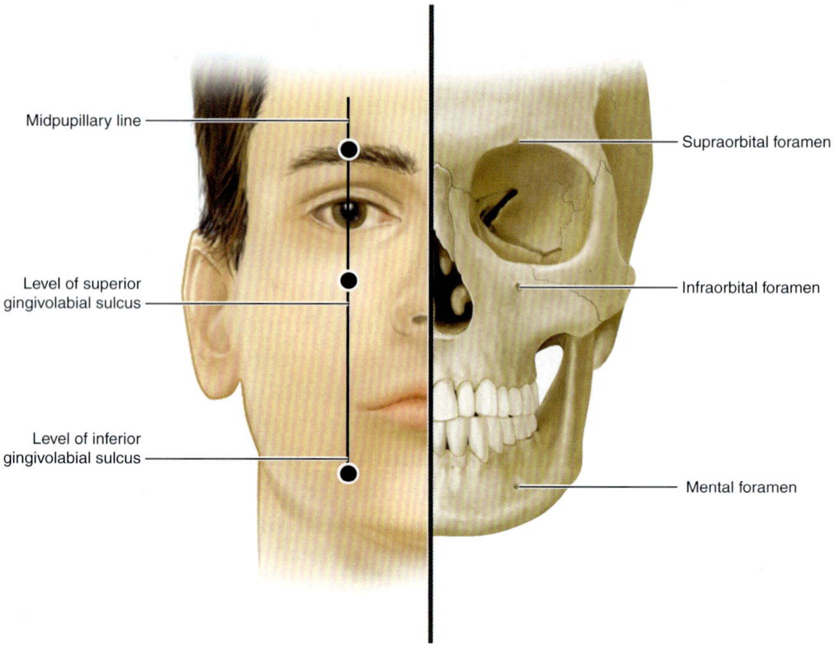


***FIGURE 3.7*** Foramina for nerve blocks.

# Supraorbital and Supratrochlear Nerve Blocks

The supraorbital and supratrochlear nerves are perhaps the easiest of the facial nerve blocks to perform. These nerves are terminal sensory branches of the ophthalmic trunk of the fifth cranial nerve. These blocks are used to administer reversible local anesthesia to the forehead. Various procedures including laceration repair, skin lesion removal, photodynamic therapy, or facial skin resurfacing of the forehead may be performed utilizing these blocks. Headache disorders including cluster, tension, and migraine headaches may also be treated by providing supraorbital, supratrochlear, infraorbital, greater occipital, and lesser occipital nerve blocks.[1,2]

**Relevant Anatomy:** (Fig. 3.8)

## PATIENT POSITION

- Supine on the examination table with the head of the bed slightly elevated.

## LANDMARKS

- With the patient supine on the examination table, the clinician stands lateral to the side of the face that is being injected.
- The supraorbital foramen is located superior (sagittal) to the center of the pupil as a subtle depression in the supraorbital ridge underneath the eyebrow.
- In an anatomic study of skulls, supraorbital foramina were found to be approximately 25 mm lateral to the midline, 30 mm medial to the temporal crest of the frontal bone, and 2 to 3 mm superior to the supraorbital rim. Additional exits for branches of the supraorbital nerve were present in 14% of skulls.[3]
- The supratrochlear nerve is located at the supraorbital ridge immediately vertical (sagittal) to the inner canthus of the eye. In most people, this is located at the medial aspect of the eyebrow.
- At sites located about 0.5 cm superior to the eyebrow at each nerve, press firmly on the skin with the retracted tip of a ballpoint pen. This indention represents the entry point for the needle.

## ANESTHESIA

- Local anesthesia of the skin in this area with use of topical vapocoolant spray is not advised due to the close proximity to the eyes. However, skin distraction techniques may be employed.

## EQUIPMENT

- 3-mL syringe
- 30-gauge, 1/2-in. needle
- 1 mL of 1% lidocaine without epinephrine
- One alcohol prep pad
- Sterile gauze pad

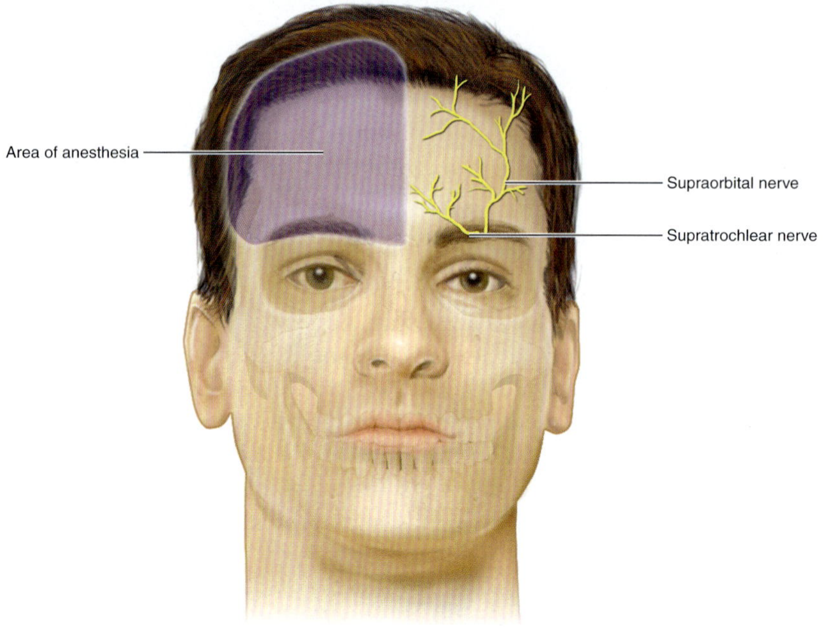


**FIGURE 3.8** Supraorbital and supratrochlear nerves and innervated areas.

## TECHNIQUE

1. Prep the insertion site with alcohol pads.
2. Position the needle at a 45-degree angle just above the eyebrow with the tip of the needle directed toward the supraorbital foramen.
3. Provide skin distraction by pinching, stretching, and rubbing adjacent skin over the eyebrow at the same time that the needle is being inserted into the skin.
4. Using the no-touch technique, quickly introduce the needle at the insertion site.
5. Advance the needle over the supraorbital foramen.
6. Inject 0.5 mL of 1% lidocaine directly over the supraorbital foramen.
7. Following injection, withdraw the needle.
8. Repeat the process for the supratrochlear nerve with the needle positioned over the supraorbital ridge immediately vertical (sagittal) to the inner canthus of the eye.

## AFTERCARE

- None needed

**CPT code:** 64400—Injection, anesthetic agent, trigeminal nerve, any division or branch

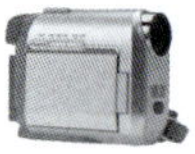

A video clip showing supraorbital/supratrochlear nerve blocks can be found in the companion eBook.

## REFERENCES

1. Blumenfeld A, Ashkenazi A, Napchan U, et al. Expert consensus recommendations for the performance of peripheral nerve blocks for headaches—A narrative review. *Headache*. 2013;53(3):437–446.
2. Ilhan Alp S, Alp R. Supraorbital and infraorbital nerve blockade in migraine patients: Results of 6-month clinical follow-up. *Eur Rev Med Pharmacol Sci*. 2013;17(13):1778–1781.
3. Gupta T. Localization of important facial foramina encountered in maxillo-facial surgery. *Clin Anat*. 2008;21(7):633–640.

# Infraorbital Nerve Block

The infraorbital nerve is a terminal sensory branch of the maxillary trunk of the fifth cranial nerve. This block is used to administer reversible local anesthesia to the central midface. Various procedures including skin laceration repair, upper lip laceration repair, photodynamic therapy, skin filler replacement, or skin lesion removal may be performed following this block. Headache disorders including cluster, tension, and migraine headaches may also be treated by providing supraorbital, supratrochlear, infraorbital, greater occipital, and lesser occipital nerve blocks.[1,2]

**Relevant Anatomy:** (Fig. 3.9)

## PATIENT POSITION

- Supine on the examination table with the head of the bed slightly elevated.

## LANDMARKS

- With the patient supine on the examination table, the clinician stands lateral to the side of the face that is being injected.
- In an anatomic study of skulls, infraorbital foramina were found to be 28.5 mm lateral to the midline and approximately 7 mm inferior to the inferior orbital rim and along a line drawn in a vertical (sagittal) orientation from the center of the patient's pupil.[3] A depression in the maxilla at the site of the foramen is difficult to palpate. To confirm the location, firm pressure directly over the foramen elicits the sensation of intense, dull pain, not found in adjacent areas.
- At that site, press firmly on the skin with the retracted tip of a ballpoint pen. This indention represents the entry point for the needle.

## ANESTHESIA

- Local anesthesia of the skin in this area with use of topical vapocoolant spray is not advised due to the close proximity to the eyes. However, skin distraction techniques may be employed.

## EQUIPMENT

- Headlamp or other light source (for intraoral approach)
- 3-mL syringe
- 30-gauge, 1/2-in. needle for transdermal and a 25-gauge 1½-in. needle for intraoral approach
- 1 mL of 1% lidocaine without epinephrine

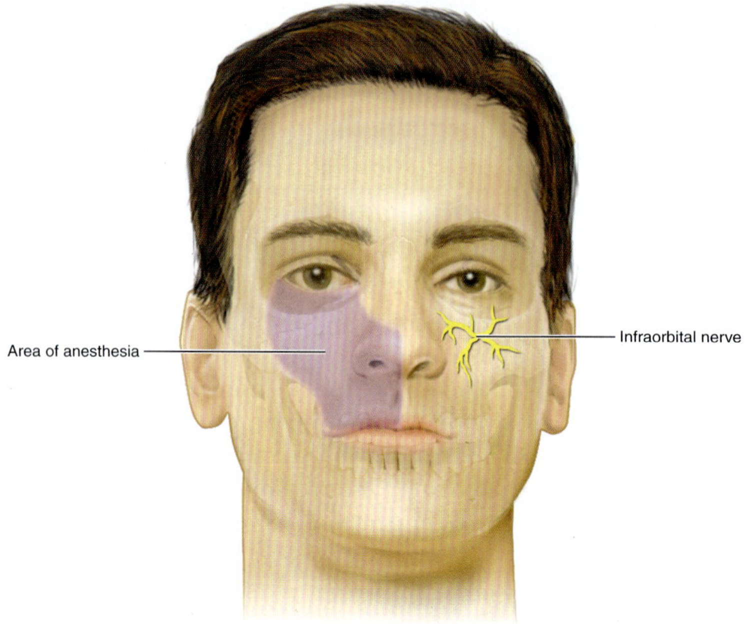


*FIGURE 3.9* ● Infraorbital nerve and innervated area.

- One alcohol prep pad (for transdermal approach)
- Sterile gauze pad

## TECHNIQUE (TRANSDERMAL)

1. Prep the insertion site with alcohol pads.
2. Position the needle perpendicularly to the skin at the location over the maxilla identified above. The tip of the needle is directed toward the infraorbital foramen.
3. Provide skin distraction by pinching, stretching, and rubbing adjacent skin at the same time that the needle is being inserted into the skin.
4. Using the no-touch technique, quickly introduce the needle at the insertion site.
5. Advance the needle over the infraorbital foramen.
6. Inject 0.5 to 1 mL of 1% lidocaine directly over the infraorbital foramen.
7. Following injection, withdraw the needle.

## TECHNIQUE (INTRAORAL)

1. Wear a headlamp to provide good illumination for the procedure.
2. Grasp the upper lip with gauze and retract it superiorly.
3. Identify the maxillary third to fourth tooth from midline (canine/first premolar). The infraorbital foramen is located just beyond the apex of the gingivolabial mucosal reflection.
4. A 1½-in. 25-gauge needle is positioned in the sagittal plane, directed toward the ipsilateral pupil.
5. The needle is quickly inserted at this point and advanced approximately 0.5 cm to a position over the infraorbital foramen.
6. Inject 1 mL of 1% lidocaine without epinephrine directly over the infraorbital foramen.
7. Following injection, withdraw the needle.

## AFTERCARE

- None needed

**CPT code:** 64400—Injection, anesthetic agent, trigeminal nerve, any division or branch

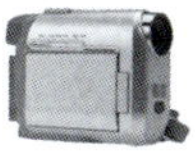

A video clip showing infraorbital nerve block can be found in the companion eBook.

## REFERENCES

1. Blumenfeld A, Ashkenazi A, Napchan, et al. Expert consensus recommendations for the performance of peripheral nerve blocks for headaches—A narrative review. *Headache*. 2013;53(3):437–446.
2. Ilhan Alp S, Alp R. Supraorbital and infraorbital nerve blockade in migraine patients: Results of 6-month clinical follow-up. *Eur Rev Med Pharmacol Sci*. 2013;17(13):1778–1781.
3. Gupta T. Localization of important facial foramina encountered in maxillo-facial surgery. *Clin Anat*. 2008;21(7):633–640.

# Mental Nerve Block

The mental nerve is a terminal sensory branch of the mandibular trunk of the fifth cranial nerve. This block is used to administer reversible local anesthesia to the lower midface. Various procedures including skin laceration repair, lower lip laceration repair, photodynamic therapy, skin filler placement, or skin lesion removal may be performed following this block.

**Relevant Anatomy:** (Fig. 3.10)

## PATIENT POSITION

- Supine on the examination table with the head of the bed slightly elevated.

## LANDMARKS

- With the patient supine on the examination table, the clinician stands lateral to the side of the face that is being injected.
- In an anatomic study of skulls, mental foramina were on average, 25.8 mm lateral to the midline and about 13 mm superior to the inferior mandibular margin and along a line drawn in a vertical (sagittal) orientation from the center of the patient's pupil.[1] A depression in the mandible at the site of the foramen is difficult to palpate. To confirm the location, firm pressure directly over the foramen elicits the sensation of intense, dull pain, not found in adjacent areas.
- At that site, press firmly on the skin with the retracted tip of a ballpoint pen. This indention represents the entry point for the needle.

## ANESTHESIA

- Usually, topical vapocoolant spray is used to decrease the pain associated with injection. Alternatively, skin distraction methods may be employed.

## EQUIPMENT

- Headlamp or other light source (for intraoral approach)
- 3-mL syringe
- 30-gauge, 1/2-in. needle for transdermal and a 25-gauge 1½-in. needle for intraoral approach
- 1 mL of 1% lidocaine without epinephrine
- One alcohol prep pad (for transdermal approach)
- Sterile gauze pad

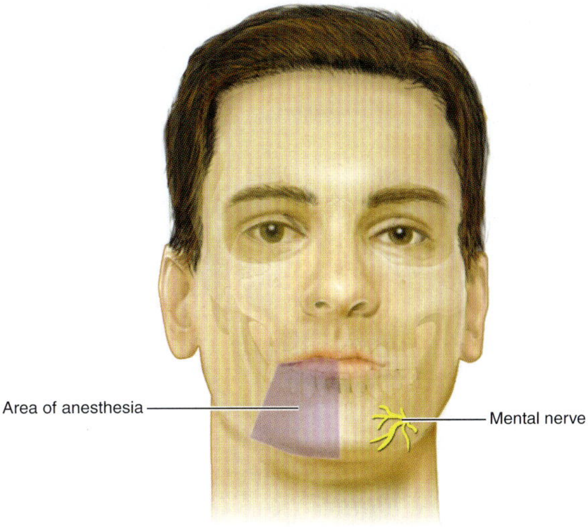


**FIGURE 3.10** ● Mental nerve and innervated area.

## TECHNIQUE (TRANSDERMAL)

1. Prep the insertion site with alcohol pads.
2. Position the needle perpendicularly to the skin at the location over the mandible identified above. The tip of the needle is directed toward the mental foramen.
3. Provide skin distraction by pinching, stretching, and rubbing adjacent skin at the same time that the needle is being inserted into the skin.
4. Using the no-touch technique, quickly introduce the needle at the insertion site.
5. Advance the needle over the mental foramen.
6. Inject 0.5 to 1 mL of 1% lidocaine directly over the mental foramen.
7. Following injection, withdraw the needle.

## TECHNIQUE (INTRAORAL)

1. Wear a headlamp to provide good illumination for the procedure.
2. Grasp the lower lip with gauze and retract it superiorly.
3. Identify the mandibular third to fourth tooth from midline (canine/first premolar). The mental foramen is located just beyond the apex of the gingivolabial mucosal reflection.
4. A 1½-in. 25-gauge needle is positioned in the sagittal plane, directed inferiorly toward the mental foramen.
5. The needle is quickly inserted at this point and advanced approximately 0.5 cm to a position over the mental foramen.
6. Inject 1 mL of 1% lidocaine without epinephrine directly over the mental foramen.
7. Following injection, withdraw the needle.

## AFTERCARE

- None needed

**CPT code:** 64400—Injection, anesthetic agent, trigeminal nerve, any division or branch

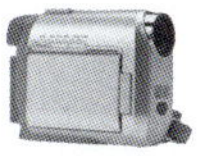

A video clip showing mental nerve block can be found in the companion eBook.

## REFERENCE

1. Gupta T. Localization of important facial foramina encountered in maxillo-facial surgery. *Clin Anat.* 2008;21(7):633–640.

# Mucosal Fold Block

Mucosal fold blocks may be placed to interrupt pain impulses from the gingival branches of the infraorbital and mental nerves. These blocks are accomplished by placing a small amount of local anesthetic into the gingival buccal reflection of each lip. A small volume of 0.1 mL of 1% lidocaine without epinephrine is injected just under the mucosa at the reflection that corresponds to the base of each tooth. This block is used to administer reversible local anesthesia to the upper lip, nasal labial fold, lower lip, and corners of the mouth. This may be given selectively to just the upper lip or right and left sides of the patient. Various procedures including lip laceration repair, skin filler replacement, or skin lesion removal may be performed following this block.

**Relevant Anatomy:** (Fig. 3.11)

## PATIENT POSITION

- Supine on the examination table with the head of the bed slightly elevated.

## LANDMARKS

- With the patient supine on the examination table, the clinician stands lateral to the side of the face that is being injected.
- Locate the mucosal reflection in the gingivobuccal sulcus that corresponds to the right or left first four teeth (medial incisor, lateral incisor, canine, and first premolar) of the maxillary or mandibular aspect of the mouth.

## ANESTHESIA

- Topical anesthesia of the mucosa in this area is usually not necessary but may be provided with a 3-minute application of viscous lidocaine or benzocaine 20% gel to the area of injection.

## EQUIPMENT

- Headlamp or other light source
- 3-mL syringe
- 25-gauge 1½-in. needle for intraoral approach
- 1 mL of 1% lidocaine without epinephrine
- Sterile gauze pad

## TECHNIQUE

1. Wear a headlamp to provide good illumination for the procedure.
2. Grasp the lip with gauze and retract the upper lip superiorly or the lower lip inferiorly.

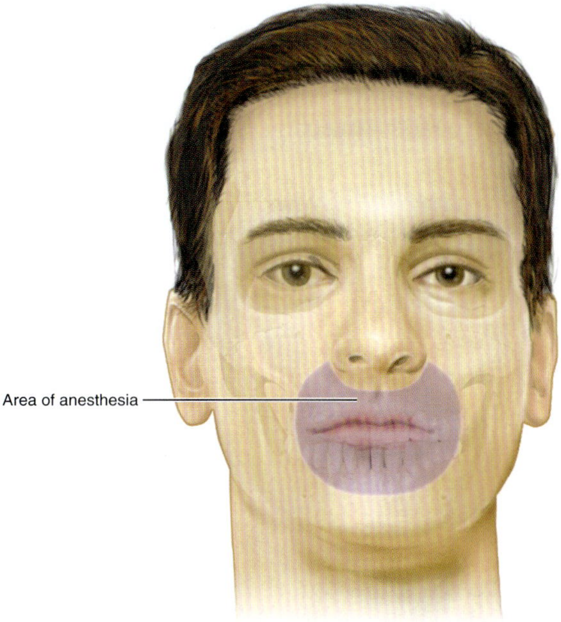


***FIGURE 3.11*** ● Mucosal nerve block innervated area.

3. Identify the mucosal reflection in the gingivobuccal sulcus that corresponds to the right or left first four teeth (medial incisor, lateral incisor, canine, and first premolar) of the maxillary or mandibular aspect of the mouth.
4. A 1½-in. 25-gauge needle is positioned in the sagittal plane, directed either superiorly in the case of the upper lip or inferiorly with the lower lip.
5. The needle is gently inserted just under the mucosa at the gingival buccal sulcus that corresponds to each of the target teeth (Fig. 3.12).
6. Inject 0.1 mL of 1% lidocaine without epinephrine directly under the mucosa at each location.
7. Following injection, withdraw the needle.

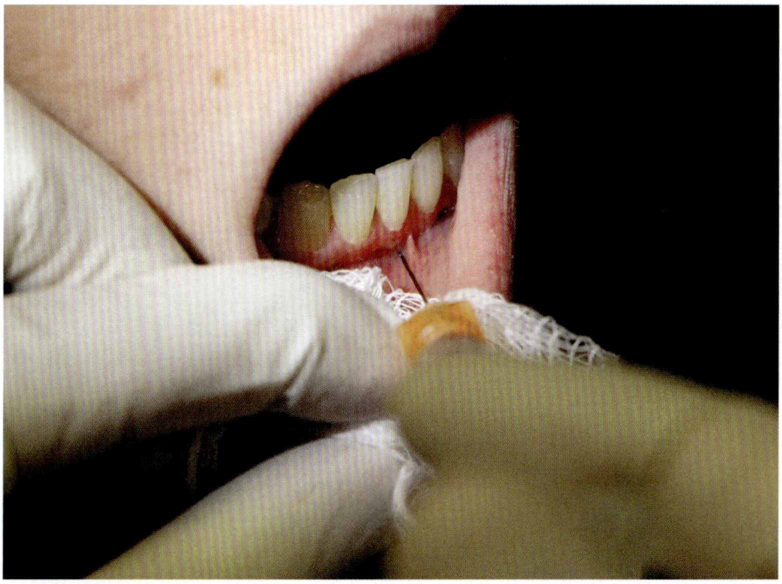

***FIGURE 3.12*** ● Mucosal nerve block.

## AFTERCARE

- None needed

**CPT code:** 64400—Injection, anesthetic agent, trigeminal nerve, any division or branch

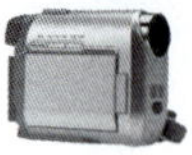

A video clip showing the mucosal fold block can be found in the companion eBook.

# 4 Chalazion

A chalazion is an acute or chronic granuloma that forms due to inflammation and obstruction in the meibomian glands (or tarsal glands) on the conjunctival surface of either the upper or the lower eyelids. The obstruction in these small sebaceous glands may occur due to allergy, acne in adolescence, or rosacea. A chalazion contains many steroid-responsive immune cells including macrophages, plasma cells, polymorphonuclear cells, and eosinophils. Patients with this condition present occasionally to the primary care office, and although considered self-limited, it may last for weeks to months before spontaneously disappearing. Traditional conservative treatment includes the application of local heat, lubricant eye drops, careful cleansing of the eyelid, and topical antibiotics (although this condition, unlike a hordeolum, is not an infectious process).

An often unrecognized procedure is the simple injection of a small amount of corticosteroid (4 mg of triamcinolone) into or around the chalazion lesion. Recent studies show that the procedure is quick, well tolerated, and safe. It results in greater than 80% resolution of the chalazion lesion within days of administration.[1–4] Response rates mirror that of surgical treatment with incision and curettage. Additional advantages of this technique over traditional I&C include its simplicity, less pain, considerably decreased cost, no requirement of special instruments, no need for postoperative eye patching, and convenience for both the provider and the patient.

| Indications | ICD-9 Code | ICD-10 Code |
|---|---|---|
| Chalazion | 373.2 | H00.19 |

**Relevant Anatomy:** (Fig. 4.1)

## PATIENT POSITION

- Supine on the examination table with the head of the bed elevated 30 degrees.
- The patient's hands are folded in his or her lap.
- The clinician stands lateral to the patient, on the same side as the chalazion.

## ANESTHESIA

- Topical corneal anesthesia is never provided so that inadvertent introduction of the needle through the eyelid, through the conjunctiva, and into the globe cannot occur.
- Topical vapocoolant spray cannot be used around the eyes, unless measures are taken to prevent inadvertent exposure to the cornea. The author uses Gebauer's Pain Ease mist spray directed onto the injection site in conjunction with a transparent

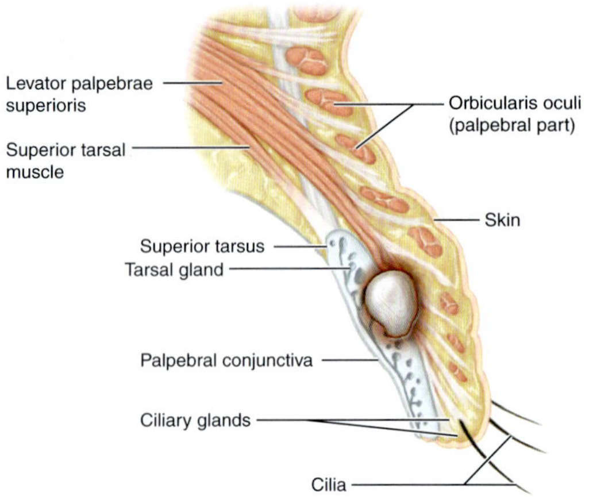


**FIGURE 4.1** Superior eyelid. The tarsus forms the skeleton of the eyelid and contains the tarsal glands. (From Tank PW, Gest TR. *Lippincott Williams & Wilkins Atlas of Anatomy*. Philadelphia, PA: Lippincott Williams & Wilkins, 2009.)

Lexan plate with a 4-mm conical opening (Brymill Cryoplate) that restricts the application and prevents overspray into the eyes. Injection of local anesthetic into the skin of the eyelid is not used. Local injection of anesthetic in this location causes swelling that obliterates the location of the chalazion.

## EQUIPMENT

- (Optional) Corneal eye shield protectors (Kolberg Optical Supplies, Inc. http://www.corneaprotectors.com/)
- (Optional) Cryoplate (Brymill Cryogenic Systems. 105 Windermere Ave. Ellington, CT 06029. http://brymill.com/)
- (Optional) Gebauer's Pain Ease mist topical vapocoolant spray
- 3-mL or a tuberculin syringe
- 30-gauge, 1/2-in. needle
- 0.1 mL of the steroid solution (40 mg/mL of triamcinolone acetonide)
- One alcohol prep pad
- Two povidone–iodine prep pads
- Sterile gauze pads

## TECHNIQUE

1. (Optional) Corneal eye shield protectors may be used to protect the cornea and globe.
2. Identify the injection site a few millimeter lateral to the chalazion. Prep the insertion site with alcohol followed by the povidone–iodine pads.
3. (Optional) A chalazion clamp may also be used, if desired, to stabilize the lesion. However, use of this instrument requires both infiltration local anesthesia and topical corneal anesthesia.
4. (Optional) At the injection site, firmly place the Brymill Cryoplate 4-mm conical opening onto the skin and then direct Gebauer's Pain Ease mist spray for several seconds until a white flash is observed on the skin surface. Stop spraying and remove the plate.
5. With your fingertips, apply lateral traction to the eyelid to stretch and fix the skin.
6. Approach the eyelid from a lateral to a medial direction.
7. To ensure safety, make sure that the needle is oriented parallel to the surface of the globe of the eye.

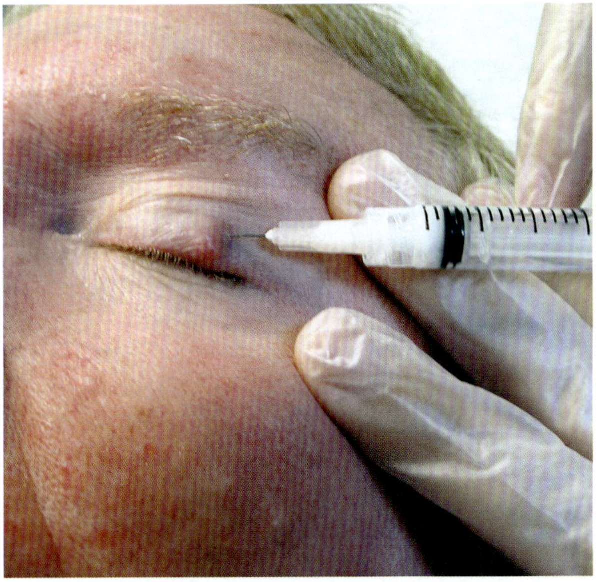

***FIGURE 4.2*** • Chalazion injection.

8. Using the no-touch technique, insert the needle through the skin external to the eyelid about 0.5 cm lateral to the chalazion (Fig. 4.2).
9. Advance it slowly and carefully into the center of the lesion.
10. After insertion into the chalazion, confirm accurate placement by moving the needle slightly from side to side to ensure that the lesion moves with the needle.
11. Inject 0.1 mL (4 mg) of the steroid solution (40 mg/mL of triamcinolone acetonide) into the chalazion.
12. Remove the needle and apply direct pressure with the gauze pad.

## AFTERCARE

- None needed.
- Consider follow-up examination in 1 week.

**CPT code:** 68200—Subconjunctival injection

## PEARLS

- After the needle has been inserted into the chalazion, confirm accurate placement by moving the needle slightly from side to side to ensure that the nodule moves with the needle.
- One-third of the cases may require a second injection.
- If the chalazion continues to recur after two injections, it should be evaluated for malignancy. In this case, more aggressive traditional measures should be used, including curettage through a cruciform incision, primary excision, or excision/destruction using radiofrequency surgery.
- Potential complications may include inadvertent corneal injury, penetration of the globe, cataract from administration of steroid in the globe, and skin depigmentation.

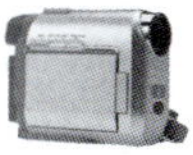

A video clip showing a chalazion injection can be found in the companion eBook.

## REFERENCES

1. Wong MY, Yau GS, Lee JW, Yuen CY. Intralesional triamcinolone acetonide injection for the treatment of primary chalazions. *Int Ophthalmol.* 2014 Jan 19. [Epub ahead of print].
2. Ben Simon GJ, Rosen N, Rosner M, et al. Intralesional triamcinolone acetonide injection versus incision and curettage for primary chalazia: A prospective, randomized study. *Am J Ophthalmol.* 2011;151(4): 714–718.
3. Goawalla A, Lee V. A prospective randomized treatment study comparing three treatment options for chalazia: triamcinolone acetonide injections, incision and curettage and treatment with hot compresses. *Clin Experiment Ophthalmol.* 2007;35(8):706–712.
4. Chung CF, Lai JS, Li PS. Subcutaneous extralesional triamcinolone acetonide injection versus conservative management in the treatment of chalazion. *Hong Kong Med J.* 2006;12(4):278–281.

# Keloid Scar

Keloid scars occur as the result of an abnormal overgrowth of dense fibrous tissue that develops in areas of prior skin trauma. The tissue elevates above the surface of the surrounding skin, extends beyond the borders of the original wound, does not regress spontaneously, and often recurs after excision. Keloids usually occur during the second and third decades of life, with a higher prevalence in those with darker pigmented skin. They are most commonly asymptomatic but can present with itching and pain if they become inflamed or enlarge.

Since primary surgical excision commonly results in worsening of the keloid scar, many other therapeutic modalities for keloids and hypertrophic scars are currently used in clinical practice. Intralesional injection is the most commonly used treatment. Medication options include intralesional injections of corticosteroids and antineoplastic agents, including 5-fluorouracil. Other modalities include silicone gel application, photodynamic therapy, cryosurgery, and laser ablation. Corticosteroids reduce excessive scarring by decreasing collagen synthesis, suppressing vascular endothelial growth factor and decreasing production of inflammatory mediators and fibroblast proliferation during wound healing. Complications of repeated corticosteroid injections may include skin atrophy, telangiectasia formation, hypopigmentation, and a depressed scar.

Combinations of various therapies have been shown to produce an even greater benefit. In vitro molecular studies show that triamcinolone suppresses cell proliferation and induces G1 cell cycle arrest but not apoptosis. In contrast, 5-fluorouracil induces G2 cell cycle arrest and apoptosis.[1] Other clinical studies demonstrate that triamcinolone used in combination with 5-flurouracil results in improved scar regression and reduced recurrence of keloids.[2,3] Combination therapy with different types of corticosteroids,[4] intralesional cryosurgery followed by injected steroids,[5] and surgical excision followed by corticosteroid injections[6–8] have also been shown to be effective. However, recent reviews agree that there is a lack of high-quality, blinded, randomized, controlled clinical trials and that more research is needed to conclusively guide therapy.[9,10]

| Indications | ICD-9 Code | ICD-10 Code |
|---|---|---|
| Keloid scar | 701.4 | L91.0 |

## PATIENT POSITION

- Supine on the examination table.
- Rotate the patient's head away from the side that is being injected. This minimizes anxiety and pain perception.
- The clinician stands on the side of the patient that allows best access to the keloid scar.

## ANESTHESIA

- Local anesthesia of the injection site with topical vapocoolant spray.

## EQUIPMENT

- 3-mL syringe
- 25-gauge, 1- or 1½-in. needle depending on the size of the keloid
- 0.25 to 1 mL of the steroid solution (40 mg/mL of triamcinolone acetonide)
- (Optional) 0.25 to 1 mL of 5-fluorouracil solution (50 mg/mL)
- One alcohol prep pad
- Two povidone–iodine prep pads
- Sterile gauze pads
- Sterile adhesive bandage

## TECHNIQUE

1. Prep the insertion site with alcohol followed by the povidone–iodine pads.
2. Achieve good local anesthesia by using topical vapocoolant spray.
3. Position the needle and syringe parallel to the surface of the skin at the edge of the keloid with the tip of the needle directed toward the center of the keloid scar.
4. Using the no-touch technique, introduce the needle at the edge of the keloid (Fig. 4.3).
5. Advance the needle into the lesion.
6. Perform a uniform injection of 0.25 to 1 mL of steroid solution (10 to 40 mg of triamcinolone acetonide) (and optionally, 0.25 to 1 mL [12.5 to 50 mg] of 5-fluorouracil solution) into the substance of the keloid at a depth that is half the thickness of the keloid.
7. Avoid injection into the subcutaneous fat or surrounding normal skin.
8. Following injection, withdraw the needle.
9. Apply a sterile adhesive bandage.

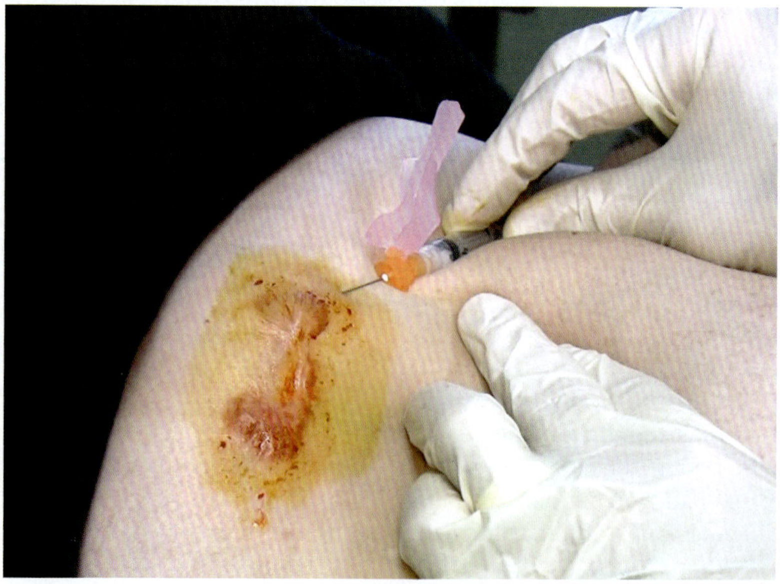

***FIGURE 4.3*** ● Keloid injection.

## AFTERCARE

- None needed
- Follow-up examination in 4 to 6 weeks

**CPT code:** Intralesional injections—11900 (one to seven lesions) and 11901 (greater than seven lesions)

## PEARLS

- If the keloid continues to recur after several injections, more aggressive measures may be used, as noted above.
- Avoid superficial injections as they may increase the likelihood of dermal complications.

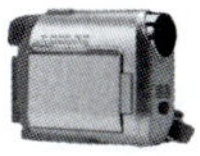

A video clip showing a keloid scar injection can be found in the companion eBook.

## REFERENCES


1. Huang L, Cai YJ, Lung I, et al. A study of the combination of triamcinolone and 5-fluorouracil in modulating keloid fibroblasts in vitro. *J Plast Reconstr Aesthet Surg*. 2013;66(9):e251–e259.
2. Davison SP, Dayan JH, Clemens MW, et al. Efficacy of intralesional 5-fluorouracil and triamcinolone in the treatment of keloids. *Aesthet Surg J*. 2009;29(1):40–46.
3. Darougheh A, Asilian A, Shariati F. Intralesional triamcinolone alone or in combination with 5-fluorouracil for the treatment of keloid and hypertrophic scars. *Clin Exp Dermatol*. 2009;34(2):219–223.
4. Syed F, Bayat A. Superior effect of combination vs. single steroid therapy in keloid disease: A comparative in vitro analysis of glucocorticoids. *Wound Repair Regen*. 2013;21(1):88–102.
5. Weshahy AH, Abdel Hay R. Intralesional cryosurgery and intralesional steroid injection: A good combination therapy for treatment of keloids and hypertrophic scars. *Dermatol Ther*. 2012;25(3):273–276.
6. Hayashi T, Furukawa H, Oyama A, et al. A new uniform protocol of combined corticosteroid injections and ointment application reduces recurrence rates after surgical keloid/hypertrophic scar excision. *Dermatol Surg*. 2012;38(6):893–897.
7. Park TH, Seo SW, Kim JK, et al. Clinical characteristics of facial keloids treated with surgical excision followed by intra- and postoperative intralesional steroid injections. *Aesthetic Plast Surg*. 2012;36(1):169–173.
8. Park TH, Seo SW, Kim JK, et al. Management of chest keloids. *J Cardiothorac Surg*. 2011;6:49.
9. Ledon JA, Savas J, Franca K, et al. Intralesional treatment for keloids and hypertrophic scars: A review. *Dermatol Surg*. 2013;39(12):1745–1757.
10. Ud-Din S, Bayat A. Strategic management of keloid disease in ethnic skin: A structured approach supported by the emerging literature. *Br J Dermatol*. 2013;169(Suppl 3):71–81.

# Common Warts

Patients very commonly present to the primary care office for evaluation of common warts. These verrucous structures are the focal dermal expression of human papillomavirus infections. Common warts may be treated with various modalities, including cryosurgery, electrosurgery, laser ablation, cautery, curettage, and injection therapy.

Immunotherapy achieved by injecting *Candida* or mumps antigen at the edge of a wart incites a host immune response that is mediated through stimulation of T helper-1 cell cytokines.[1] This commonly results in spontaneous regression of the treated warts. In addition, an HPV-directed cell-mediated immune response plays a role in the resolution of distant untreated warts. There is a small body of literature that documents effectiveness and safety of intralesional and/or perilesional injection therapy with *Candida* and mumps antigens.[1–6] A single study documents the effectiveness of *Candida* antigen in the treatment of molluscum.[7] The antineoplastic chemotherapy drug, bleomycin, inhibits DNA synthesis in cells and viruses. This causes acute tissue necrosis and may also stimulate an immune response. Adverse effects include pain, swelling, and redness. Necrosis of skin may cause scarring, pigment change, or nail damage. Bleomycin has also demonstrated similar effectiveness to antigens when injected intralesionally.[8–10] In a recent meta-analysis of five randomized controlled trials, cure rates ranged from 16% to 94%.[11]

*Candida* antigen is available as "Candin" (Allermed Labs, 7203 Convoy Court, San Diego, CA 92111, phone: 1–800–221–2748, web site: http://www.allermed.com/candin/) or the generic (Hollister Stier Labs Inc. 3525 N. Regal, Spokane, WA 99207, phone: 1–800–992–1120, web site: http://www.hsallergy.com/).

| Indications | ICD-9 Code | ICD-10 Code |
|---|---|---|
| Common warts | 078.10 | B07.8 |
| Genital warts | 078.11 | A63.0 |
| Plantar warts | 078.12 | B07.0 |

## PATIENT POSITION

- Supine on the examination table.
- Rotate the patient's head away from the side that is being injected. This minimizes anxiety and pain perception.

## ANESTHESIA

- Local anesthesia of the skin using topical vapocoolant spray.

## EQUIPMENT

- 3-mL syringe
- 25-gauge, 1/2-in. needle

- Up to 1 mL of the *Candida* antigen
- Up to 1 mL of 1% lidocaine without epinephrine
- One alcohol prep pad
- Sterile gauze pads
- Sterile adhesive bandage
- Nonsterile, clean chucks pad

## TECHNIQUE

1. Prepare the injection solution: Mix equal parts of up to 1 mL of *Candida* antigen and up to 1 mL of 1% lidocaine without epinephrine.
2. Prep the insertion site(s) with alcohol pads.
3. Achieve good local anesthesia by using topical vapocoolant spray.
4. Position the needle and syringe at a 10-degree angle to the surface of the skin at the edge of the wart with the tip of the needle directed toward the wart.
5. Using the no-touch technique, introduce the needle about 5 mm from the edge of the wart (Fig. 4.4).
6. Advance the needle into the dermis at the edge of the wart.
7. Perform an intradermal injection immediately adjacent to the wart using 0.1 to 0.3 mL of the solution per wart. Limit total amount at any one visit to 1 mL of the *Candida* antigen.
8. Avoid injection into the subcutaneous tissues.
9. Following injection of the solution, withdraw the needle.
10. Apply a sterile adhesive bandage.

## AFTERCARE

- None needed.
- Instruct the patient to expect these local symptoms following injection as the immune system is reacting to the antigen: localized erythema, itching, drying of the wart,

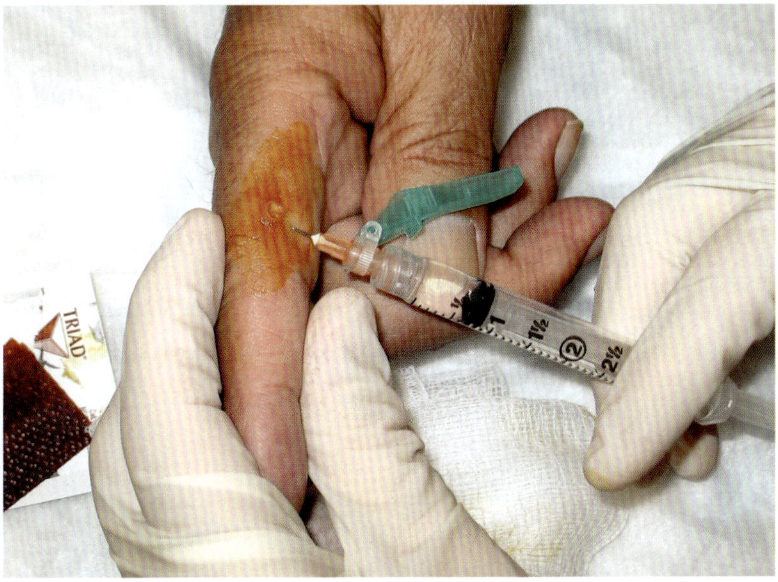


**FIGURE 4.4** • Common wart injection.

lesion turning a black color, peeling of the treated tissue, or simply spontaneous regression.
- Adverse reactions may also include rash, adenopathy, and persistence of wart(s).
- Consider follow-up examination in 2 to 4 weeks.

**CPT code:** Intralesional injections—11900 (one to seven lesions) and 11901 (greater than seven lesions)

## PEARLS

- *Candida* antigen should not be used after a previous unacceptable adverse reaction such as extreme hypersensitivity or allergy to this antigen or to a similar product.
- Repeat injection in 1 month if there is any residual wart.
- Sixty-five to seventy-five percent of warts treated with *Candida* antigen injection resolve after the first injection.
- Fifty percent of the remaining warts respond after a second injection.
- Antigen injection of warts is an "off-label" use of *Candida* and mumps antigens, and there is no J code listed for these antigens. Thus, insurance companies do not provide reimbursement for the antigen used in this procedure. Unfortunately, the injection code does not include this cost, and the antigen itself is more expensive than the payment for the procedure. Therefore, if providing this treatment, consider asking the patient to fill a prescription at a reputable pharmacy, bring the unopened injectable to the office, and then perform the procedure.

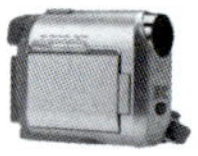

A video clip showing a common wart injection can be found in the companion eBook.

## REFERENCES

1. Nofal A, Salah E, Nofal E, et al. Intralesional antigen immunotherapy for the treatment of warts: Current concepts and future prospects. *Am J Clin Dermatol.* 2013;14(4):253–260.
2. Horn TD, Johnson SM, Helm RM, et al. Intralesional immunotherapy of warts with mumps, Candida, and Trichophyton skin test antigens: A single-blinded, randomized, and controlled trial. *Arch Dermatol.* 2005;141(5):589–594.
3. Johnson SM, Horn TD. Intralesional immunotherapy for warts using a combination of skin test antigens: A safe and effective therapy. *J Drugs Dermatol.* 2004;3(3):263–265.
4. Clifton MM, Johnson SM, Roberson PK, et al. Immunotherapy for recalcitrant warts in children using intralesional mumps or Candida antigens. *Pediatr Dermatol.* 2003;20(3):268–271.
5. Signore RJ. Candida albicans intralesional injection immunotherapy of warts. *Cutis.* 2002;70(3):185–192.
6. Johnson SM, Roberson PK, Horn TD. Intralesional injection of mumps or Candida skin test antigens: A novel immunotherapy for warts. *Arch Dermatol.* 2001;137(4):451–455.
7. Enns LL, Evans MS. Intralesional immunotherapy with Candida antigen for the treatment of molluscum contagiosum in children. *Pediatr Dermatol.* 2011;28(3):254–258.
8. Alghamdi KM, Khurram H. Successful treatment of plantar warts with very diluted bleomycin using a translesional multipuncture technique: Pilot prospective study. *J Cutan Med Surg.* 2012;16(4):250–256.
9. Saitta P, Krishnamurthy K, Brown LH. Bleomycin in dermatology: A review of intralesional applications. *Dermatol Surg.* 2008;34(10):1299–1313.
10. Soni P, et al. Efficacy of intralesional bleomycin in palmo-plantar and periungual warts. *J Cutan Aesthet Surg.* 2011;4(3):188–191.
11. Kwok CS, Gibbs S. Topical treatments for cutaneous warts. *Cochrane Database Syst Rev.* 2012;9:CD001781.

# Granuloma Annulare and Other Thin, Benign, Inflammatory Dermatoses

Granuloma annulare is an example of a *thin* benign inflammatory dermatosis. It is a relatively common disorder of unknown etiology occurring in children and young adults. In the most common localized form, this presents as skin-colored or erythematous dermal papules and ring-shaped lesions up to 5 cm in diameter (Fig. 4.5). Localized granuloma annulare has a predilection for the feet, ankles, lower limbs, and wrists. Localized granuloma annulare is usually asymptomatic and usually resolves spontaneously within 2 years. Treatment is not evidence based and is determined by provider preference, expert opinion, and case reports. Topical potent corticosteroids or intralesional corticosteroids are most commonly utilized. There are a myriad of other treatment options, including liquid nitrogen cryosurgery, photodynamic therapy, hydroxychloroquine, dapsone, tacrolimus, pimecrolimus, and imiquimod.[1]

| Indications | ICD-9 Code | ICD-10 Code |
|---|---|---|
| Alopecia areata | 704.01 | L63.9 |

## PATIENT POSITION

- Supine on the examination table with the head of the bed elevated 30 degrees.
- The patient's hands are folded in his or her lap.
- The clinician stands lateral to or behind the patient, on the same side as the affected area.

## ANESTHESIA

- Local anesthesia of the injection site with topical vapocoolant spray.

## EQUIPMENT

- 0.5-mL insulin syringe with its attached 8-mm, 31-gauge needle
- Steroid solution (10 mg/mL of triamcinolone acetonide)
- Gebauer's Pain Ease mist topical vapocoolant spray
- One alcohol prep pad
- Sterile gauze pads
- Sterile adhesive bandage
- Nonsterile, clean chucks pad

## TECHNIQUE

1. Over the lesion, plot out a grid at 1-cm intervals using a ruler and surgical marking pen.
2. Prep the site with an alcohol pad.
3. Achieve good local anesthesia by using Gebauer's Pain Ease mist topical vapocoolant spray (Fig. 4.6).

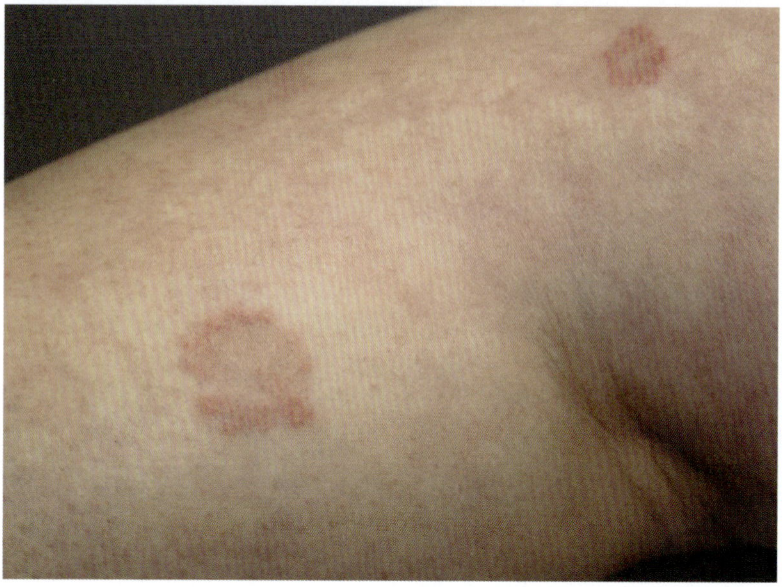

**FIGURE 4.5** ● Granuloma annulare lesion.

4. Position the needle and syringe at a 30-degree angle to the surface of the skin at each injection site.
5. Using the no-touch technique, quickly introduce the needle into the skin.
6. Advance the needle to a depth of approximately 2 mm.
7. Inject 0.01 to 0.05 mL of the steroid solution (10 mg/mL of triamcinolone acetonide) (Fig. 4.7).
8. Repeat the injections to cover the entire lesion.
9. Following the injections of the corticosteroid solution, withdraw the needle, and apply direct pressure with the gauze pad.
10. Apply a sterile adhesive bandage.
11. The injections may be repeated every 4 to 6 weeks until the lesion resolves (Fig. 4.8).

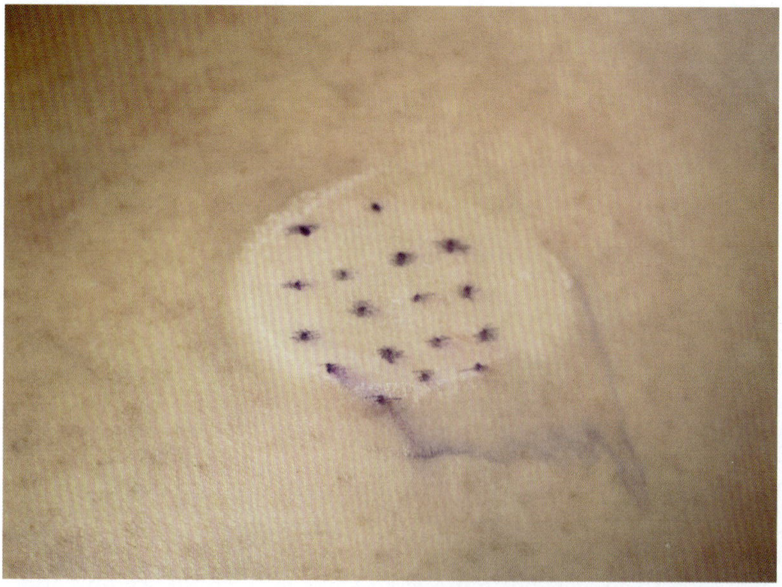

**FIGURE 4.6** ● Granuloma annulare lesion with 1-cm grid markings—immediately after Pain Ease mist topical vapocoolant spray.

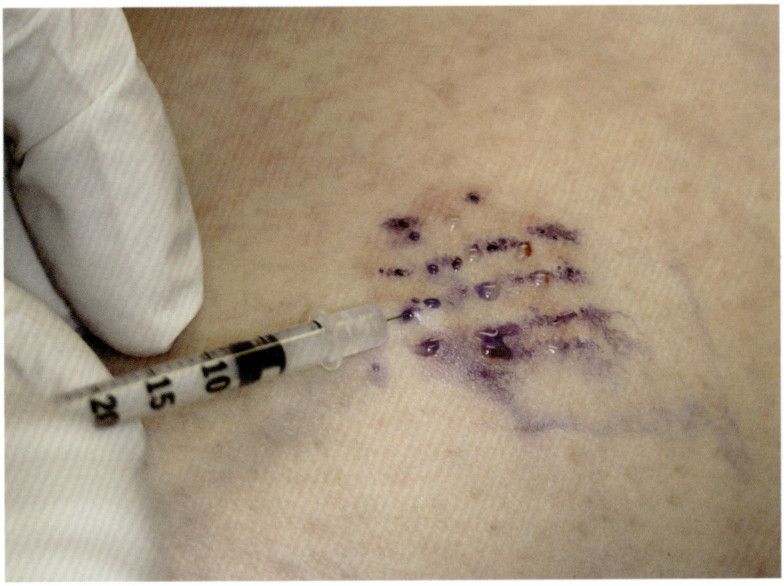


*FIGURE 4.7* • Injections of granuloma annulare lesion using an insulin syringe/needle with small volumes of triamcinolone.

## AFTERCARE

- None needed.
- Schedule follow-up examination in 4 to 6 weeks.

**CPT code:** Intralesional injections—11900 (one to seven lesions) and 11901 (greater than seven lesions)

## PEARLS

- Avoid injection into the epidermis or subcutaneous tissues.

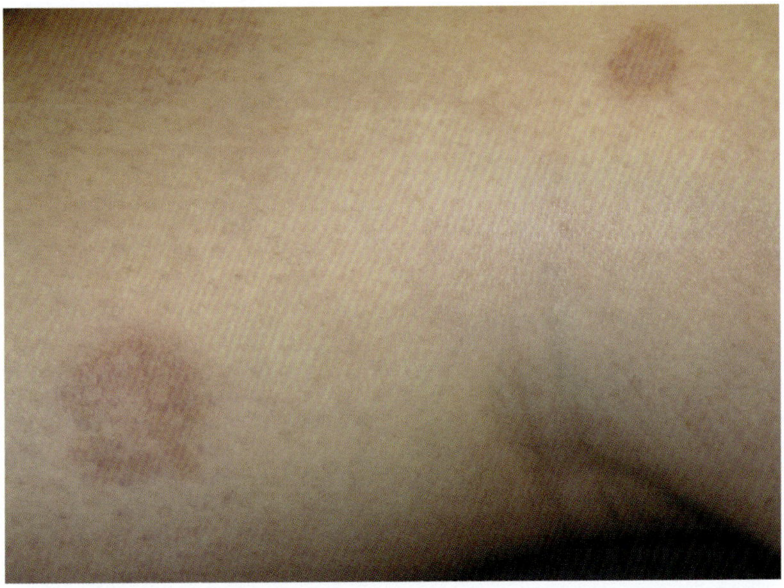

*FIGURE 4.8* • Resolving granuloma annulare lesion 7 days after corticosteroid injection.

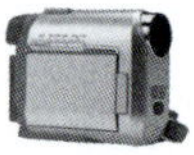

A video clip showing injection for thin, benign, inflammatory dermatoses can be found in the companion eBook.

## REFERENCE

1. Thornsberry LA, English JC III. Etiology, diagnosis, and therapeutic management of granuloma annulare: An update. *Am J Clin Dermatol*. 2013;14(4):279–290.

# Prurigo Nodularis and Other Thick, Benign, Inflammatory Dermatoses

Prurigo nodularis is an example of a *thick* benign inflammatory dermatosis. It is a chronic, highly pruritic condition characterized by the presence of generally symmetric, hyperkeratotic, excoriated, hyperpigmented or purpuric, firm, intensely pruritic nodules. Chronic and repetitive scratching or picking of the nodules causes permanent changes, including nodular lichenification, hyperkeratosis, hyperpigmentation, and skin thickening. Unhealed, excoriated lesions are often scaling and crusted. They can involve any part of the body, but generally begin on the arms and legs. Recent findings suggest a neuropathic origin, with alterations in the dermal and epidermal small diameter nerve fibers.[1] No reliable data exist about incidence and prevalence of this in the general population, but it seems to be more frequent and more intense in females. Prurigo nodularis may be associated with many dermatologic and nondermatologic comorbidities, including psychiatric disease. The diagnosis is based on the physical features of the nodules and the presence of itching. A skin biopsy is often performed to exclude other diseases.

Prurigo nodularis often has a tremendous impact on the quality of life. Unfortunately, few randomized controlled trials are available to guide therapy.[1] Therapeutic options include topical and intralesional steroids, cryosurgery, thalidomide, and UVB light. Intralesional steroids are highly effective, and triamcinolone acetonide is commonly used. Concentrations as low as 2.5 mg/mL may be effective, although most scarred pruriginous lesions require higher concentrations. A total dose of up to 20 mg for adults may need to be repeated monthly for a maximum of 4 months to achieve a good clinical result.[2] Regardless of the intervention, effective management of this condition involves consideration of the associated psychological factors.[3]

| Indications | ICD-9 Code | ICD-10 Code |
|---|---|---|
| Prurigo nodularis | 698.2 | L28.1 |

## PATIENT POSITION

- Supine on the examination table.
- Rotate the patient's head away from the side that is being injected. This minimizes anxiety and pain perception.
- The clinician stands on the side of the patient that allows best access to the prurigo nodularis lesion.

## ANESTHESIA

- Local anesthesia of the injection site with topical vapocoolant spray.

## EQUIPMENT

- 3-mL syringe
- 25-gauge, 1-in. needle
- 0.25 to 1 mL of the steroid solution (10 to 40 mg/mL of triamcinolone acetonide)
- One alcohol prep pad
- Two povidone–iodine prep pads
- Sterile gauze pads
- Sterile adhesive bandage

## TECHNIQUE

1. Prep the insertion site with alcohol.
2. Achieve good local anesthesia by using topical vapocoolant spray.
3. Position the needle and syringe at a 0- to 45-degree angle to the surface of the skin at the edge of the lesion with the tip of the needle directed toward the center of the nodule.
4. Using the no-touch technique, introduce the needle at the edge of the lesion (Fig. 4.9).
5. Advance the needle into the lesion.
6. Perform injection(s) of 0.1 mL to a maximum of 1 mL (40 mg/mL of triamcinolone acetonide) into the base of the lesion to uniformly cover the entire lesion.
7. Avoid injection into the epidermis or subcutaneous tissues.
8. Following the injection of the corticosteroid solution, withdraw the needle.
9. Apply a sterile adhesive bandage.

## AFTERCARE

- None needed.
- Schedule follow-up examination in 4 to 6 weeks.

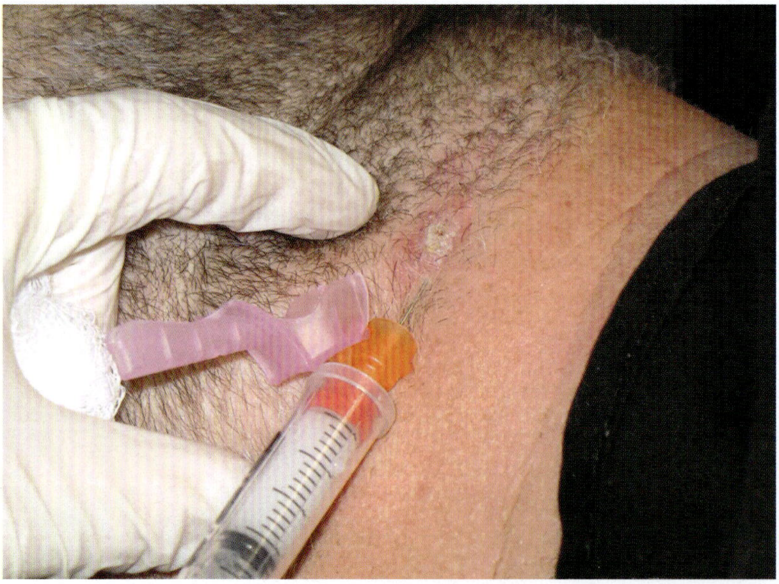

**FIGURE 4.9** ● Injection of prurigo nodularis lesion using a 25-gauge needle with triamcinolone.

**CPT code:** Intralesional injections—11900 (one to seven lesions) and 11901 (greater than seven lesions)

## PEARLS

- Avoid injection into the epidermis or subcutaneous tissues.

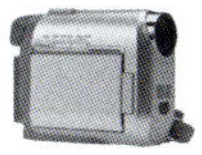

A video clip showing injection for thin, benign, inflammatory dermatoses can be found in the companion eBook.

## REFERENCES

1. Fostini AC, Girolomoni G, Tessari G. Prurigo nodularis: An update on etiopathogenesis and therapy. *J Dermatolog Treat*. 2013;24(6):458–462.
2. Richards RN. Update on intralesional steroid: Focus on dermatoses. *J Cutan Med Surg*. 2010;14(1):19–23.
3. Lotti T, Buggiani G, Prignano F. Prurigo nodularis and lichen simplex chronicus. *Dermatol Ther*. 2008;21(1):42–46.

5

# Temporomandibular Joint

Patients commonly present to the primary care office for evaluation of jaw pain from temporomandibular joint (TMJ) dysfunction and/or arthritis. Injection of corticosteroid into the TMJ space is an effective treatment option for this difficult-to-treat condition.[1] Although the Food and Drug Administration has not approved hyaluronic acid for clinical use in this joint, research demonstrates safe and effective treatment using hyaluronic acid injections.[2,3] Ultrasound guidance of the procedure improves the localization of the injections, especially in the pediatric population.[4,5] Trials examining the use of botulinum toxin injections have had mixed results.[6,7] As with many musculoskeletal injections, more high-quality research is needed.

| Indications | ICD-9 Code | ICD-10 Code |
|---|---|---|
| TMJ dysfunction | 524.60 | M26.60 |
| TMJ arthritis, unspecified | 716.98 | M26.62 |

**Relevant Anatomy:** (Fig. 5.1)

## PATIENT POSITION

- Sitting on the exam table.
- The patient's hands are folded in his or her lap.

## LANDMARKS

1. With the patient seated on the exam table, the clinician stands lateral and posterior to the affected jaw.
2. Palpate the TMJ with the mouth in the closed and then the fully open positions.
3. Identify the sulcus that forms with jaw opening and mark that spot with ink.
4. At that site, press firmly on the skin with the retracted tip of a ballpoint pen. This indention represents the entry point for the needle.
5. After the landmarks are identified, the patient should not move the jaw.
6. The patient must keep his or her mouth open until the completion of the procedure.

## ANESTHESIA

- Local anesthesia of the skin using topical vapocoolant spray may be used but is not necessary in most patients. If using a spray, make sure that "overspray" of the vapocoolant chemical does not enter the patient's eyes or external ear canal.

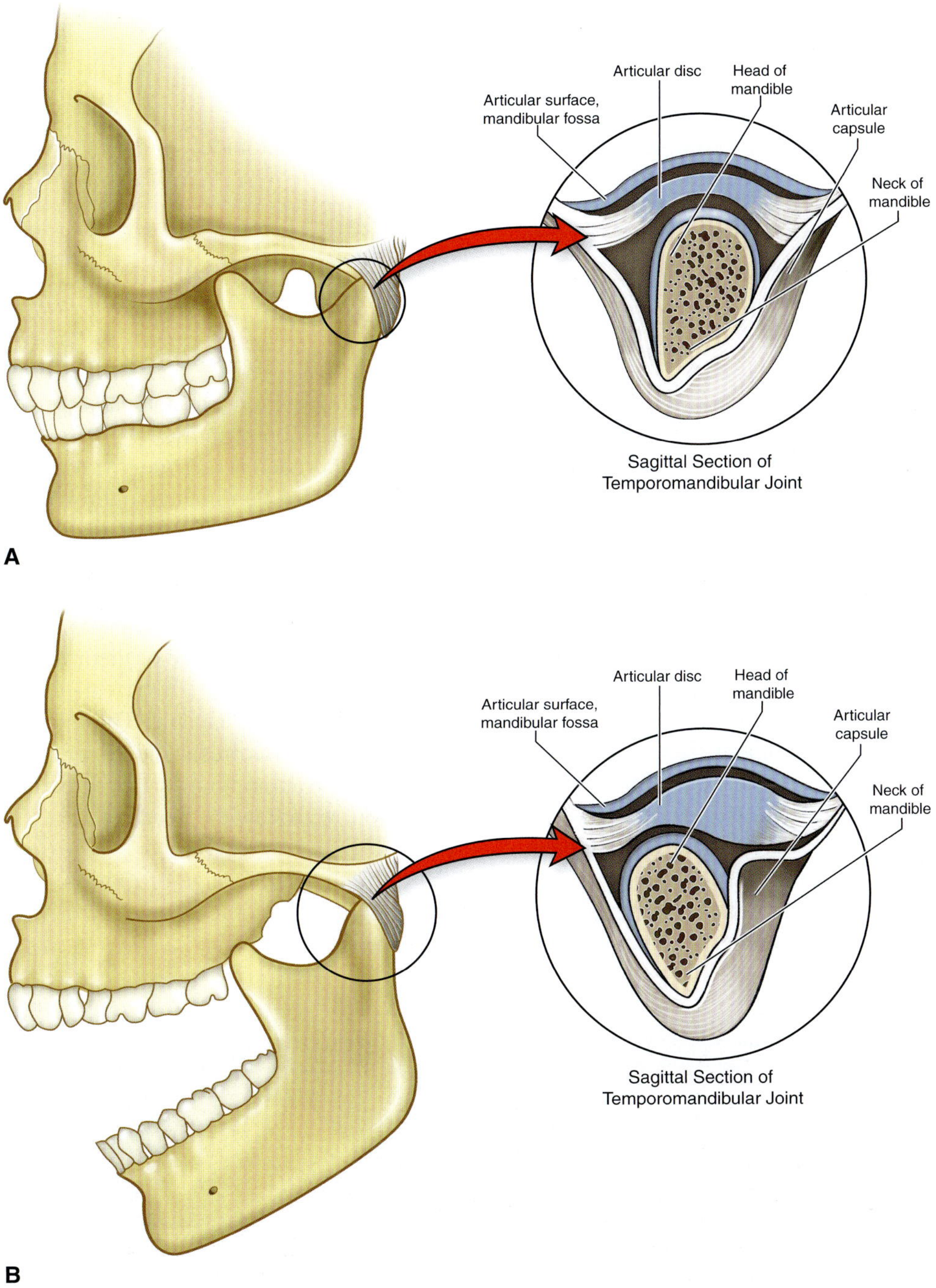


***FIGURE 5.1*** ● Sagittal view of the temporomandibular joint. **A:** Jaw closed. **B:** Jaw open. (From Tank PW, Gest TR. *Lippincott Williams & Wilkins Atlas of Anatomy*. Philadelphia, PA: Lippincott Williams & Wilkins, 2009.)

## EQUIPMENT

- 3-mL syringe
- 25-gauge, 1-in. needle
- 0.5 mL of 1% lidocaine without epinephrine
- 0.5 mL of the steroid solution (20 mg of triamcinolone acetonide)
- One alcohol prep pad
- Two povidone–iodine prep pads
- Sterile gauze pads
- Sterile adhesive bandage

## TECHNIQUE

1. Prep the insertion site with alcohol followed by the povidone–iodine pads.
2. Achieve good local anesthesia by using topical vapocoolant spray.
3. Position the needle and syringe from a posterior approach at a 30-degree angle to the sagittal plane into the sulcus with the tip of the needle directed anteromedial toward the posterior aspect of the TMJ.
4. Using the no-touch technique, introduce the needle at the insertion site (Fig. 5.2).
5. Advance the needle toward the joint until the needle tip is located in the joint capsule. There will be a decrease in resistance when entering the joint capsule. After entering the joint space, the needle will touch the articular surface or the articular disk. Back up the needle 1 to 2 mm.
6. Inject the steroid solution as a bolus into the TMJ articular capsule. The injected solution should flow smoothly into the space. If increased resistance is encountered, advance or withdraw the needle slightly before attempting further injection.
7. Following injection of the corticosteroid solution, withdraw the needle.
8. Apply a sterile adhesive bandage.
9. Instruct the patient to move his or her jaw through its full range of motion. This movement distributes the steroid solution throughout the joint capsule.
10. Reexamine the TMJ in 5 min to confirm pain relief.

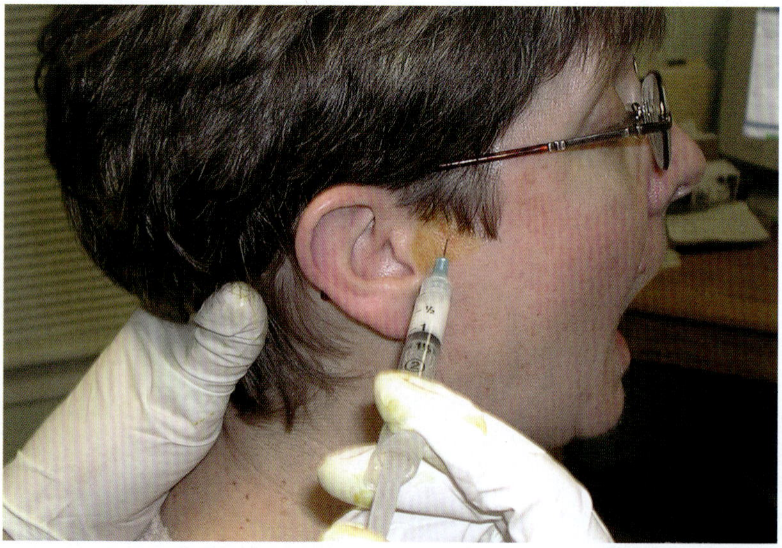

**FIGURE 5.2** ● Temporomandibular joint injection.

## AFTERCARE

- Avoid excessive use of the jaw by avoiding chewing gum, chewing tough foods, and excessive talking over the next 2 weeks.
- Nonsteroidal anti-inflammatory drugs (NSAIDs), ice, and/or physical therapy as indicated.
- Consider follow-up examination in 2 weeks.

**CPT code:** 20605—Arthrocentesis, aspiration, and/or injection of the intermediate joint or bursa

## PEARLS

- Be aware that there are reports of articular degeneration following corticosteroid joint injections.

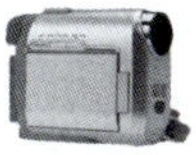

A video clip showing a TMJ injection can be found in the companion eBook.

## REFERENCES

1. Machado E, Bonotto D, Cunali PA. Intra-articular injections with corticosteroids and sodium hyaluronate for treating temporomandibular joint disorders: A systematic review. *Dental Press J Orthod.* 2013;18(5):128–133.
2. Manfredini D, Piccotti F, Guarda-Nardini L. Hyaluronic acid in the treatment of TMJ disorders: A systematic review of the literature. *Cranio.* 2010;28(3):166–176.
3. Guarda-Nardini L, Cadorin C, Frizziero A, et al. Comparison of 2 hyaluronic acid drugs for the treatment of temporomandibular joint osteoarthritis. *J Oral Maxillofac Surg.* 2012;70(11):2522–2530.
4. Young CM, Shiels WE II, Coley BD. Ultrasound-guided corticosteroid injection therapy for juvenile idiopathic arthritis: 12-year care experience. *Pediatr Radiol.* 2012;42(12):1481–1489.
5. Habibi S, Ellis J, Strike H, et al. Safety and efficacy of US-guided CS injection into temporomandibular joints in children with active JIA. *Rheumatology (Oxford).* 2012;51(5):874–877.
6. Sidebottom AJ, Patel AA, Amin J. Botulinum injection for the management of myofascial pain in the masticatory muscles. A prospective outcome study. *Br J Oral Maxillofac Surg.* 2013;51(3):199–205.
7. Ernberg M, Hedenberg-Magnusson B, List T, et al. Efficacy of botulinum toxin type A for treatment of persistent myofascial TMD pain: A randomized, controlled, double-blind multicenter study. *Pain.* 2011;152(9):1988–1996.

# Greater Occipital Neuralgia

Patients occasionally present to the primary care office for the treatment of headaches caused by greater occipital neuralgia. The greater occipital nerve, which is composed of C2 sensory fibers, can become entrapped as it passes through the aponeurotic attachments of the trapezius and semispinalis capitis muscles to the occipital bone. Typically, the pain of occipital neuralgia begins in the neck and then spreads to the vertex, ear, frontal area, or even the eyes. The International Headache Society diagnostic criteria for occipital neuralgia include paroxysmal stabbing pain, with or without persistent aching between paroxysms, in the distribution(s) of the greater, lesser, and/or third occipital nerves; tenderness over the affected nerve; and pain is eased temporarily by local anesthetic block of the nerve.[1]

A double-blind, controlled trial of cluster headache has demonstrated that injectable steroids with local anesthetics benefit cluster headache patients. A double-blind, controlled trial of nerve blocks in occipital neuralgia, which may have actually been chronic migraine, was positive.[2] A recent review of the available literature was generally positive for injection management, but there are methodologic limitations of the available studies. The procedures were generally well tolerated. There is a need to perform more rigorous clinical trials to clarify the role of occipital nerve blocks in the management of various headache disorders and to standardize the injection techniques.[3]

| Indications | ICD-9 Code | ICD-10 Code |
|---|---|---|
| Occipital neuralgia | 723.8 | M54.81 |

**Relevant Anatomy:** (Fig. 5.3)

## PATIENT POSITION

- Sitting on an exam stool with neck flexed and leaning forward with arms resting on the exam table.

## LANDMARKS

1. With the patient seated on the exam stool, the clinician stands directly behind the patient.
2. Find the external occipital protuberance of the occipital bone in the midline.
3. The point of injection of the greater occipital nerve is 2 cm lateral to the external occipital protuberance along the superior nuchal line and then 2 cm inferior (caudal).[4] At the point where the greater occipital nerve courses over the occipital bone, pressure over the nerve will elicit pain. Mark that spot with an ink pen.
4. At that site, press firmly on the skin with the retracted tip of a ballpoint pen. This indention represents the entry point for the needle.
5. After the landmarks are identified, the patient should not move the neck.

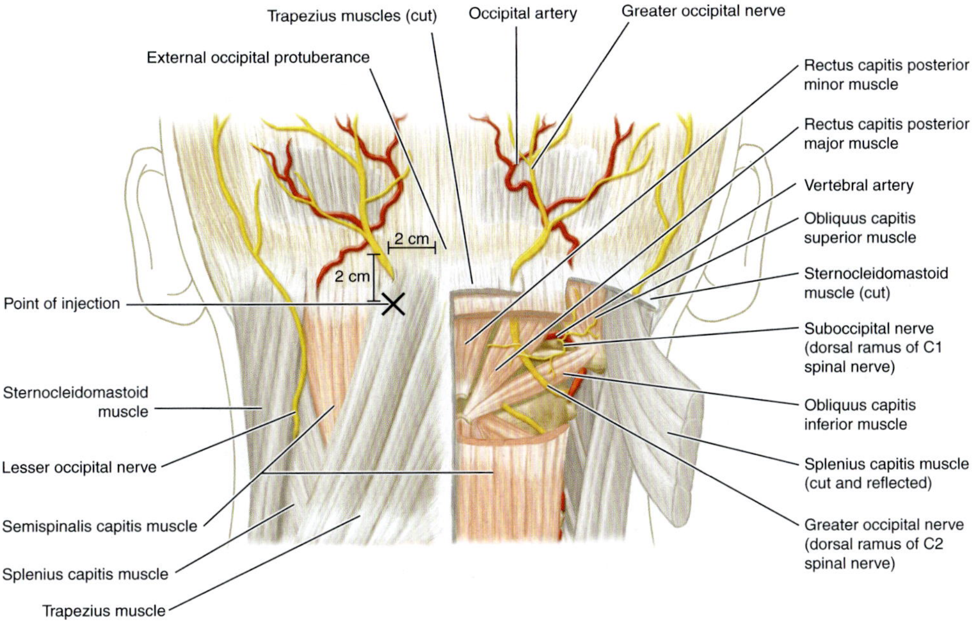


**FIGURE 5.3** • Suboccipital region. (From Tank PW, Gest TR. *Lippincott Williams & Wilkins Atlas of Anatomy*. Philadelphia, PA: Lippincott Williams & Wilkins, 2009.)

## ANESTHESIA

- Local anesthesia of the skin with topical vapocoolant spray may be used but is not necessary in most patients.

## EQUIPMENT

- 3-mL syringe
- 25-gauge, 1-in. needle
- 1 mL of 1% lidocaine without epinephrine
- 1 mL of the steroid solution (40 mg of triamcinolone acetonide)
- One alcohol prep pad
- Two povidone–iodine prep pads
- Sterile gauze pads
- Sterile adhesive bandage

## TECHNIQUE

1. Part the hair and prep the insertion site with alcohol followed by the povidone–iodine pads.
2. Achieve good local anesthesia by using topical vapocoolant spray (optional).
3. Position the needle and syringe perpendicular to the skin with the tip of the needle directed anteriorly toward the nuchal line of the occiput.
4. Using the no-touch technique, introduce the needle at the insertion site (Fig. 5.4).
5. Advance the needle toward the location of the greater occipital nerve until the needle tip contacts the occiput at the superior nuchal line. Back up the needle 1 to 2 mm.

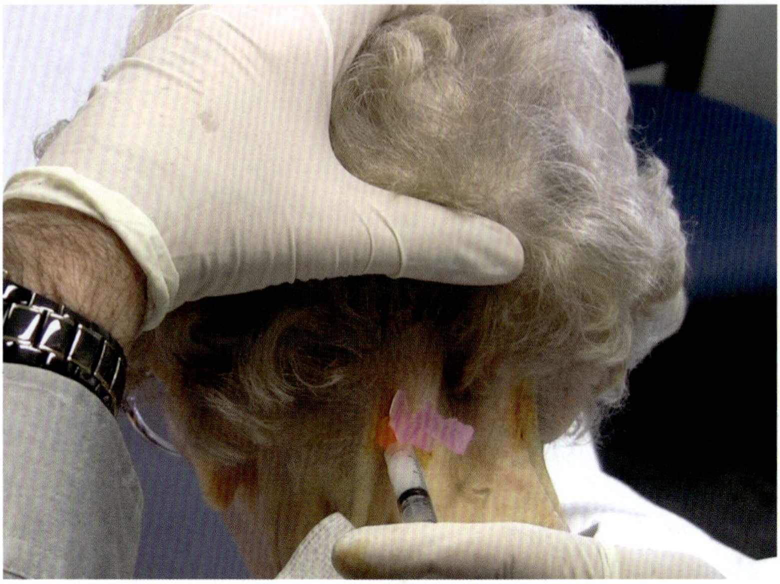

*FIGURE 5.4* ● Greater occipital neuralgia injection.

6. Inject the steroid solution as a bolus around the greater occipital nerve. The injected solution should flow smoothly into the tissues. If increased resistance is encountered, advance or withdraw the needle slightly before attempting further injection.
7. Following injection of the corticosteroid solution, withdraw the needle.
8. Apply a sterile adhesive bandage.
9. Instruct the patient to gently massage the area with a piece of gauze. This movement distributes the steroid solution around the nerve.
10. Reexamine the greater occipital nerve in 5 min to confirm pain relief.

## AFTERCARE

- Muscle relaxants, ice, physical therapy, chiropractic manipulation, or other modalities as indicated.
- Consider follow-up examination in 2 weeks.

**CPT code:** 64405—Injection of greater occipital nerve

## PEARLS

- Occipital neuralgia must be distinguished from occipital referral of pain from the atlantoaxial or upper zygapophyseal joints or from tender trigger points in neck muscles or their insertions.[1]

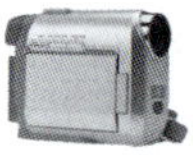

A video clip showing a greater occipital neuralgia injection can be found in the companion eBook.

## REFERENCES

1. http://ihs-classification.org/en/02_klassifikation/04_teil3/13.08.00_facialpain.html. Accessed on May 25, 2014.
2. Young WB. Blocking the greater occipital nerve: Utility in headache management. *Curr Pain Headache Rep*. 2010;14(5):404–408.
3. Ashkenazi A, Blumenfeld A, Napchan U, et al. Peripheral nerve blocks and trigger point injections in headache management—A systematic review and suggestions for future research. *Headache*. 2010;50(6):943–952.
4. Loukas M, El-Sedfy A, Tubbs RS, et al. Identification of greater occipital nerve landmarks for the treatment of occipital neuralgia. *Folia Morphol (Warsz)*. 2006;65(4):337–342.

# Cervical Strain and Sprain

Patients very commonly present to the primary care office for evaluation and treatment of neck strain and sprain. These conditions are the result of acute injury or chronic repetitive motion. Depending on the biomechanics involved, any of the neck muscles shown below in the anatomic plates may be injured. Intramuscular injections of anesthetic may be helpful in cases where the diagnosis is unclear. Corticosteroid injections are not indicated for the treatment of acute trauma. However, they may play a role in managing inappropriate inflammation causing chronic pain. They may also allow patients to more fully participate in rehabilitative therapy. Botulinum toxin A injections have utility when injected into cervical trigger points in the treatment of whiplash-associated headache pain. Epidural, nerve root, and facet joint injections are outside the scope of this text.

| Indications | ICD-9 Code | ICD-10 Code |
|---|---|---|
| Cervical sprain and strain | 847.0 | S16.1 |

**Relevant Anatomy:** (Figs. 5.5 and 5.6)

## PATIENT POSITION

- Sitting on an exam stool with the neck flexed and leaning forward with the arms resting on the exam table.

## LANDMARKS

1. With the patient seated on the exam stool, the clinician stands directly behind the patient.
2. Locate the cervical spinous processes of the posterior neck.
3. Palpate the area of maximal tenderness in the muscles of the posterior neck. Direct pressure over this area will elicit pain and is often associated with muscle spasm. Mark the spot(s) with an ink pen.
4. At the injection site(s), press firmly on the skin with the retracted tip of a ballpoint pen. The indention(s) represents the entry point for the needle.
5. After the landmarks are identified, the patient should not move the neck.

## ANESTHESIA

- Local anesthesia of the skin with topical vapocoolant spray may be used as needed but is not mandatory.

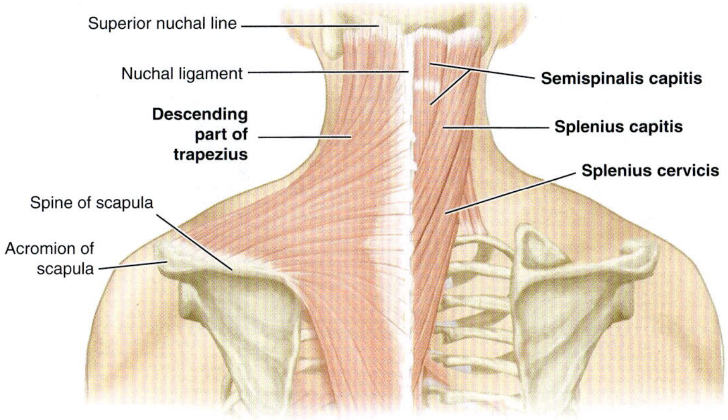


*FIGURE 5.5* • Posterior cervical region: Trapezius. (From Tank PW, Gest TR. *Lippincott Williams & Wilkins Atlas of Anatomy*. Philadelphia, PA: Lippincott Williams & Wilkins, 2009.)

## EQUIPMENT

- 3-mL syringe
- 25-gauge, 1½-in. needle
- 1 mL of 1% lidocaine without epinephrine
- 0.5 to 1 mL of the steroid solution (20 to 40 mg of triamcinolone acetonide)
- One alcohol prep pad
- Two povidone–iodine prep pads
- Sterile gauze pads
- Sterile adhesive bandage

## TECHNIQUE

1. Prep the insertion site with alcohol followed by the povidone–iodine pads.
2. Achieve good local anesthesia by using topical vapocoolant spray.
3. Position the needle and syringe perpendicular to the skin with the tip of the needle directed toward the target muscle.
4. Using the no-touch technique, introduce the needle at the insertion site (Fig. 5.7).

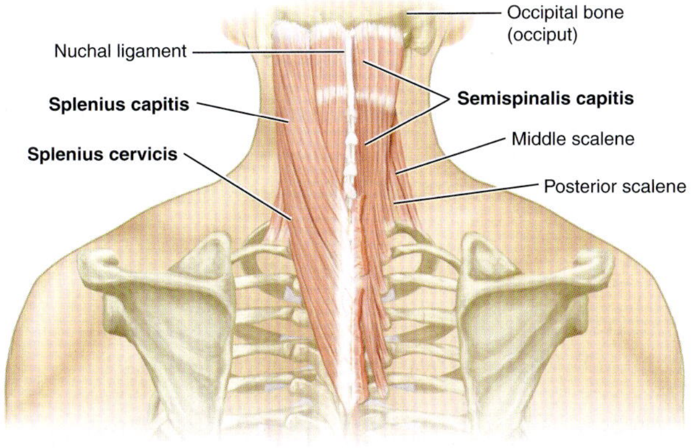


*FIGURE 5.6* • Posterior cervical region: Semispinalis. (From Tank PW, Gest TR. *Lippincott Williams & Wilkins Atlas of Anatomy*. Philadelphia, PA: Lippincott Williams & Wilkins, 2009.)

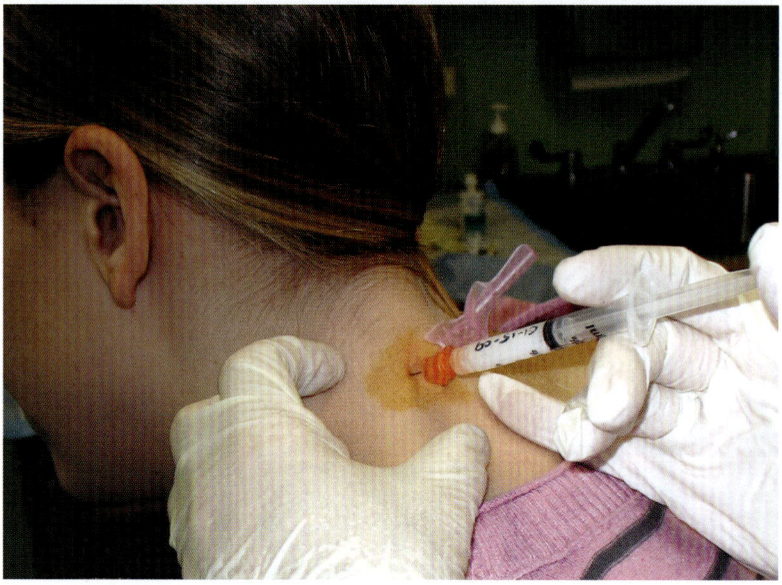

***FIGURE 5.7*** Cervical strain and sprain injection.

5. Advance the needle into the body of each muscle, delivering the full volume of the syringe divided between all of the sites. If only one site is located, then only give half of the volume of the syringe into that spot.
6. Following injection of the corticosteroid solution, withdraw the needle.
7. Apply a sterile adhesive bandage.
8. Instruct the patient to massage the area and move his or her neck slowly through its full range of motion. This movement distributes the steroid solution in the injected muscles.
9. Reexamine the neck in 5 min to confirm pain relief.

## AFTERCARE

- Avoid excessive use of the neck over the next 2 weeks.
- Consider the use of a cervical collar.
- NSAIDs, muscle relaxants, ice, and/or physical therapy as indicated.
- Consider follow-up examination in 2 weeks.

### CPT codes

20552—Injection of trigger point(s) in 1 to 2 muscle groups
20553—Injection of trigger point(s) in 3+ muscle groups
These codes are used only once each session, regardless of the number of injections.

## PEARLS

- When injecting into neck structures, always make certain to aspirate before giving the injection because of the rich network of blood vessels.

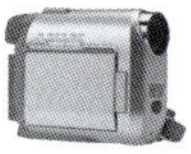

A video clip showing a cervical strain injection can be found in the companion eBook.

# 6 Subacromial Space Injection—Posterior Approach

Patients commonly present to the primary care office for evaluation of shoulder pain. Almost all shoulder disorders that can be treated by injection therapy involve the rotator cuff complex. These disorders are either primary from acute injury—usually superimposed on chronic degeneration—or secondary to impingement. Since the subacromial space encompasses the rotator cuff complex as well as the proximal aspect of the biceps tendon, it allows easy access to these structures for corticosteroid treatment. In patients with long-standing degenerative disease, the subacromial bursa commonly perforates into the glenohumeral (GH) joint creating an open communication between the two structures.

The posterior approach to the subacromial space is the easiest to perform and is well accepted by patients. Since they cannot see the approaching needle, anxiety is diminished. Of the three standard portals, it holds an additional advantage over the anterior and lateral approaches. When using the posterior approach, the needle is directed cephalad piercing the supraspinatus muscle/tendon, entering the subacromial space, and then impacting the underside of the acromion. Therefore, accurate placement is confirmed. When utilizing the anterior and lateral approaches, the operator cannot be assured that the corticosteroid is not being deposited into the supraspinatus muscle/tendon. However, a longer needle must be used in the posterior approach.[1] A small-diameter needle is appropriate as this technique is only used to inject anesthetic and/or steroid solution into the subacromial space. A large-diameter needle is usually not necessary since fluid typically does not collect in the space. The posterior approach is considered a safe procedure since there are no major arteries or nerves in the immediate path of the needle.

Available literature indicates that corticosteroid injections in the subacromial space are effective in the short- to medium-term treatment of rotator cuff disorders[2,3] and for the treatment of adhesive capsulitis.[4,5] Safety has also been established as use in patients with subacromial impingement does not result in an increase in rotator cuff tears.[6] Hyaluronic acid viscosupplementation has been studied and shown to be effective at 12 weeks.[7–9] However, this has not been approved by the FDA for use outside of osteoarthritis of the knee. The use of ultrasound improves the accuracy of injection,[10] although the clinical significance does not seem to be affected.[11]

A subacromial injection performed using local anesthetic without steroid can help the clinician differentiate the cause of vague shoulder pain. The injected lidocaine removes pain from subacromial impingement as a confounding factor and allows the clinician to physically test the integrity of the rotator cuff complex by asking the patient to abduct the shoulder. This is known as the "impingement test." Injection of local anesthetic does not cause muscle weakness and therefore does not affect the validity of this test.[12]

| Indications | ICD-9 Code | ICD-10 Code |
|---|---|---|
| Shoulder pain | 719.41 | M25.519 |
| Rotator cuff sprain | 840.4 | S43.42 |
| Impingement syndrome | 726.1 | M75.40 |
| Rotator cuff tendonitis | 726.10 | M75.50 |

**Relevant Anatomy:** (Figs. 6.1 and 6.2)

## PATIENT POSITION

- Sitting on the examination table.
- The patient's hands are folded in his or her lap with fingers interlaced.
- This allows consistency of positioning of the shoulder so that the landmarks do not change from the time that they are identified and marked until the time of injection.

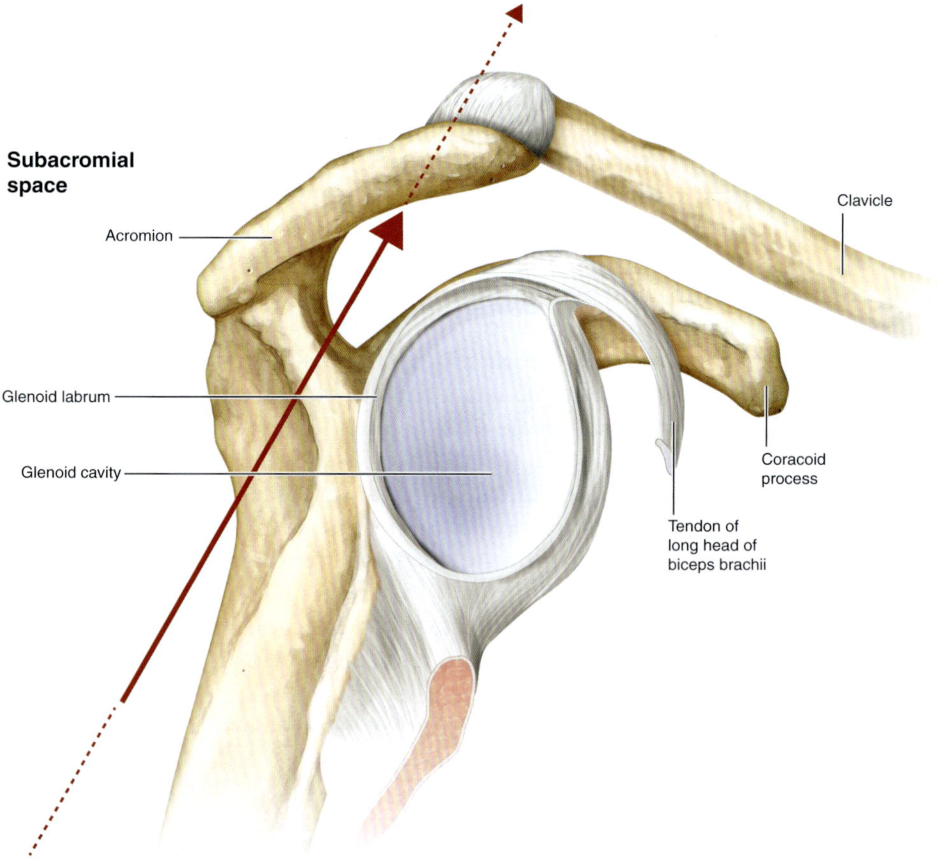


**FIGURE 6.1** Lateral aspect of right shoulder (*red arrow* indicates path of the needle). (From Tank PW, Gest TR. *Lippincott Williams & Wilkins Atlas of Anatomy*. Philadelphia, PA: Lippincott Williams & Wilkins, 2009.)

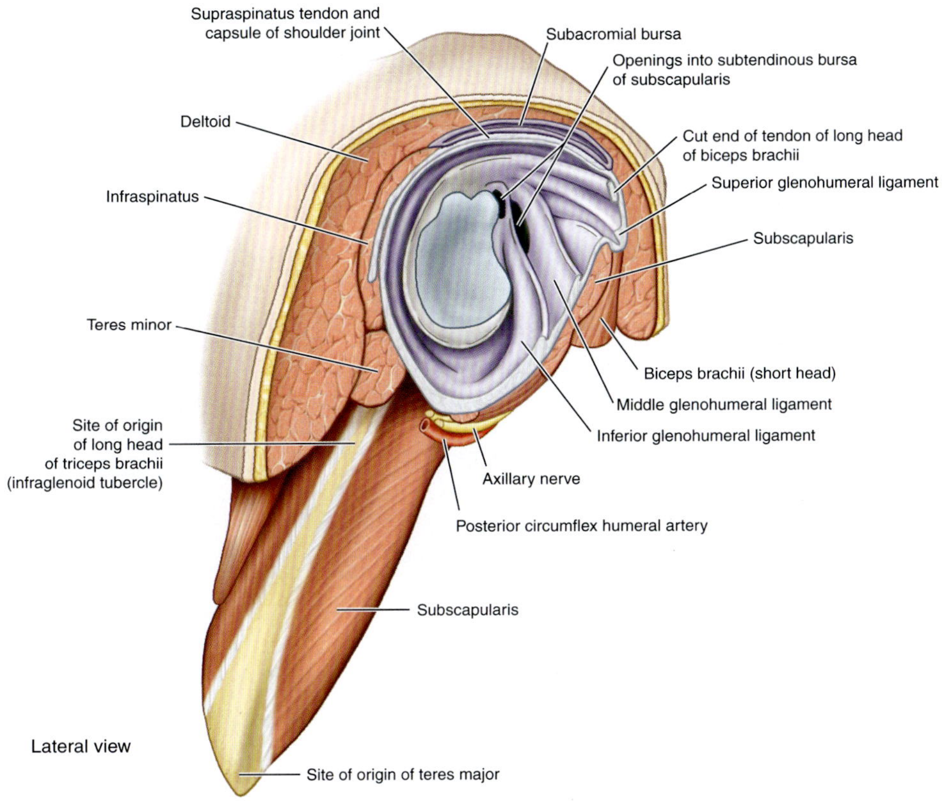


**FIGURE 6.2** • Interior of right shoulder. (From Tank PW, Gest TR. *Lippincott Williams & Wilkins Atlas of Anatomy*. Philadelphia, PA: Lippincott Williams & Wilkins, 2009.)

## LANDMARKS

1. With the patient seated on the examination table, the clinician stands lateral and posterior to the affected shoulder.
2. Find the lateral edge of the acromion, and mark it with an ink pen.
3. Palpate the posterior edge of the acromion and mark that.
4. Having identified the posterior lateral corner of the acromion, drop a vertical line down from that point and mark a spot 2 cm below the posterior lateral corner.
5. At that site, press firmly with the retracted tip of a ballpoint pen. This indention represents the entry point for the needle.
6. Next, identify the target site by placing the index finger of your nondominant hand over the superior aspect of the acromion posterior to the acromioclavicular (AC) joint. This will be the target for the tip of the needle (Fig. 6.3). If your index finger is at the target site—on top of the acromion—it will be protected from accidental needlestick.
7. After the landmarks are identified, the patient should not move the shoulder or arm.

## ANESTHESIA

- Tactile skin distraction is administered by firmly stroking the skin outside of the injection point as the needle is quickly introduced into the skin. Topical vapocoolant spray or injection of a local anesthetic is unnecessary in almost all patients.

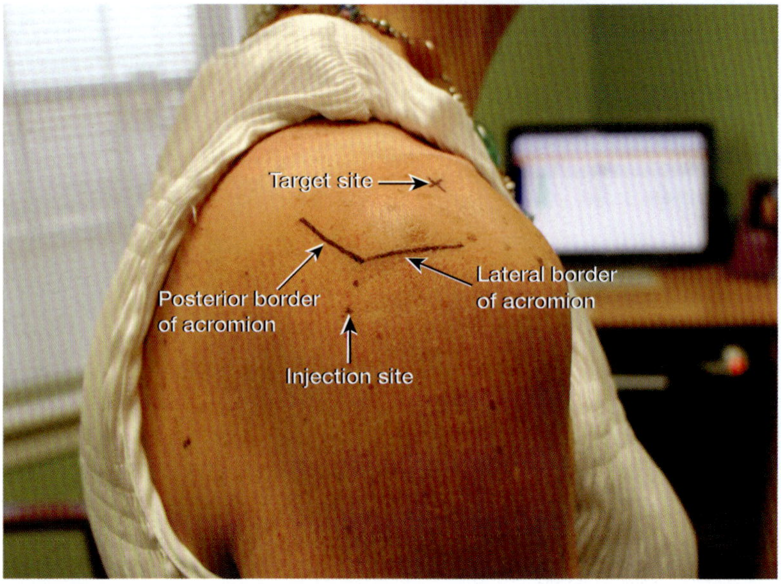


*FIGURE 6.3* Right shoulder injection landmarks.

## EQUIPMENT

- 5-mL syringe
- 25-gauge, 2-in. needle (Consider a 3½ in., 25-gauge needle in large individuals.)
- 3 mL of 1% lidocaine without epinephrine
- 1 mL of the steroid solution (40 mg of triamcinolone acetonide)
- One alcohol prep pad
- Two povidone–iodine prep pads
- Sterile gauze pads
- Sterile adhesive bandage

## TECHNIQUE

1. Prep the insertion site with alcohol followed by the povidone–iodine pads.
2. Position the needle and syringe at about a 30-degree angle to the skin with the needle tip directed cephalad toward the acromion.
3. Using the no-touch technique, introduce the needle at the insertion site (Fig. 6.4).
4. Direct the needle underneath the acromion, and advance it toward the target until the needle tip touches the undersurface of the acromion. Back up the needle 1 to 2 mm.
5. Inject the steroid solution as a bolus into the subacromial space. The injected solution should flow smoothly into the space. Increased resistance may indicate that the injected fluid is entering the supraspinatus muscle or tendon. In that case, advance or withdraw the needle slightly before attempting further injection.
6. Following injection of the corticosteroid solution, withdraw the needle.
7. Apply a sterile adhesive bandage.
8. Instruct the patient to move his or her shoulder through its full range of motion. This movement distributes the steroid solution throughout the subacromial space.
9. Reexamine the shoulder in 5 min to confirm pain relief.

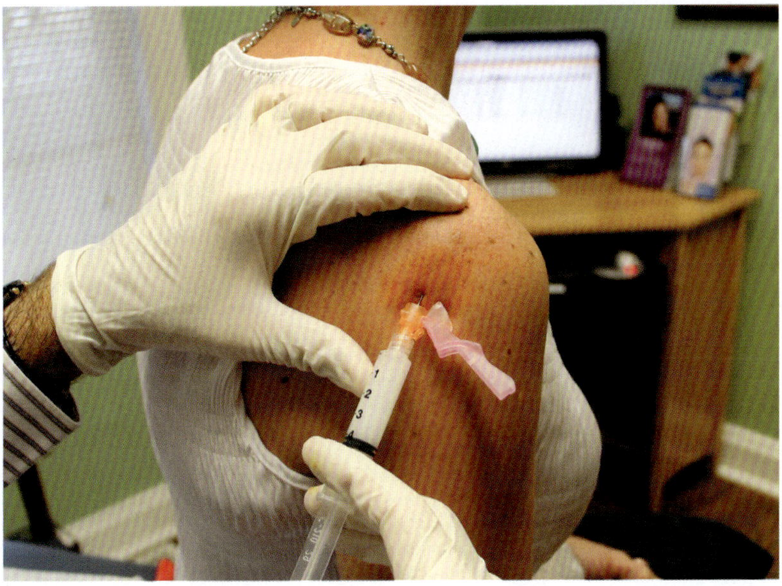

*FIGURE 6.4* ● Right shoulder subacromial space injection.

## AFTERCARE

- Avoid excessive use of the shoulder over the next 2 weeks.
- Consider the use of an arm sling.
- Nonsteroidal anti-inflammatory drugs (NSAIDs), ice, and/or physical therapy as indicated.
- Consider follow-up examination in 2 weeks.

**CPT code:** 20610—Injection of major joint or bursa

## PEARLS

- The correct identification of the acromion landmarks is more difficult than many primary care providers realize. Make sure to take your time and recheck the landmarks before proceeding with the injection.
- When palpating to determine the location of the acromion, use the tips of your index, middle, and ring fingers. Gently and methodically move in a distal-to-proximal direction. Mark the site where your fingers meet the bone.
- Use a 2-in., 25-gauge needle for this injection.
- Ensure that the needle is underneath the acromion before advancing it toward the target finger.
- Always keep your target finger over the acromion to protect it from accidental needlestick.

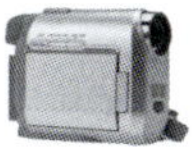

A video clip showing a subacromial space injection can be found in the companion eBook.

## REFERENCES


1. Sardelli M, Burks RT. Distances to the subacromial bursa from 3 different injection sites as measured arthroscopically. *Arthroscopy*. 2008;24(9):992–996.
2. Gialanella B, Prometti P. Effects of corticosteroids injection in rotator cuff tears. *Pain Med*. 2011;12(10):1559–1565.
3. Karthikeyan S, Kwong HT, Upadhyay PK, et al. A double-blind randomised controlled study comparing subacromial injection of tenoxicam or methylprednisolone in patients with subacromial impingement. *J Bone Joint Surg Br*. 2010;92(1):77–82.
4. Shin SJ, Lee SY. Efficacies of corticosteroid injection at different sites of the shoulder for the treatment of adhesive capsulitis. *J Shoulder Elbow Surg*. 2013;22(4):521–527.
5. Oh JH, Oh CH, Choi JA, et al. Comparison of glenohumeral and subacromial steroid injection in primary frozen shoulder: a prospective, randomized short-term comparison study. *J Shoulder Elbow Surg*. 2011;20(7):1034–1040.
6. Bhatia M, Singh B, Nicolaou N, et al. Correlation between rotator cuff tears and repeated subacromial steroid injections: a case-controlled study. *Ann R Coll Surg Engl*. 2009;91(5):414–416.
7. Kim YS, Park JY, Lee CS, et al. Does hyaluronate injection work in shoulder disease in early stage? A multicenter, randomized, single blind and open comparative clinical study. *J Shoulder Elbow Surg*. 2012;21(6):722–727.
8. Merolla G, Bianchi P, Porcellini G. Ultrasound-guided subacromial injections of sodium hyaluronate for the management of rotator cuff tendinopathy: a prospective comparative study with rehabilitation therapy. *Musculoskelet Surg*. 2013;97(Suppl 1):49–56.
9. Noël E, Hardy P, Hagena FW, et al. Efficacy and safety of Hylan G-F 20 in shoulder osteoarthritis with an intact rotator cuff. Open-label prospective multicenter study. *Joint Bone Spine*. 2009;76(6):670–673.
10. Daley EL, Bajaj S, Bisson LJ, et al. Improving injection accuracy of the elbow, knee, and shoulder: does injection site and imaging make a difference? A systematic review. *Am J Sports Med*. 2011;39(3):656–662.
11. Bloom JE, Rischin A, Johnston RV, et al. Image-guided versus blind glucocorticoid injection for shoulder pain. *Cochrane Database Syst Rev*. 2012;8:CD009147.
12. Farshad M, Jundt-Ecker M, Sutter R, et al. Does subacromial injection of a local anesthetic influence strength in healthy shoulders? A double-blinded, placebo-controlled study. *J Bone Joint Surg Am*. 2012;94(19):1751–1755.

# Glenohumeral Joint—Posterior Approach

The GH joint is a relatively uncommon injection site for most primary care physicians. Successful injection can be difficult because of the limited space available in patients with adhesive capsulitis. Both anterior and posterior approaches can be used. For reasons listed in the previous chapter, the posterior approach is preferred. One uses the same injection site identified above in the "Subacromial Space Injection" chapter. Since the long head of the biceps tendon has its origin within the joint capsule, a GH joint injection offers an approach to tendonitis of this structure.

A small-diameter needle is appropriate as this technique is used to inject steroid solution into the joint space. A large-diameter needle is usually not necessary since a significant amount of fluid typically does not collect in the joint capsule.

| Indications | ICD-9 Code | ICD-10 Code |
|---|---|---|
| Shoulder pain | 719.41 | M25.519 |
| Shoulder adhesive capsulitis | 726.0 | M75.00 |
| GH joint arthritis, unspecified | 716.91 | M12.9 |
| GH joint osteoarthritis, primary | 715.11 | M19.019 |
| GH joint arthrosis, posttraumatic | 716.11 | M19.119 |
| GH joint arthrosis, secondary | 715.21 | M19.219 |

**Relevant Anatomy:** (Figs. 6.5 and 6.6)

## PATIENT POSITION

- Sitting on the examination table.
- The patient's hands are folded in his or her lap with fingers interlaced.
- This allows consistency of positioning of the shoulder so that the landmarks do not change from the time that they are identified and marked until the time of injection.

## LANDMARKS

1. With the patient seated on the examination table, the clinician stands lateral and posterior to the affected shoulder.
2. Find the lateral edge of the acromion, and mark it with an ink pen.
3. Palpate the posterior edge of the acromion and mark that.
4. Having identified the posterior lateral corner of the acromion, drop a vertical line down from that point and mark a spot 2 cm below the posterior lateral corner.
5. At that site, press firmly with the retracted tip of a ballpoint pen. This indention represents the entry point for the needle.
6. Next, identify the target site by placing the index finger of your nondominant hand over the coracoid process. This will be the target for the tip of the needle.
7. After the landmarks are identified, the patient should not move the shoulder or arm.

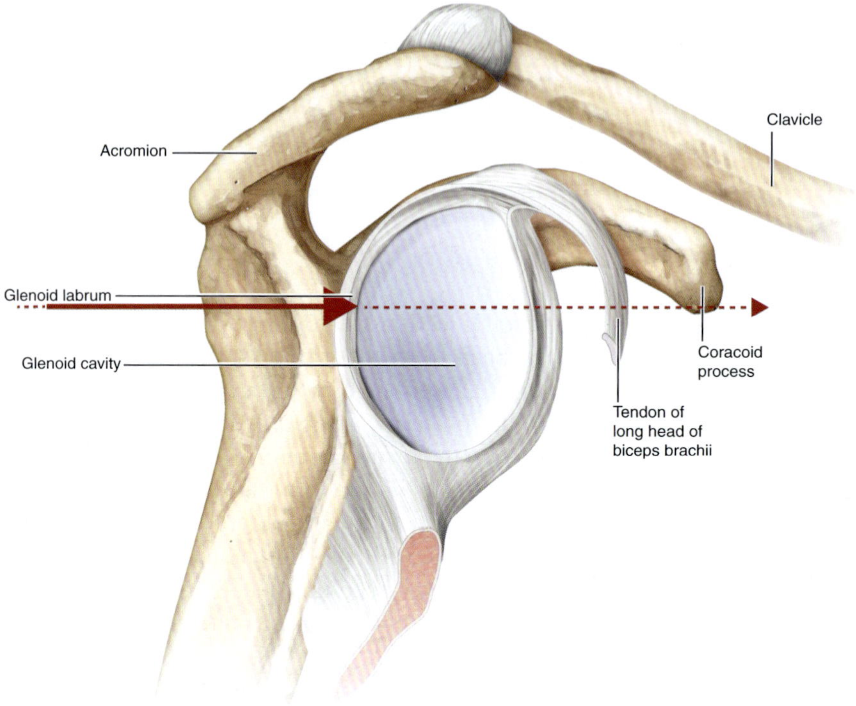


**FIGURE 6.5** Lateral aspect of right shoulder (*red arrow* indicates path of the needle). (From Tank PW, Gest TR. *Lippincott Williams & Wilkins Atlas of Anatomy*. Philadelphia, PA: Lippincott Williams & Wilkins, 2009.)

## ANESTHESIA

- Tactile skin distraction is administered by firmly stroking the skin outside of the injection point as the needle is quickly introduced into the skin. Topical vapocoolant spray or injection of a local anesthetic is unnecessary in almost all patients.

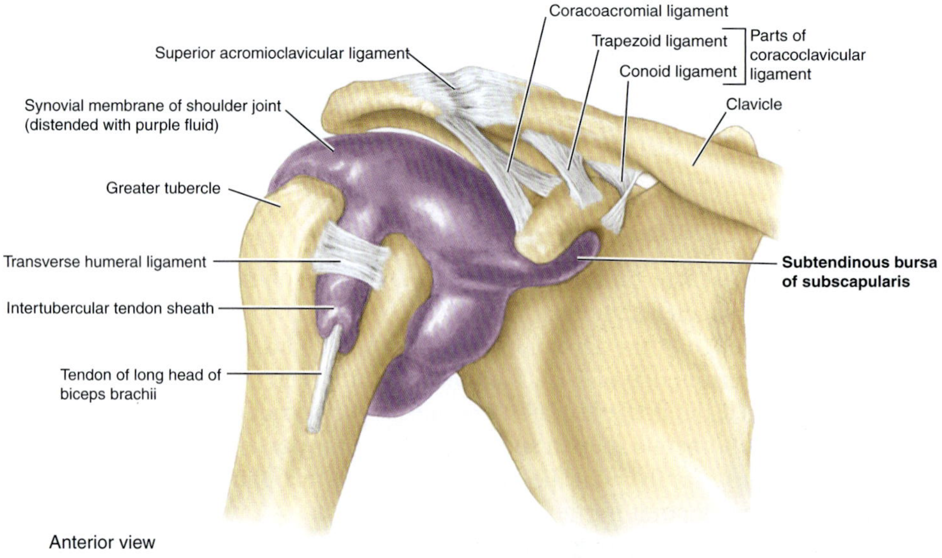


**FIGURE 6.6** Right glenohumeral joint capsule. (From Tank PW, Gest TR. *Lippincott Williams & Wilkins Atlas of Anatomy*. Philadelphia, PA: Lippincott Williams & Wilkins, 2009.)

## EQUIPMENT

- 3-mL syringe
- 25-gauge, 1½ in. needle
- 1 mL of 1% lidocaine without epinephrine
- 1 mL of the steroid solution (40 mg of triamcinolone acetonide)
- One alcohol prep pad
- Two povidone–iodine prep pads
- Sterile gauze pads
- Sterile adhesive bandage

## TECHNIQUE

1. Prep the insertion site with alcohol followed by the povidone–iodine pads.
2. Position the needle and syringe perpendicular to the skin with the needle tip directed anterior toward the coracoid process.
3. Using the no-touch technique, introduce the needle at the insertion site (Fig. 6.7).
4. Advance the needle toward the target until the needle tip touches the humeral head. Back up the needle 1 to 2 mm.
5. Inject the steroid solution as a bolus into the GH joint. The injected solution should flow smoothly into the joint space. If increased resistance is encountered, advance or withdraw the needle slightly before attempting further injection.
6. Following injection of the corticosteroid solution, withdraw the needle.
7. Apply a sterile adhesive bandage.
8. Instruct the patient to move his or her shoulder through its full range of motion. This movement distributes the steroid solution throughout the subacromial space.
9. Reexamine the shoulder in 5 min to confirm pain relief.

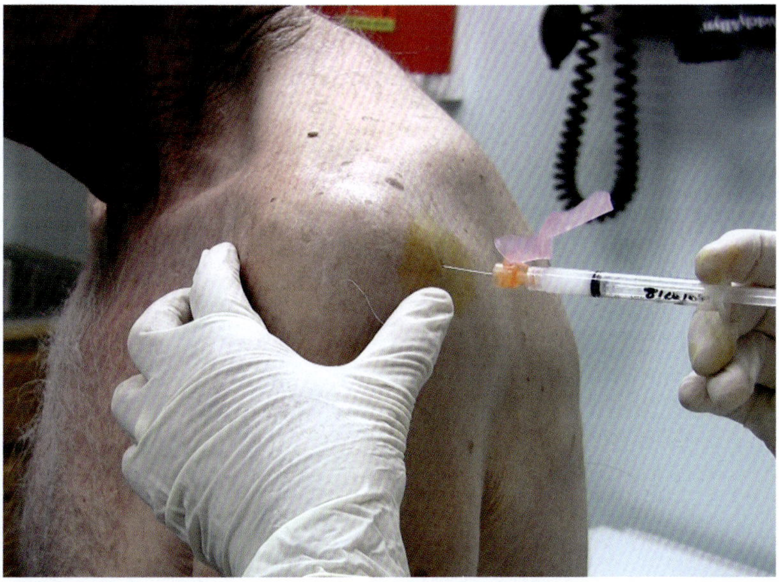

*FIGURE 6.7* • Glenohumeral joint injection—posterior approach.

## AFTERCARE

- Avoid excessive use of the shoulder over the next 2 weeks.
- Consider the use of an arm sling.
- NSAIDs, ice, and/or physical therapy as indicated.
- Consider follow-up examination in 2 weeks.

**CPT code:** 20610—Injection of major joint or bursa

## PEARLS

- The correct identification of the acromion landmarks is more difficult than many primary care providers realize. Make sure to take your time and recheck the landmarks before proceeding with the injection.
- When palpating to determine the location of the acromion, use the fingertips of your index, middle, and ring fingers. Gently and methodically move in a distal-to-proximal direction. Mark the site where your fingers meet the bone.
- A smaller volume of lidocaine is used in this injection compared to the subacromial space injection because the joint capsule is frequently contracted—especially in patients with adhesive capsulitis.

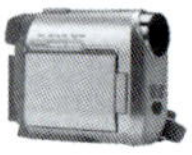

A video clip showing a GH joint injection can be found in the companion eBook.

## REFERENCES

Please consult references listed in the preceding section.

# Glenohumeral Joint—Anterior Approach

The GH joint is a relatively uncommon injection site for most primary care physicians. Successful injection can be difficult because of the limited space available in patients with adhesive capsulitis. Because the physician is operating in front of the patient, this technique generates much more patient anxiety and perceived pain. For these reasons, the posterior approach is preferred. Since the long head of the biceps tendon has its origin within the joint capsule, a GH joint injection offers an approach to tendonitis of this structure.

A small-diameter needle is appropriate as this technique is used to inject steroid solution into the joint space. A large-diameter needle is usually not necessary since a significant amount of fluid usually typically does not collect in the joint capsule.

| Indications | ICD-9 Code | ICD-10 Code |
|---|---|---|
| Shoulder pain | 719.41 | M25.519 |
| Shoulder adhesive capsulitis | 726.0 | M75.00 |
| GH joint arthritis, unspecified | 716.91 | M12.9 |
| GH joint osteoarthritis, primary | 715.11 | M19.019 |
| GH joint osteoarthritis, posttraumatic | 716.11 | M19.119 |
| GH joint osteoarthritis, secondary | 715.21 | M19.219 |

**Relevant Anatomy:** (Figs. 6.8 and 6.9)

## PATIENT POSITION

- Sitting or supine on the examination table.
- The patient's hands are folded in his or her lap with fingers interlaced.
- This allows consistency of positioning of the shoulder so that the landmarks do not change from the time that they are identified and marked until the time of injection.
- Rotate the patient's head away from the side that is being injected. This minimizes anxiety and pain perception.

## LANDMARKS

1. With the patient seated on the examination table, the clinician stands lateral and anterior to the affected shoulder.
2. Identify the coracoid process. This is the hard and somewhat tender knob of bone immediately medial to the humeral head.
3. The injection point is 1 cm lateral to the coracoid process.
4. At that site, press firmly on the skin with the retracted tip of a ballpoint pen. This indention represents the entry point for the needle.
5. Find the lateral edge of the acromion, and mark it with an ink pen.
6. Palpate the posterior edge of the acromion and mark that.

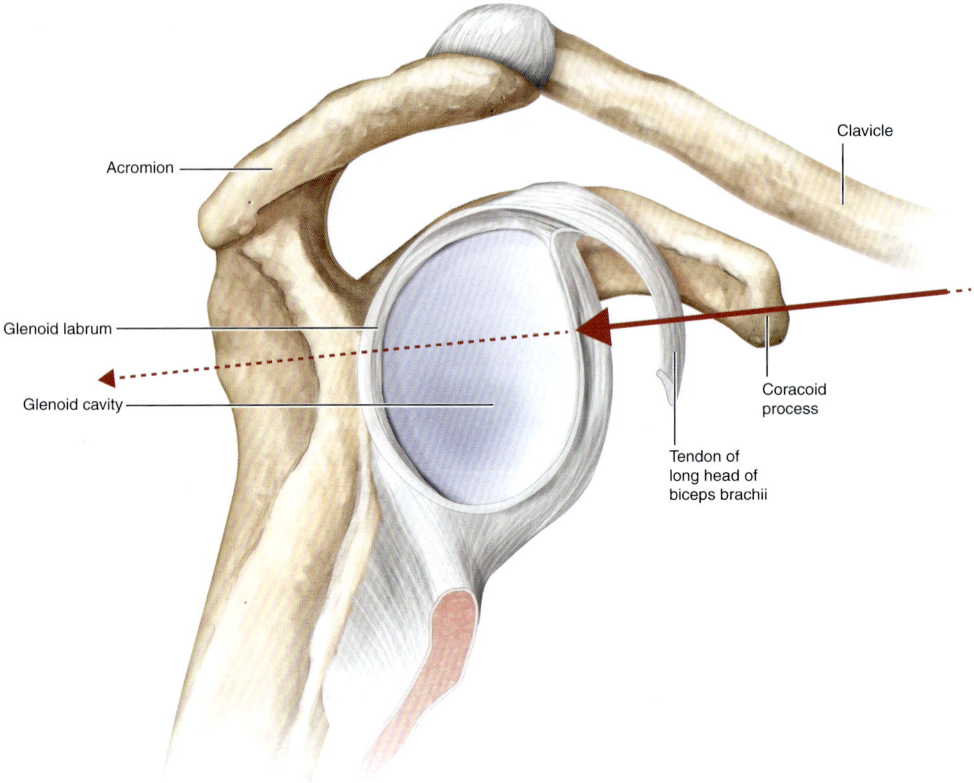


**FIGURE 6.8** Lateral aspect of right shoulder (*red arrow* indicates path of the needle). (From Tank PW, Gest TR. *Lippincott Williams & Wilkins Atlas of Anatomy*. Philadelphia, PA: Lippincott Williams & Wilkins, 2009.)

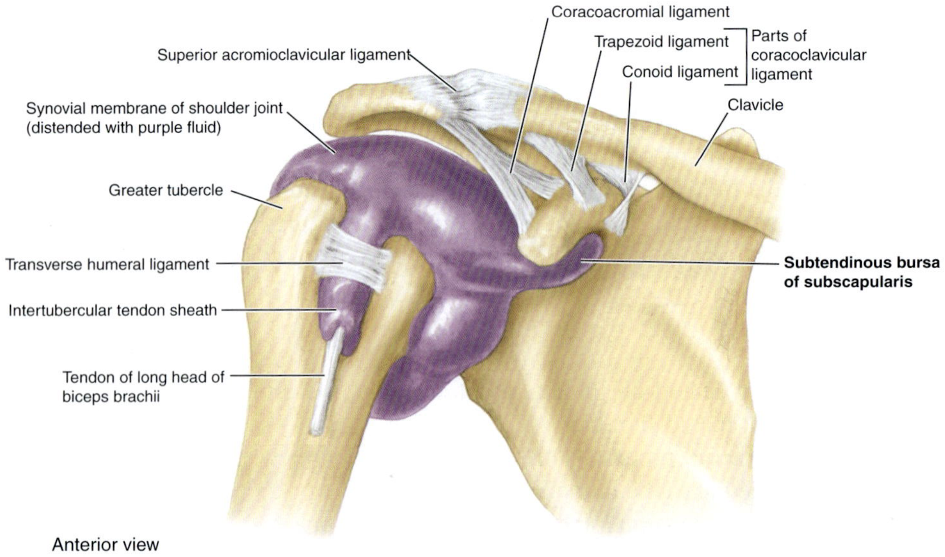


**FIGURE 6.9** Right glenohumeral joint capsule. (From Tank PW, Gest TR. *Lippincott Williams & Wilkins Atlas of Anatomy*. Philadelphia, PA: Lippincott Williams & Wilkins, 2009.)

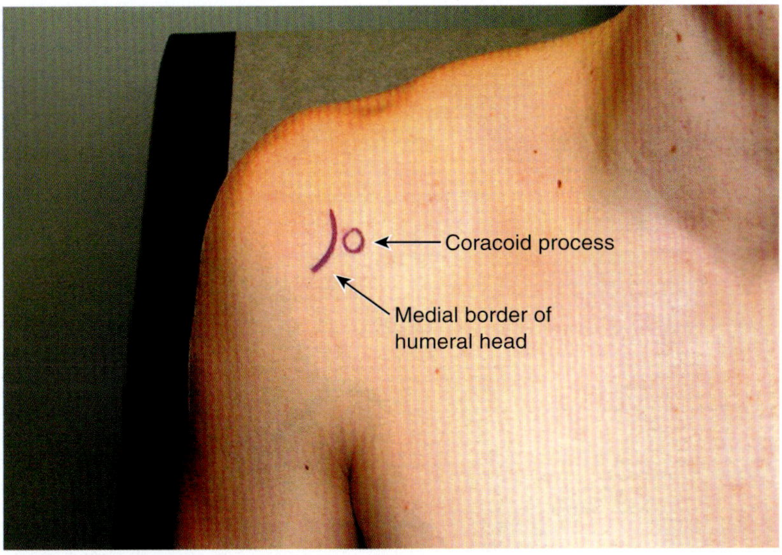


*FIGURE 6.10* • Anterior right shoulder landmarks.

7. Having identified the posterior lateral corner of the acromion, drop a vertical line down from that point and mark a spot 2 cm below the posterior lateral corner. This will be the target for the tip of the needle (Fig. 6.10).
8. Once the landmarks are identified, the patient should not move the shoulder or arm.

## ANESTHESIA

- Local anesthesia of the skin using topical vapocoolant spray.

## EQUIPMENT

- 3-mL syringe
- 25-gauge, 1½ in. needle (Consider longer, 25-gauge needles in large individuals.)
- 1 mL of 1% lidocaine without epinephrine
- 1 mL of the steroid solution (40 mg of triamcinolone acetonide)
- One alcohol prep pad
- Two povidone–iodine prep pads
- Sterile gauze pads
- Sterile adhesive bandage

## TECHNIQUE

1. Prep the insertion site with alcohol followed by the povidone–iodine pads.
2. Position the needle and syringe perpendicular to the skin with the needle tip directed posterior toward the target site 2 cm caudad to the posterior lateral corner of the acromion.
3. Using the no-touch technique, introduce the needle at the insertion site (Fig. 6.11).
4. Advance the needle toward the target until the needle tip touches the humeral head. Back up the needle 1 to 2 mm.
5. Inject the steroid solution as a bolus into the GH joint. The injected solution should flow smoothly into the joint space. If increased resistance is encountered, advance or withdraw the needle slightly before attempting further injection.
6. Following injection of the corticosteroid solution, withdraw the needle.

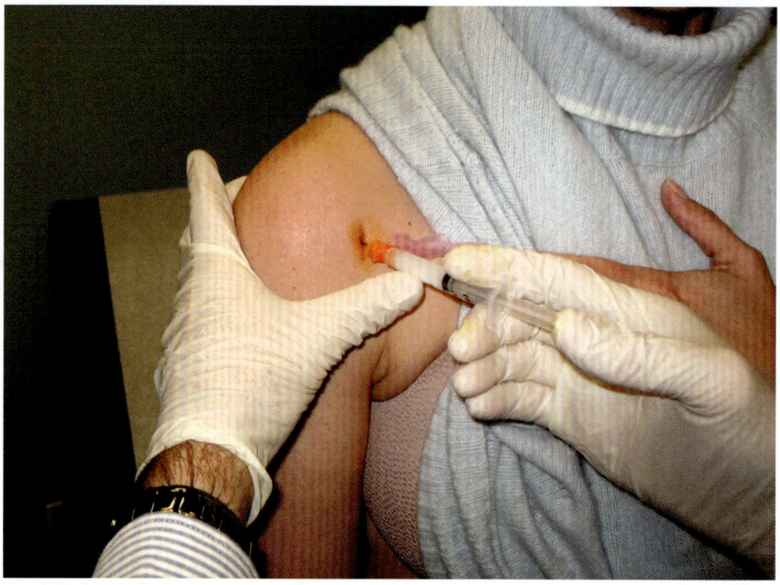

**FIGURE 6.11** ● Glenohumeral joint injection—anterior approach.

7. Apply a sterile adhesive bandage.
8. Instruct the patient to move his or her shoulder through its full range of motion. This movement distributes the steroid solution throughout the subacromial space.
9. Reexamine the shoulder in 5 min to confirm pain relief.

## AFTERCARE

- Avoid excessive use of the shoulder over the next 2 weeks.
- Consider use of an arm sling.
- NSAIDs, ice, and/or physical therapy as indicated.
- Consider follow-up examination in 2 weeks.

**CPT code:** 20610—Injection of major joint or bursa

## PEARLS

- When palpating to determine the location of the coracoid, use the fingertips of your index, middle, and ring fingers. Firmly palpate the humeral head and methodically move in a lateral-to-medial direction. Mark the site where your fingers meet the coracoid.
- When palpating to determine the location of the acromion, use the fingertips of your index, middle, and ring fingers. Gently and methodically move in a distal-to-proximal direction. Mark the site where your fingers meet the bone.
- A smaller volume of lidocaine is used in this injection compared to the subacromial space injection because the joint capsule may be stenosed—especially in patients with adhesive capsulitis.

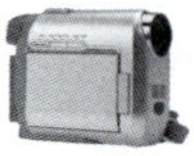

A video clip showing a GH joint injection can be found in the companion eBook.

## REFERENCES

Please consult references listed in the preceding section.

# Acromioclavicular Joint

The AC joint is a relatively uncommon injection site for most primary care physicians. Successful injection can be difficult because of the small joint space. A small-diameter needle is appropriate as this technique is only used to inject steroid solution into the AC joint.

Clinical trials demonstrate effectiveness of the corticosteroid injection into the AC joint in only a minority of patients.[1] But those do respond typically have a sustained effect.[2] Multiple studies show that this is a difficult injection to perform successfully. Only about 40% of injections reached the intended intra-articular target.[3] Ultrasound greatly improves accuracy to nearly 100%.[4–6] However, clinically, there appears to be little difference in outcomes whether the injection was intra-articular or periarticular.[7]

| Indications | ICD-9 Code | ICD-10 Code |
|---|---|---|
| AC joint pain | 719.41 | M25.519 |
| AC joint sprain | 840.0 | S43.50 |
| AC joint subluxation/dislocation | 831.04 | S43.10 |
| AC joint arthritis, unspecified | 716.91 | M12.9 |
| AC joint osteoarthritis, primary | 715.11 | M19.019 |
| AC joint osteoarthritis, posttraumatic | 716.11 | M19.119 |
| AC joint osteoarthritis, secondary | 715.21 | M19.219 |

**Relevant Anatomy:** (Fig. 6.12)

## PATIENT POSITION

- Sitting or lying supine on the examination table.
- The patient's hands are folded in his or her lap with fingers interlaced.
- This allows consistency of positioning of the shoulder so that the landmarks do not change from the time that they are identified and marked until the time of injection.
- Rotate the patient's head away from the side that is being injected. This minimizes anxiety and pain perception.

## LANDMARKS

1. With the patient seated or lying supine on the examination table, the clinician stands lateral and anterior to the affected shoulder.
2. Identify the AC joint. Palpate the clavicle in a medial-to-lateral direction. At the lateral aspect of the clavicle, there is a small depression that will be tender in the above conditions.
3. The injection point is located directly over the AC joint. At that site, press firmly with the retracted tip of a ballpoint pen. This indention represents the entry point for the needle.
4. Once the landmarks are identified, the patient should not move the chest or shoulder.

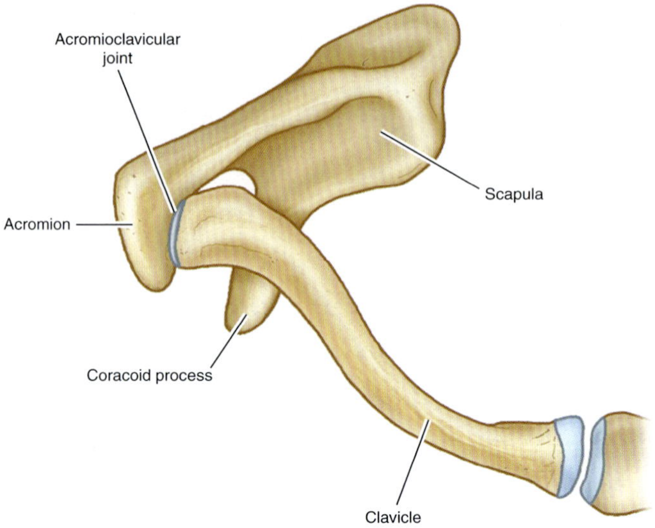


**FIGURE 6.12** Right AC joint. (From Tank PW, Gest TR. *Lippincott Williams & Wilkins Atlas of Anatomy*. Philadelphia, PA: Lippincott Williams & Wilkins, 2009.)

## ANESTHESIA

- Local anesthesia of the skin using topical vapocoolant spray.

## EQUIPMENT

- 3-mL syringe
- 25-gauge, 5/8-in. needle
- 0.5 mL of 1% lidocaine without epinephrine
- 0.5 mL of the steroid solution (20 mg of triamcinolone acetonide)
- One alcohol prep pad
- Two povidone–iodine prep pads
- Sterile gauze pads
- Sterile adhesive bandage

## TECHNIQUE

1. Prep the insertion site with alcohol followed by the povidone–iodine pads.
2. Achieve good local anesthesia by using topical vapocoolant spray.
3. Position the needle and syringe perpendicular to the skin with the needle tip directed caudad.
4. Using the no-touch technique, introduce the needle at the insertion site (Fig. 6.13).
5. Advance the needle into the AC joint. If the needle does not "drop" into the AC joint, then "walk" the needle in the area until it does so.
6. Inject the steroid solution as a bolus into the AC joint. The injected solution should flow smoothly into the space. If increased resistance is encountered, advance or withdraw the needle slightly before attempting further injection. If the needle will not drop into the joint, then perform a periarticular injection.
7. Following injection of the corticosteroid solution, withdraw the needle.
8. Apply a sterile adhesive bandage.
9. Instruct the patient to move his or her shoulder through its full range of motion. This movement distributes the steroid solution throughout the AC joint.
10. Reexamine the shoulder in 5 min to confirm pain relief.

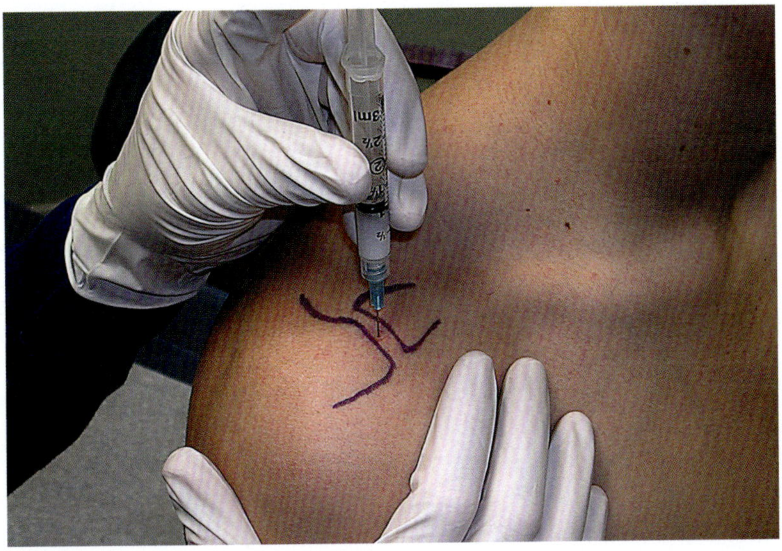

**FIGURE 6.13** • Right AC joint injection with landmarks.

## AFTERCARE

- Avoid excessive use of the shoulder over the next 2 weeks.
- Consider the use of an arm sling.
- NSAIDs, ice, and/or physical therapy as indicated.
- Consider follow-up examination in 2 weeks.

**CPT code:** 20600—Injection of small joint

## PEARLS

- The AC joint is superficial. Depositing corticosteroid in the subcutaneous tissues can result in the complication of skin atrophy and hypopigmentation. Avoid the development of a subdermal wheal while performing all injections of corticosteroid solutions. Perform the "pinch technique" as described in the "Lateral Epicondylitis" chapter.

## REFERENCES


1. van Riet RP, Goehre T, Bell SN. The long term effect of an intra-articular injection of corticosteroids in the acromioclavicular joint. *J Shoulder Elbow Surg*. 2012;21(3):376–379.
2. Hossain S, Jacobs LG, Hashmi R. The long-term effectiveness of steroid injections in primary acromioclavicular joint arthritis: a five-year prospective study. *J Shoulder Elbow Surg*. 2008;17(4):535–538.
3. Wasserman BR, Pettrone S, Jazrawi LM, et al. Accuracy of acromioclavicular joint injections. *Am J Sports Med*. 2013;41(1):149–152.
4. Borbas P, Kraus T, Clement H, et al. The influence of ultrasound guidance in the rate of success of acromioclavicular joint injection: an experimental study on human cadavers. *J Shoulder Elbow Surg*. 2012;21(12):1694–1697.
5. Peck E, Lai JK, Pawlina W, et al. Accuracy of ultrasound-guided versus palpation-guided acromioclavicular joint injections: a cadaveric study. *PM R*. 2010;2(9):817–821.
6. Sabeti-Aschraf M, Lemmerhofer B, Lang S, et al. Ultrasound guidance improves the accuracy of the acromioclavicular joint infiltration: a prospective randomized study. *Knee Surg Sports Traumatol Arthrosc*. 2011;19(2):292–295.
7. Sabeti-Aschraf M, Stotter C, Thaler C, et al. Intra-articular versus periarticular acromioclavicular joint injection: a multicenter, prospective, randomized, controlled trial. *Arthroscopy*. 2013;29(12):1903–1910.

# Sternoclavicular Joint

The sternoclavicular (SC) joint is an uncommon injection site for most primary care physicians. Successful injection can be difficult because of the small joint space. Except for a single study that described CT-guided injections,[1] no research studies are available that describe injections into the SC joint.

A small-diameter needle is appropriate as this technique is only used to inject steroid solution into the SC joint.

| Indications | ICD-9 Code | ICD-10 Code |
|---|---|---|
| SC joint pain | 719.41 | M25.519 |
| SC joint sprain | 848.41 | S23.420 |
| SC joint subluxation | 739.61 | S43.20 |
| SC joint arthritis, unspecified | 716.91 | M12.9 |
| SC joint osteoarthritis, primary | 715.11 | M19.019 |
| SC joint osteoarthritis, posttraumatic | 716.11 | M19.119 |
| SC joint osteoarthritis, secondary | 715.21 | M19.219 |

**Relevant Anatomy:** (Fig. 6.14)

## PATIENT POSITION

- Supine on the examination table.
- The patient's hands are folded in his or her lap with fingers interlaced.
- Rotate the patient's head away from the side that is being injected. This minimizes anxiety and pain perception.

## LANDMARKS

1. With the patient supine on the examination table, the clinician stands to the patient's side.
2. Identify the SC joint. Palpate the clavicle in a lateral-to-medial direction. At the medial aspect of the clavicle, there is a small depression that represents the SC joint. This structure will be tender.
3. It may be helpful to rotate the ipsilateral shoulder in order to more easily identify the SC joint.
4. The injection point is directly over the SC joint.
5. At that site, press firmly on the skin with the retracted tip of a ballpoint pen. This indention represents the entry point for the needle.
6. After the landmarks are identified, the patient should not move the chest or shoulder.

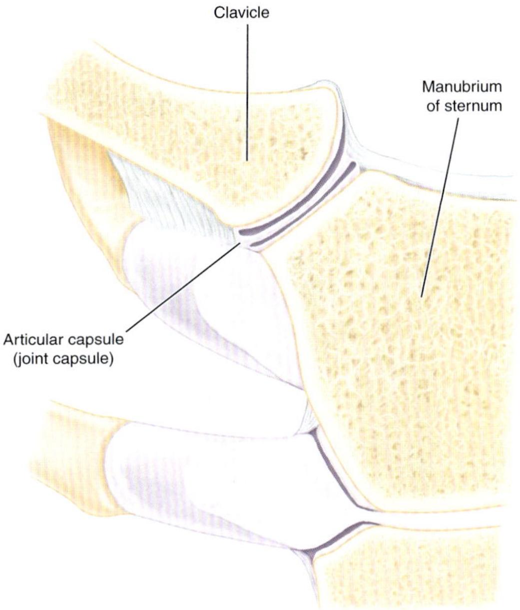


*FIGURE 6.14* • Sternoclavicular joint. (From Tank PW, Gest TR. *Lippincott Williams & Wilkins Atlas of Anatomy.* Philadelphia, PA: Lippincott Williams & Wilkins, 2009.)

## ANESTHESIA

- Local anesthesia of the skin using topical vapocoolant spray.

## EQUIPMENT

- 3-mL syringe
- 25-gauge, 1-in. needle
- 0.5 mL of 1% lidocaine without epinephrine
- 0.5 mL of the steroid solution (20 mg of triamcinolone acetonide)
- One alcohol prep pad
- Two povidone–iodine prep pads
- Sterile gauze pads
- Sterile adhesive bandage

## TECHNIQUE

1. Prep the insertion site with alcohol followed by the povidone–iodine pads.
2. Achieve good local anesthesia by using topical vapocoolant spray.
3. Position the needle and syringe perpendicular to the skin with the needle tip directed posteriorly.
4. Using the no-touch technique, introduce the needle at the insertion site (Fig. 6.15).
5. Advance the needle into the SC joint space.
6. Inject the steroid solution as a bolus into the SC joint. The injected solution should flow smoothly into the space. If increased resistance is encountered, advance or withdraw the needle slightly before attempting further injection.
7. Following injection of the corticosteroid solution, withdraw the needle.
8. Apply a sterile adhesive bandage.
9. Instruct the patient to move his or her shoulder through its full range of motion. This movement distributes the steroid solution throughout the SC joint.
10. Reexamine the SC joint in 5 min to confirm pain relief.

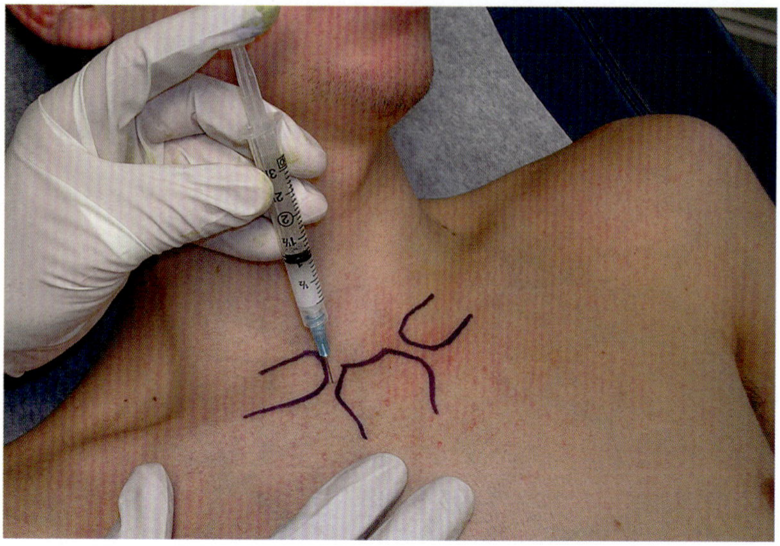

**FIGURE 6.15** ● Sternoclavicular joint injection with landmarks.

## AFTERCARE

- Avoid excessive use of the shoulder over the next 2 weeks.
- Consider use of an arm sling.
- NSAIDs, ice, and/or physical therapy as indicated.
- Consider follow-up examination in 2 weeks.

**CPT code:** 20600—Injection of small joint

## PEARLS

- The SC joint is superficial. Depositing corticosteroid in the subcutaneous tissues can result in the complication of skin atrophy and hypopigmentation. Avoid the development of a subdermal wheal while performing all injections of corticosteroid solutions.

## REFERENCE

1. Peterson CK, Saupe N, Buck F, et al. CT-guided sternoclavicular joint injections: description of the procedure, reliability of imaging diagnosis, and short-term patient responses. *AJR Am J Roentgenol.* 2010;195(6):W435–W439.

# Bicipital Tenosynovitis—Long Head

Patients occasionally present to the primary care office for evaluation and treatment of bicipital tendonitis. This is an inflammatory and degenerative condition more frequently seen in the long head than the short head of the biceps brachii muscle. It develops either from direct acute trauma or chronic overuse in throwing athletes and nonathletes who use their arms to do repetitive biceps contraction, resisted forearm supination, or overhead work. Bicipital tendinitis is frequently diagnosed in association with rotator cuff disease as a component of the impingement syndrome or secondary to intra-articular pathology, such as labral tears. Local tenderness is usually located over the bicipital groove of the humerus. Conservative management of biceps tendonitis consists of rest, ice, oral analgesics, physical therapy, or corticosteroid injections.

As demonstrated in the literature, physicians have difficulty correctly identifying the intertubercular groove that contains the long head of the biceps tendon. Localization attempts are usually far medial of its actual location.[1] Consequently, clinicians should exercise caution when relying on clinical palpation to perform a bicipital tendon sheath injection. Ultrasound guidance of this injection significantly improves the accuracy rate.[2,3]

| Indication | ICD-9 Code | ICD-10 Code |
|---|---|---|
| Bicipital tenosynovitis | 726.12 | M75.20 |

**Relevant Anatomy:** (Fig. 6.16)

## PATIENT POSITION

- Supine on the examination table with the head of the bed elevated 30 degrees.
- The patient's hands are placed in a position of supination at his or her side with slight external rotation of the arm.
- Rotate the patient's head away from the side that is being injected. This minimizes anxiety and pain perception.

## LANDMARKS

1. With the patient lying supine on the examination table, the clinician stands lateral and posterior to the affected arm.
2. Instruct the patient to flex the elbow and contract the biceps muscle.
3. Palpate the course of the long head of the bicipital tendon over the anterior aspect of the upper arm.
4. Determine the location of maximal tenderness, which will most likely be under the edge of the pectoralis major muscle. Mark that spot with an ink pen.

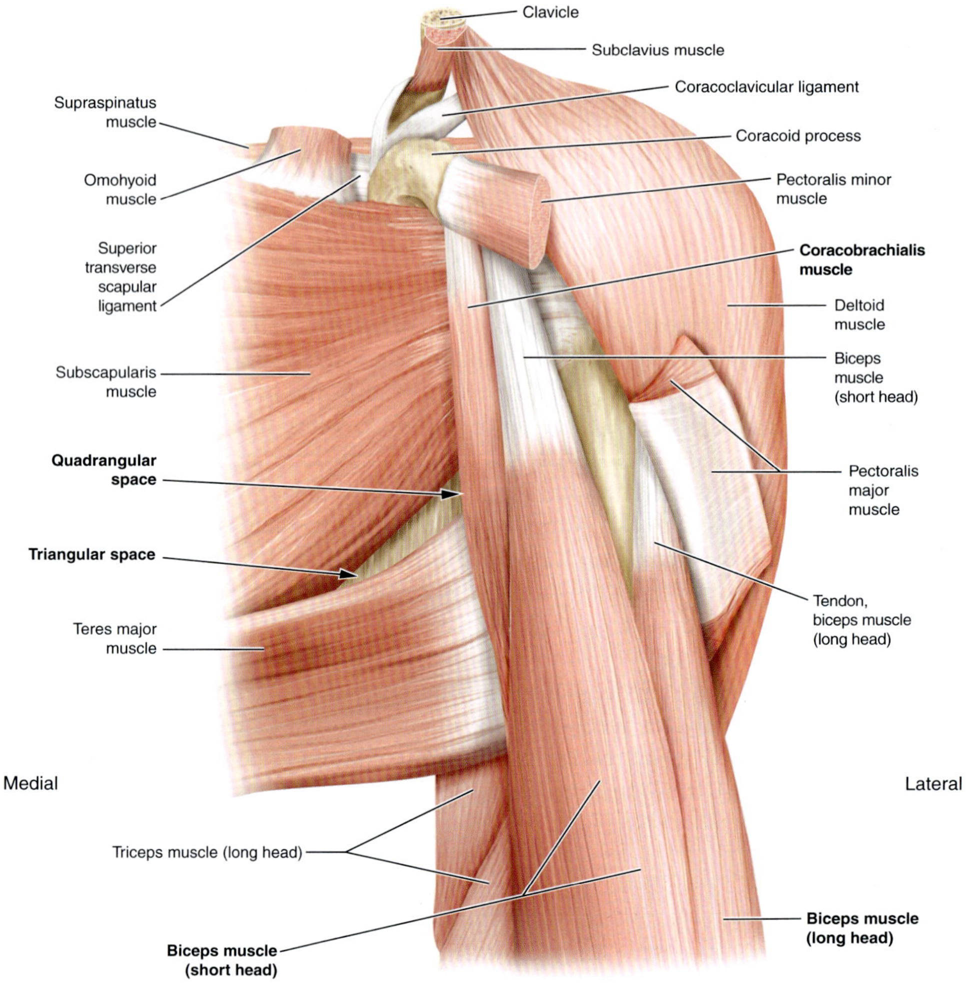


**FIGURE 6.16** Muscles of anterior left arm. (From Tank PW, Gest TR. *Lippincott Williams & Wilkins Atlas of Anatomy*. Philadelphia, PA: Lippincott Williams & Wilkins, 2009.)

5. At that site, press firmly on the skin with the retracted tip of a ballpoint pen. This indention represents the entry point for the needle.
6. After the landmarks are identified, the patient should not move the shoulder or arm.

## ANESTHESIA

- Local anesthesia of the skin using topical vapocoolant spray.

## EQUIPMENT

- 3-mL syringe
- 25-gauge, 1½ in. needle
- 1 mL of 1% lidocaine without epinephrine
- 0.5 to 1 mL of the steroid solution (20 to 40 mg of triamcinolone acetonide)
- One alcohol prep pad
- Two povidone–iodine prep pads

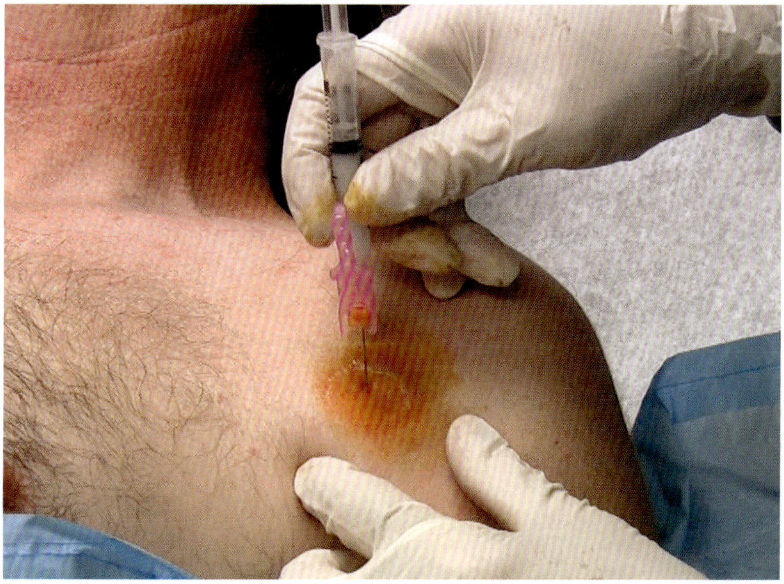

***FIGURE 6.17*** • Bicipital tendosynovitis injection.

- Sterile gauze pads
- Sterile adhesive bandage
- Nonsterile, clean chucks pad

## TECHNIQUE

1. Prep the insertion site with alcohol followed by the povidone–iodine pads.
2. Achieve good local anesthesia by using topical vapocoolant spray.
3. Position the needle and syringe at a 45-degree angle to the skin with the needle tip directed proximally.
4. Using the no-touch technique, introduce the needle at the insertion site (Fig. 6.17).
5. Advance the needle until the needle tip touches the tendon. (An increase in resistance will be detected.) Back up the needle 1 to 2 mm.
6. Inject the steroid solution as a bolus around the bicipital tendon. The injected solution should flow smoothly into the tenosynovial sheath. If increased resistance is encountered, advance or withdraw the needle slightly before attempting further injection.
7. Following injection of the corticosteroid solution, withdraw the needle.
8. Apply a sterile adhesive bandage.
9. Instruct the patient to move his or her biceps muscle and shoulder through their full range of motion. This movement distributes the steroid solution throughout the tenosynovial sheath.
10. Reexamine the arm in 5 min to confirm pain relief.

## AFTERCARE

- Avoid all throwing and excessive use of the arm and shoulder over the next 2 weeks.
- NSAIDs, ice, and/or physical therapy as indicated.
- Consider follow-up examination in 2 weeks.

**CPT code:** 20550—Injection of single tendon sheath

## PEARLS

- Failure to recognize or treat this condition may lead to rupture of the long head of the biceps brachii tendon.
- Make sure to place the injection around the tendon and not into the substance of the tendon in order to prevent iatrogenic degeneration of the tendon and rupture.
- Subacromial or GH joint steroid injections are recommended for persistent cases of bicipital tendinitis.

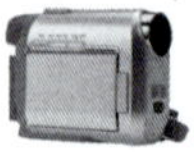

A video clip showing a bicipital tenosynovitis injection can be found in the companion eBook.

## REFERENCES

1. Gazzillo GP, Finnoff JT, Hall MM, et al. Accuracy of palpating the long head of the biceps tendon: an ultrasonographic study. *PM R*. 2011;3(11):1035–1040.
2. Hashiuchi T, Sakurai G, Morimoto M, et al. Accuracy of the biceps tendon sheath injection: ultrasound-guided or unguided injection? A randomized controlled trial. *J Shoulder Elbow Surg*. 2011;20(7): 1069–1073.
3. Zhang J, Ebraheim N, Lause GE. Ultrasound-guided injection for the biceps brachii tendinitis: results and experience. *Ultrasound Med Biol*. 2011;37(5):729–733.

# Cubital Tunnel Syndrome

Cubital tunnel syndrome is an uncommon condition encountered by primary care physicians. It occurs when the ulnar nerve becomes entrapped in the cubital tunnel posterior to the medial epicondyle. Treatment of this usually involves conservative measures including avoidance of predisposing repetitive movements, nighttime application of an elbow brace, and NSAIDs. Corticosteroid injection of the cubital tunnel may bring pain relief. However, there are no studies reported in the literature regarding this injection site. The practitioner may want to consider ultrasound guidance in order to avoid injury to the ulnar nerve. Successful treatment may require surgical transposition of the nerve over the medial epicondyle.

| Indication | ICD-9 Code | ICD-10 Code |
|---|---|---|
| Cubital tunnel syndrome | 354.2 | G56.20 |

**Relevant Anatomy:** (Fig. 6.18)

## PATIENT POSITION

- Supine on the examination table with the head of the bed elevated 30 degrees.
- Shoulder at 30 degrees of abduction and full external rotation.
- The affected elbow is flexed at 90 degrees.
- The wrist is in a neutral position.
- The elbow is supported with the placement of chucks pads or towels.
- Rotate the patient's head away from the side that is being injected. This minimizes anxiety and pain perception.

## LANDMARKS

1. With the patient supine on the examination table, the clinician stands lateral to the affected elbow.
2. Identify and mark the medial epicondyle of the humerus.
3. Identify and mark the course of the ulnar nerve in the ulnar groove posterior to the medial epicondyle.
4. Mark the point of maximal tenderness over the ulnar nerve. This is usually just posterior to the medical epicondyle.
5. At that site, press firmly on the skin with the retracted tip of a ballpoint pen. This indention represents the entry point for the needle.
6. After the landmarks are identified, the patient should not move the elbow.

## ANESTHESIA

- Local anesthesia of the skin using topical vapocoolant spray.

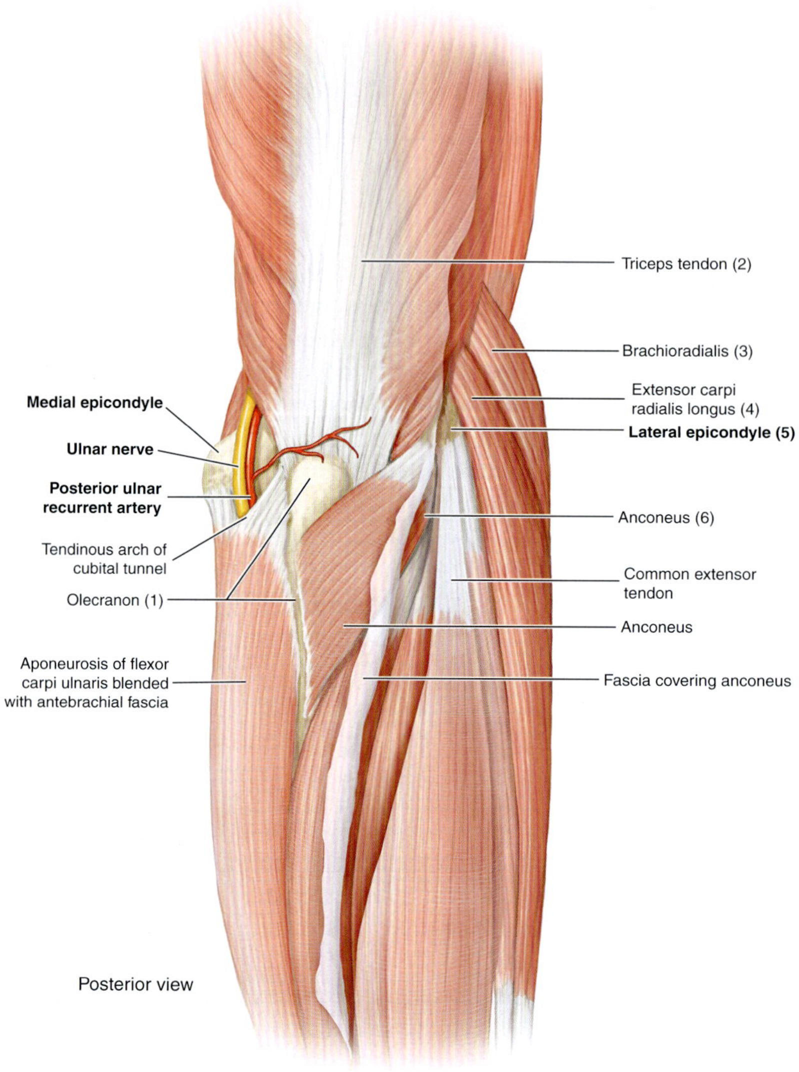


**FIGURE 6.18** ● Posterior aspect of right elbow. (From Tank PW, Gest TR. *Lippincott Williams & Wilkins Atlas of Anatomy*. Philadelphia, PA: Lippincott Williams & Wilkins, 2009.)

## EQUIPMENT

- 3-mL syringe
- 25-gauge, 1-in. needle
- 1 mL of 1% lidocaine without epinephrine
- 1 mL of the steroid solution (40 mg of triamcinolone acetonide)
- One alcohol prep pad
- Two povidone–iodine prep pads
- Sterile gauze pads
- Sterile adhesive bandage
- Nonsterile, clean chucks pad

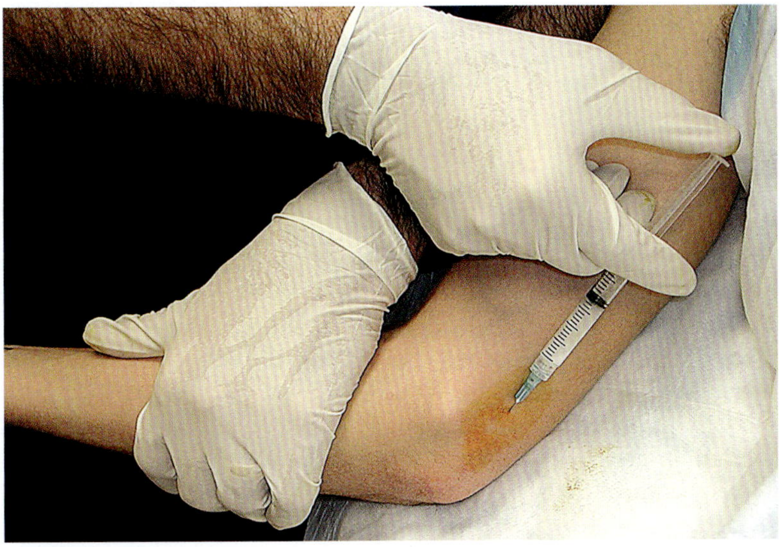

***FIGURE 6.19*** ● Right cubital tunnel injection.

## TECHNIQUE

1. Prep the insertion site with alcohol followed by the povidone–iodine pads.
2. Achieve good local anesthesia by using topical vapocoolant spray.
3. Position the needle and syringe at a 30-degree angle to the skin with the tip of the needle directed distally along the ulnar nerve.
4. Using the no-touch technique, introduce the needle at the insertion site (Fig. 6.19).
5. Advance the needle slowly at a shallow angle to a position just along the side of the ulnar nerve.
6. If any pain, paresthesias, or numbness is encountered, withdraw the needle slightly and redirect the needle tip using a slightly different angle.
7. When the needle is placed along the ulnar nerve, slowly deposit the steroid solution as a bolus around that structure.
8. Inject the steroid solution steadily into this area. If increased resistance is encountered, advance or withdraw the needle slightly before attempting further injection.
9. Following injection of the corticosteroid solution, withdraw the needle.
10. Apply a sterile adhesive bandage.
11. Instruct the patient to move his or her wrist and elbow through their full range of motion.
12. Reexamine the elbow in 5 min to confirm pain relief and the development of numbness in the distribution of the ulnar nerve from the local anesthetic.

## AFTERCARE

- Avoid further overuse mechanisms of injury.
- Use an elbow extension brace while sleeping to avoid excessive elbow flexion.
- NSAIDs, ice, and/or physical therapy as indicated.
- Consider follow-up examination in 2 weeks.

**CPT code:** 64450—Injection, nerve block, therapeutic, other peripheral nerve or branch

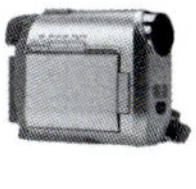

A video clip showing a cubital tunnel syndrome injection can be found in the companion eBook.

# Elbow Joint

Aspiration and injection of the elbow joint are uncommon procedures in most primary care practices. Tense collections of blood distending the elbow joint develop with fractures of the radial head. Significant pain relief follows aspiration. Arthritis in the elbow most commonly occurs due to rheumatoid arthritis, gout, and osteoarthritis. This may respond to corticosteroid injection, but this aspiration and injection procedure is not described in any clinical trials.

| Indications | ICD-9 Code | ICD-10 Code |
|---|---|---|
| Elbow pain | 729.5 | M25.529 |
| Elbow sprain | 841.9 | S53.40 |
| Elbow joint arthritis, unspecified | 716.92 | M12.9 |
| Elbow joint osteoarthritis, primary | 715.12 | M19.029 |
| Elbow joint osteoarthritis, posttraumatic | 716.12 | M19.129 |
| Elbow joint osteoarthritis, secondary | 715.22 | M19.229 |

**Relevant Anatomy:** (Fig. 6.20)

## PATIENT POSITION

- Supine on the examination table with the head of the bed elevated 30 degrees.
- The elbow is positioned at 45 degrees of extension.
- The wrist is in a neutral position.
- The elbow is supported with the placement of chucks pads or towels.
- Rotate the patient's head away from the side that is being injected. This minimizes anxiety and pain perception.

## LANDMARKS

1. With the patient supine on the examination table, the clinician stands lateral to the affected elbow.
2. Locate the radial head by palpating over the lateral aspect of the elbow while supinating and pronating the wrist.
3. Find the depression immediately proximal to the radial head and mark it with ink.
4. At that site, press firmly on the skin with the retracted tip of a ballpoint pen. This indention represents the entry point for the needle.
5. After the landmarks are identified, the patient should not move the elbow.

## ANESTHESIA

- Local anesthesia of the skin using topical vapocoolant spray.

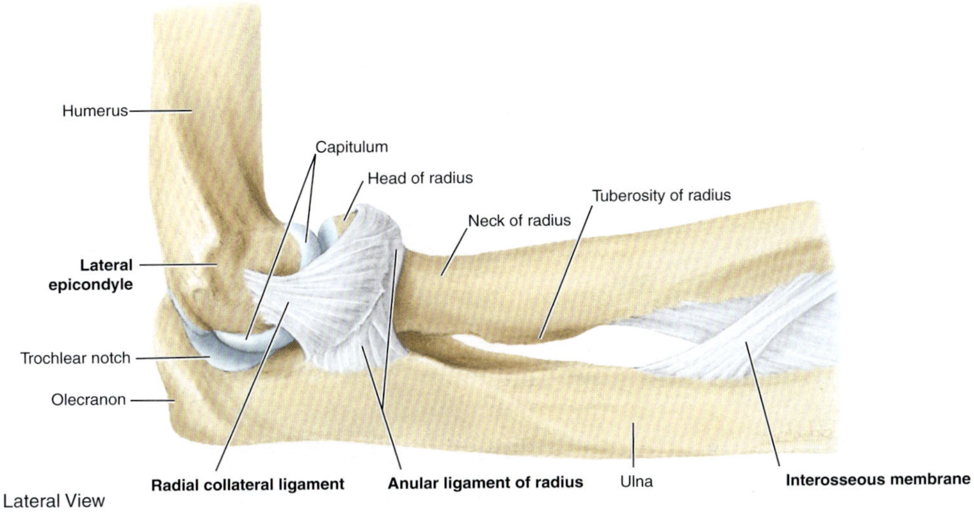


*FIGURE 6.20* • Right lateral elbow joint. (From Tank PW, Gest TR. *Lippincott Williams & Wilkins Atlas of Anatomy*. Philadelphia, PA: Lippincott Williams & Wilkins, 2009.)

## EQUIPMENT

- 3-mL syringe
- 10-mL syringe—for optional aspiration
- 25-gauge, 1-in. needle
- 20-gauge, 1-in. needle—for optional aspiration
- 0.5 mL of 1% lidocaine without epinephrine
- 0.5 mL of the steroid solution (20 mg of triamcinolone acetonide)
- One alcohol prep pad
- Two povidone–iodine prep pads
- Sterile gauze pads
- Sterile adhesive bandage
- Nonsterile, clean chucks pad

## TECHNIQUE

1. Prep the insertion site with alcohol followed by the povidone–iodine pads.
2. Achieve good local anesthesia by using topical vapocoolant spray.
3. Position the needle and syringe perpendicular to the skin with the needle tip directed medially toward the elbow joint.
4. Using the no-touch technique, introduce the needle at the insertion site (Fig. 6.21).
5. Advance the needle into the elbow joint. This places the needle tip between the humeral lateral condyle and the radial head.
6. If aspirating, withdraw fluid using a 20-gauge, 1-in. needle with the 10-mL syringe.
7. If injection of corticosteroid is to follow the aspiration, grasp the needle firmly, remove the 10-mL syringe from the 20-gauge needle, and then attach the 3-mL syringe filled with the steroid–lidocaine mixture.
8. If only injecting the steroid mixture, use a 25-gauge, 1-in. needle with the 3-mL syringe.
9. Inject the steroid solution as a bolus into the elbow joint. The injected solution should flow smoothly into the space. If increased resistance is encountered, advance or withdraw the needle slightly before attempting further injection.
10. Following injection of the corticosteroid solution, withdraw the needle.

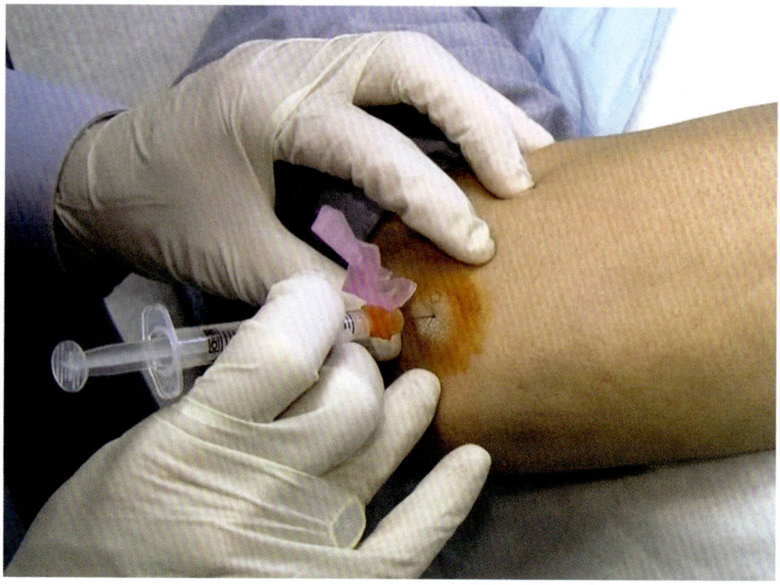

**FIGURE 6.21** ● Left elbow joint injection.

11. Apply a sterile adhesive bandage.
12. Instruct the patient to move his or her elbow through its full range of motion. This movement distributes the steroid solution throughout the elbow joint.
13. Reexamine the elbow in 5 min to confirm pain relief.

## AFTERCARE

- Do not brace or rest the elbow. A recent study showed a significantly higher rate of synovitis relapse in patients following corticosteroid injection who were rested for 48 hours in an elbow sling versus normal activity without restrictions.[1]
- Consider use of a neoprene elbow sleeve.
- Avoid vigorous use of the elbow over the next 2 weeks.
- NSAIDs, ice, and/or physical therapy as indicated.
- Consider follow-up examination in 2 weeks.

**CPT code:** 20605—Arthrocentesis, aspiration, and/or injection of intermediate joint or bursa

## PEARLS

- The joint space at the radial head can be "opened up" by extending the elbow.
- Since the elbow has a narrow joint space, a 20-gauge needle is used for aspiration instead of the larger diameter, 18-gauge needle.
- If a fracture is suspected, do not inject corticosteroid.

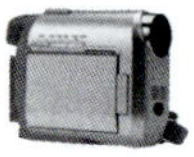

A video clip showing an elbow joint injection can be found in the companion eBook.

## REFERENCE

1. Weitoft T, Forsberg C. Importance of immobilization after intraarticular glucocorticoid treatment for elbow synovitis: a randomized controlled study. *Arthritis Care Res (Hoboken)*. 2010;62(5):735–737.

# Olecranon Bursitis

Olecranon bursitis is a relatively common aspiration and injection site for primary care physicians. Successful aspiration is usually accomplished because the location of the bursa is readily evident. The subcutaneous olecranon bursa may become inflamed and accumulate fluid when subjected to repeated excessive pressure or friction. The fluid may consist of blood in acute trauma, thick proteinaceous mucoid fluid after repetitive injury, or purulent fluid if infected. Corticosteroids should never be administered if an infectious bursitis is suspected.

An 18-gauge needle is used to aspirate a large volume of fluid. Occasionally, the clinician may elect to inject a steroid solution if the fluid recollects—but only when an infection is excluded.

| Indication | ICD-9 Code | ICD-10 Code |
|---|---|---|
| Olecranon bursitis | 726.33 | M70.20 |

**Relevant Anatomy:** (Fig. 6.22)

## PATIENT POSITION

- Supine on the examination table with the head of the bed elevated 30 degrees.
- The affected elbow is maximally flexed.
- The elbow is supported with the placement of chucks pads or towels.
- Rotate the patient's head away from the side that is being injected. This minimizes anxiety and pain perception.

## LANDMARKS

1. With the patient supine on the examination table, the clinician stands lateral to the affected elbow.
2. The point of maximal fluctuance is identified.
3. At that site, press firmly on the skin with the retracted tip of a ballpoint pen. This indention represents the entry point for the needle.
4. After the landmarks are identified, the patient should not move the elbow.

## ANESTHESIA

- Local anesthesia of the skin using topical vapocoolant spray.

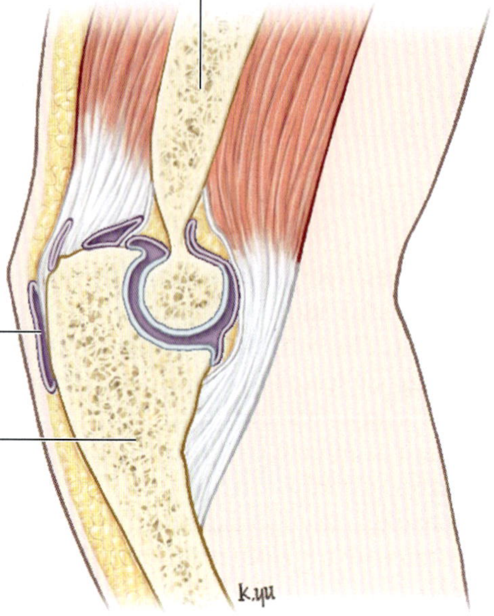


*FIGURE 6.22* ● Lateral aspect of left elbow. (From Tank PW, Gest TR. *Lippincott Williams & Wilkins Atlas of Anatomy*. Philadelphia, PA: Lippincott Williams & Wilkins, 2009.)

## EQUIPMENT

- 20-mL syringe—for aspiration
- 3-mL syringe—for optional injection
- 18-gauge, 1½ in. needle
- 1 mL of 1% lidocaine without epinephrine—for optional injection
- 1 mL of the steroid solution (40 mg of triamcinolone acetonide)—for optional injection
- One alcohol prep pad
- Two povidone–iodine prep pads
- Sterile gauze pads
- Sterile adhesive bandage
- Nonsterile, clean chucks pad

## TECHNIQUE

1. Prep the insertion site with alcohol followed by the povidone–iodine pads.
2. Achieve good local anesthesia by using topical vapocoolant spray.
3. Position the 18-gauge needle and syringe with the needle tip directed toward the area of maximal fluid collection.
4. Using the no-touch technique, introduce the needle at the insertion site (Fig. 6.23).
5. Advance the needle into the center of the bursa.
6. Aspiration should be easy accomplished. Use multiple syringes if the effusion is large.
7. If injection following aspiration is elected, grasp the hub of the needle, remove the large syringe, and then attach the 3-mL syringe filled with the steroid solution.

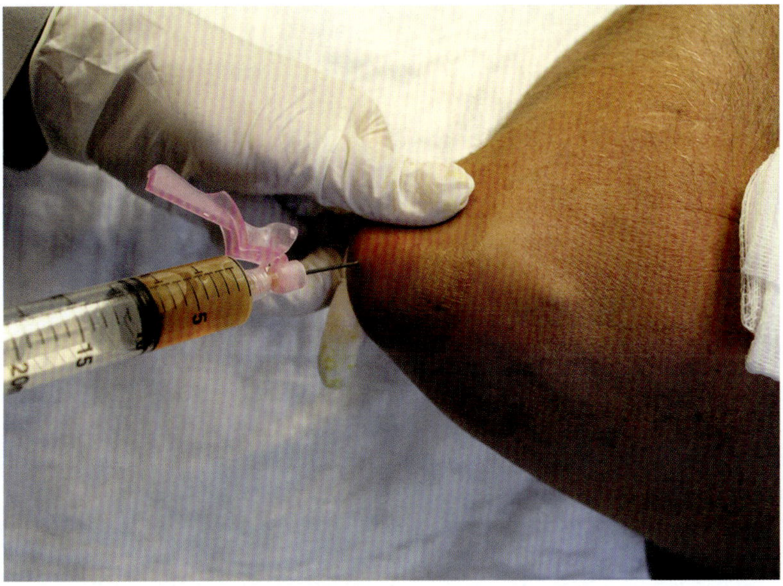


***FIGURE 6.23*** • Olecranon bursa aspiration.

8. The injected solution should flow smoothly into the space. If increased resistance is encountered, advance or withdraw the needle slightly before attempting further injection.
9. Following complete aspiration, and possible injection of corticosteroid solution, withdraw the needle.
10. Apply a sterile adhesive bandage followed by a compressive elastic bandage.
11. Reexamine the elbow in 5 min to confirm pain relief.

## AFTERCARE

- Avoid excessive use of the elbow over the next 2 weeks.
- Consider the use of a neoprene elbow sleeve or elastic compression bandage.
- NSAIDs, ice, and/or physical therapy as indicated.
- Consider follow-up examination in 2 weeks.

**CPT code:** 20605—Aspiration and/or injection of intermediate bursa

## PEARLS

- If the olecranon bursitis is due to an infection or acute hemorrhagic event, do not follow aspiration with corticosteroid injection.
- Injection of corticosteroid is usually reserved for recurrent bursitis.

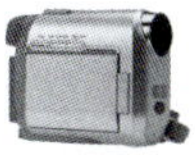

A video clip showing an olecranon bursitis aspiration can be found in the companion eBook.

# Lateral Epicondylitis

Lateral epicondylitis is one of the most common soft tissue conditions treated by primary care providers. This is a misnomer and actually involves a noninflammatory tendinosis with collagen disarray. It usually is the result of an overuse injury with microtears to the hypovascular origins of the wrist extensor and supinator muscle groups.

Injection of various substances to treat this condition has been extensively reported in the literature. Although corticosteroid injections have been used for years, it appears that they are beneficial only in the short term.[1,2] Long-term effects are no better than placebo and may in fact be worse.[2,3] Botulinum toxin has also been used with conflicting results.[4,5] Injections of platelet-rich plasma and autologous blood show more promise in the medium to long term, but further research is needed.[6] In actuality, there is no injection or physiotherapy intervention that has consistently shown treatment efficacy in the medium to long term in patients diagnosed with lateral epicondylitis.[7,8]

| Indication | ICD-9 Code | ICD-10 Code |
|---|---|---|
| Lateral epicondylitis | 726.32 | M77.10 |

**Relevant Anatomy:** (Fig. 6.24)

## PATIENT POSITION

- Supine on the examination table with the head of the bed elevated 30 degrees.
- The affected elbow is slightly flexed.
- The wrist is in a neutral to slightly pronated position.
- The elbow is supported with the placement of chucks pads or towels.
- Rotate the patient's head away from the side that is being injected. This minimizes anxiety and pain perception.

## LANDMARKS

1. With the patient supine on the examination table, the clinician stands lateral to the affected elbow.
2. Identify and mark the point of maximal tenderness adjacent to the lateral epicondyle.
3. At that site, press firmly on the skin with the retracted tip of a ballpoint pen. This indention represents the entry point for the needle.
4. After the landmarks are identified, the patient should not move the elbow.

## ANESTHESIA

- Local anesthesia of the skin using topical vapocoolant spray.

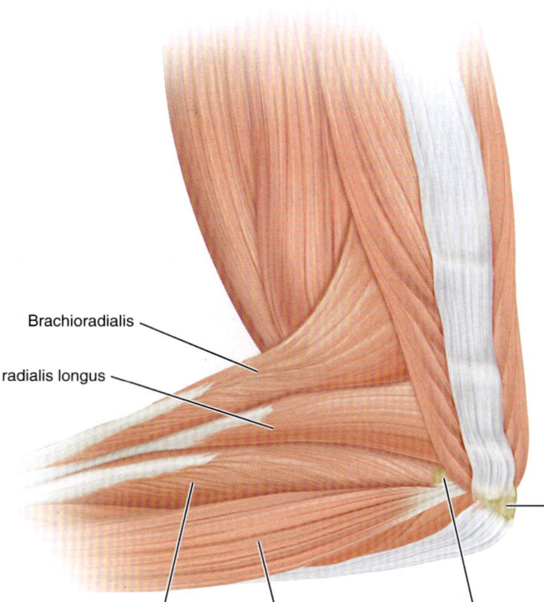


**FIGURE 6.24** • Lateral view of muscular structures at left elbow. (From Tank PW, Gest TR. *Lippincott Williams & Wilkins Atlas of Anatomy*. Philadelphia, PA: Lippincott Williams & Wilkins; 2009.)

## EQUIPMENT

- 3-mL syringe
- 25-gauge, 1-in. needle
- 1 mL of 1% lidocaine without epinephrine
- 0.5 mL of the steroid solution (20 mg of triamcinolone acetonide)
- One alcohol prep pad
- Two povidone–iodine prep pads
- Sterile gauze pads
- Sterile adhesive bandage
- Nonsterile, clean chucks pad

## TECHNIQUE

1. Prep the insertion site with alcohol followed by the povidone–iodine pads.
2. Achieve good local anesthesia by using topical vapocoolant spray.
3. Position the needle and syringe perpendicular to the skin with the needle tip directed medially toward the lateral epicondyle.
4. Using the no-touch technique, introduce the needle at the insertion site (Fig. 6.25).
5. Advance the needle to the bone of the lateral epicondyle.
6. Withdraw the needle 1 to 2 mm.
7. Perform the "pinch technique" (see description in "Pearls" section).
8. Inject the steroid solution steadily into this area. If increased resistance is encountered, advance or withdraw the needle slightly before attempting further injection.
9. Following injection of the corticosteroid solution, withdraw the needle.

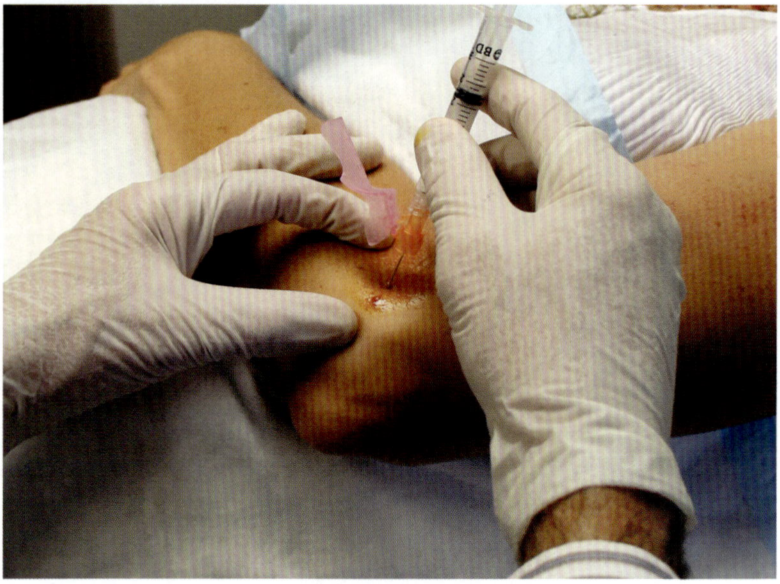

*FIGURE 6.25* ● Left elbow lateral epicondylitis injection.

10. Apply a sterile adhesive bandage.
11. Instruct the patient to move his or her wrist and elbow through their full range of motion.
12. Reexamine the elbow in 5 min to confirm pain relief.

## AFTERCARE

- Avoid excessive wrist extension and supination over the next 2 weeks.
- Consider the use of a neoprene elbow sleeve or elastic compression bandage.
- Consider the use of a wrist brace to limit wrist extension.
- NSAIDs, ice, heat, and/or physical therapy as indicated.
- Consider follow-up examination in 2 weeks.

**CPT code:** 20551—Injection of tendon origin or insertion

## PEARLS

- Entrapment of branches of the radial nerve in the elbow and forearm can mimic the pain of lateral epicondylitis. Radial tunnel syndrome is most commonly caused by entrapment of the deep radial nerve as it enters the supinator muscle at the arcade of Frohse. Pain in this condition occurs about 4 cm distal and anterior to the lateral epicondyle.
- The lateral epicondylitis injection can be superficial—especially in thin persons. Depositing corticosteroid in the subcutaneous tissues can result in the complication of skin atrophy and hypopigmentation. This particular injection is notorious for the development of this complication. Avoid the development of a subdermal wheal while performing all injections of corticosteroid solutions.
- In order to prevent this complication, one can use the pinch technique (Fig. 6.26). After insertion, gently grasp the skin on either side of the needle and pinch or pull

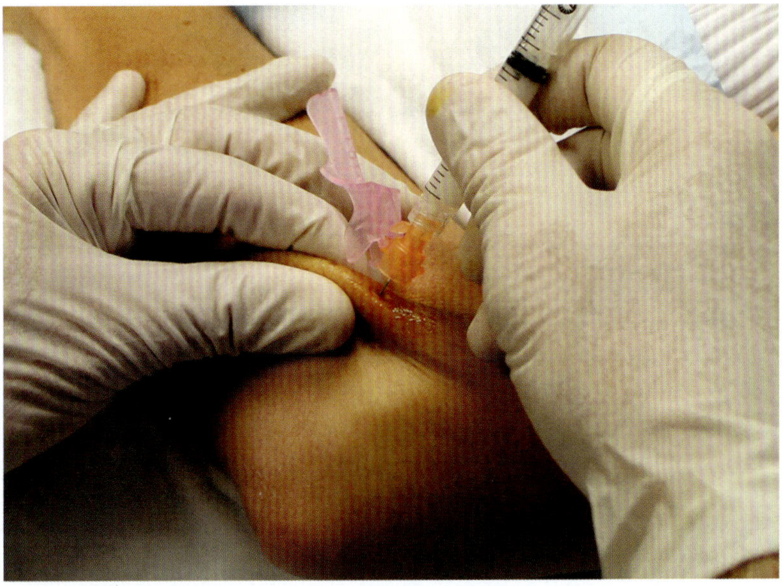

*FIGURE 6.26* ● Pinch up the tissue to avoid subcutaneous deposition of corticosteroid.

that up the needle toward the syringe. This provides a greater distance between the skin and the actual injection site, thus minimizing the chance of developing atrophy and hypopigmentation.

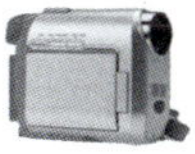

A video clip showing a lateral epicondylitis injection can be found in the companion eBook.

## REFERENCES


1. Krogh TP, Fredberg U, Stengaard-Pedersen K, et al. Treatment of lateral epicondylitis with platelet-rich plasma, glucocorticoid, or saline: a randomized, double-blind, placebo-controlled trial. *Am J Sports Med.* 2013;41(3):625–635.
2. Coombes BK, Bisset L, Vicenzino B. Efficacy and safety of corticosteroid injections and other injections for management of tendinopathy: a systematic review of randomised controlled trials. *Lancet.* 2010;376(9754):1751–1767.
3. Coombes BK, Bisset L, Brooks P, et al. Effect of corticosteroid injection, physiotherapy, or both on clinical outcomes in patients with unilateral lateral epicondylalgia: a randomized controlled trial. *JAMA.* 2013;309(5):461–469.
4. Kalichman L, Bannuru RR, Severin M, et al. Injection of botulinum toxin for treatment of chronic lateral epicondylitis: systematic review and meta-analysis. *Semin Arthritis Rheum.* 2011;40(6):532–538.
5. Lin C, Tu YK, Chen SS, et al. Comparison between botulinum toxin and corticosteroid injection in the treatment of acute and subacute tennis elbow: a prospective, randomized, double-blind, active drug-controlled pilot study. *Am J Phys Med Rehabil.* 2010;89(8):653–659.
6. Gosens T, Peerbooms JC, van Laar W, et al. Ongoing positive effect of platelet-rich plasma versus corticosteroid injection in lateral epicondylitis: a double-blind randomized controlled trial with 2-year follow-up. *Am J Sports Med.* 2011;39(6):1200–1208.
7. Krogh TP, Bartels EM, Ellingsen T, et al. Comparative effectiveness of injection therapies in lateral epicondylitis: a systematic review and network meta-analysis of randomized controlled trials. *Am J Sports Med.* 2013;41(6):1435–1446.
8. Wolf JM, Ozer K, Scott F, et al. Comparison of autologous blood, corticosteroid, and saline injection in the treatment of lateral epicondylitis: a prospective, randomized, controlled multicenter study. *J Hand Surg Am.* 2011;36(8):1269–1272.

# Medial Epicondylitis

Medial epicondylitis is a fairly common soft tissue condition encountered by primary care physicians. Pathologically similar to lateral epicondylitis, this condition also involves a noninflammatory tendinosis with collagen disarray. It usually is the result of an overuse injury with microtears to the hypovascular origins of the wrist flexor and pronator muscle groups. As with lateral epicondylitis, there is no consistent medical literature that is available to guide treatment with any injectable medication or intervention. A single study suggests short-term improvement only with use of corticosteroids.[1] Corticosteroid injections appear to be beneficial only in the short term.

| Indication | ICD-9 Code | ICD-10 Code |
|---|---|---|
| Medial epicondylitis | 726.31 | M77.00 |

**Relevant Anatomy:** (Fig. 6.27)

## PATIENT POSITION

- Supine on the examination table with the head of the bed elevated 30 degrees.
- Shoulder at 30 degrees of abduction and full external rotation.
- The affected elbow is flexed at 90 degrees.
- The wrist is in a neutral position.
- The elbow is supported with the placement of chucks pads or towels.
- Rotate the patient's head away from the side that is being injected. This minimizes anxiety and pain perception.

## LANDMARKS

1. With the patient supine on the examination table, the clinician stands lateral to the affected elbow.
2. Identify and mark the point of maximal tenderness adjacent to the medial epicondyle.
3. At that site, press firmly on the skin with the retracted tip of a ballpoint pen. This indention represents the entry point for the needle.
4. After the landmarks are identified, the patient should not move the elbow.

## ANESTHESIA

- Local anesthesia of the skin using topical vapocoolant spray.

## EQUIPMENT

- 3-mL syringe
- 25-gauge, 1-in. needle

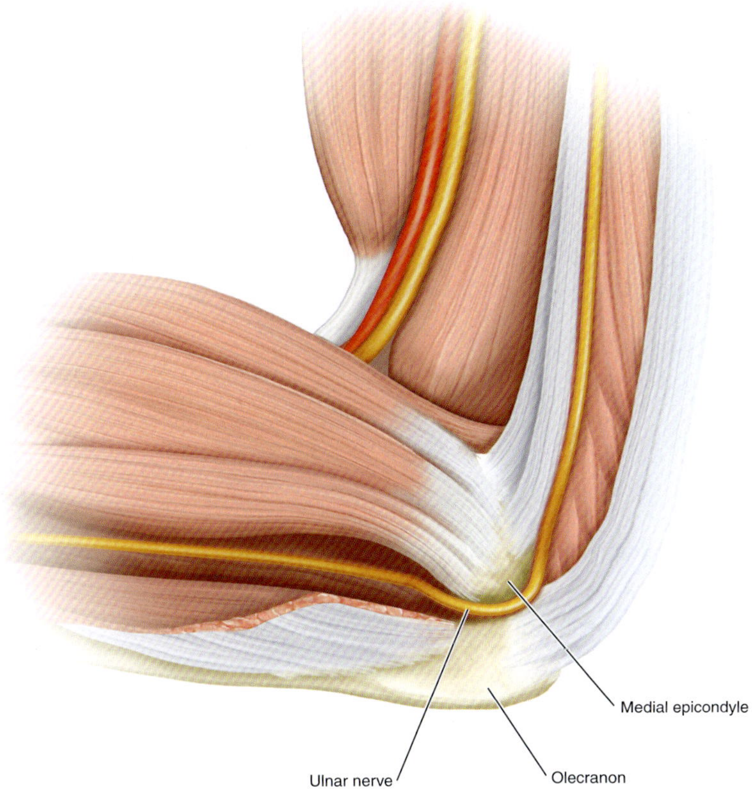


**FIGURE 6.27** • Medial view of muscular structures at right elbow. (From Tank PW, Gest TR. *Lippincott Williams & Wilkins Atlas of Anatomy*. Philadelphia, PA: Lippincott Williams & Wilkins, 2009.)

- 1 mL of 1% lidocaine without epinephrine
- 0.5 mL of the steroid solution (20 mg of triamcinolone acetonide)
- One alcohol prep pad
- Two povidone–iodine prep pads
- Sterile gauze pads
- Sterile adhesive bandage
- Nonsterile, clean chucks pad

## TECHNIQUE

1. Prep the insertion site with alcohol followed by the povidone–iodine pads.
2. Achieve good local anesthesia by using topical vapocoolant spray.
3. Position the needle and syringe perpendicular to the skin with the needle tip directed laterally toward the medial epicondyle.
4. Using the no-touch technique, introduce the needle at the insertion site (Fig. 6.28).
5. Advance the needle to the bone of the medial epicondyle.
6. Withdraw the needle 1 to 2 mm.
7. Inject the steroid solution steadily into this area. If increased resistance is encountered, advance or withdraw the needle slightly before attempting further injection.
8. Following injection of the corticosteroid solution, withdraw the needle.
9. Apply a sterile adhesive bandage.

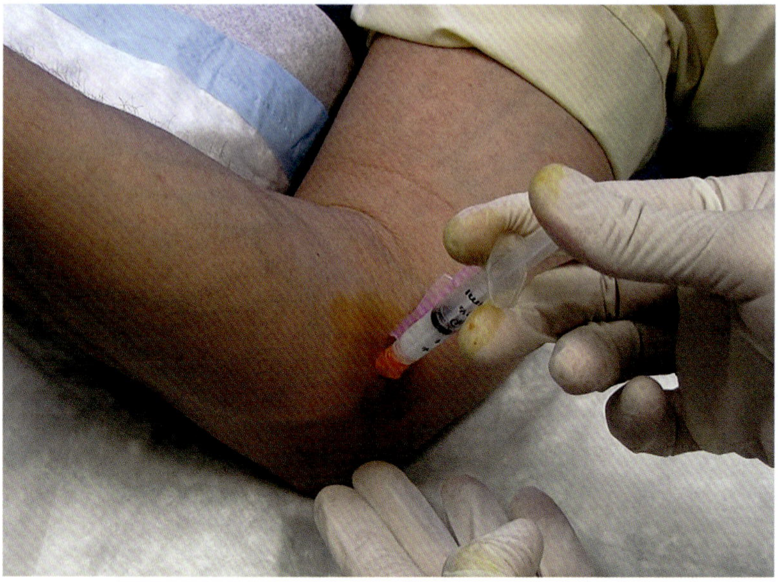

**FIGURE 6.28** ● Right elbow medial epicondylitis injection.

10. Instruct the patient to move his or her wrist and elbow through their full range of motion.
11. Reexamine the elbow in 5 min to confirm pain relief.

## AFTERCARE

- Avoid excessive wrist flexion or pronation over the next 2 weeks.
- Consider the use of a neoprene elbow sleeve or elastic compression bandage.
- Consider the use of a wrist brace to limit wrist flexion.
- NSAIDs, ice, heat, and/or physical therapy as indicated.
- Consider follow-up examination in 2 weeks.

**CPT code:** 20551—Injection of tendon origin or insertion

## PEARLS

- The ulnar nerve travels in close proximity to this injection. It courses just posterior and inferior to the medial epicondyle. On occasion, the local anesthetic spreading out from a properly placed injection may involve the ulnar nerve. The patient should be warned that transient numbness might occur in the lateral aspect of the hand as well as the ring and little fingers.

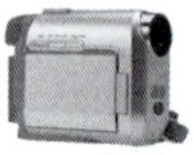

A video clip showing a medial epicondylitis injection can be found in the companion eBook.

## REFERENCE

1. Stahl S, Kaufman T. The efficacy of an injection of steroids for medial epicondylitis: a prospective study of sixty elbows. *J Bone Joint Surg Am*. 1997;79(11):1648–1652.

# Radial Nerve Entrapment

Patients uncommonly present to the primary care office for treatment of radial nerve entrapment in the forearm. This syndrome is caused by entrapment of the deep branch of the radial nerve (posterior interosseous nerve) as it enters the supinator muscle at the arcade of Frohse. Compression or scarring of the posterior interosseous nerve may cause denervation of extensor/supinator muscles and numbness or paresthesias in the distribution of the radial sensory nerve. The result can be pain, weakness, and dysfunction. Pain in this condition occurs about 4 cm distal to the lateral epicondyle. A nerve block injection utilizing local anesthetic can be given to help confirm diagnosis, and corticosteroid may be added for conservative management. Successful treatment often requires surgical release.

| Indication | ICD-9 Code | ICD-10 Code |
|---|---|---|
| Radial nerve entrapment syndrome | 354.2 | G56.30 |

**Relevant Anatomy:** (Fig. 6.29)

## PATIENT POSITION

- Supine on the examination table with the head of the bed elevated 30 degrees.
- The affected elbow is slightly flexed.
- The wrist is in a neutral to slightly pronated position.
- The elbow is supported with the placement of chucks pads or towels.
- Rotate the patient's head away from the side that is being injected. This minimizes anxiety and pain perception.

## LANDMARKS

1. With the patient supine on the examination table, the clinician stands lateral to the affected forearm.
2. Identify the lateral epicondyle.
3. The point of maximal tenderness is usually located about 4 cm distal and anterior to the lateral epicondyle.
4. Identify and mark the point of maximal tenderness.
5. At that site, press firmly on the skin with the retracted tip of a ballpoint pen. This indention represents the entry point for the needle.
6. After the landmarks are identified, the patient should not move the elbow.

## ANESTHESIA

- Local anesthesia of the skin using topical vapocoolant spray.

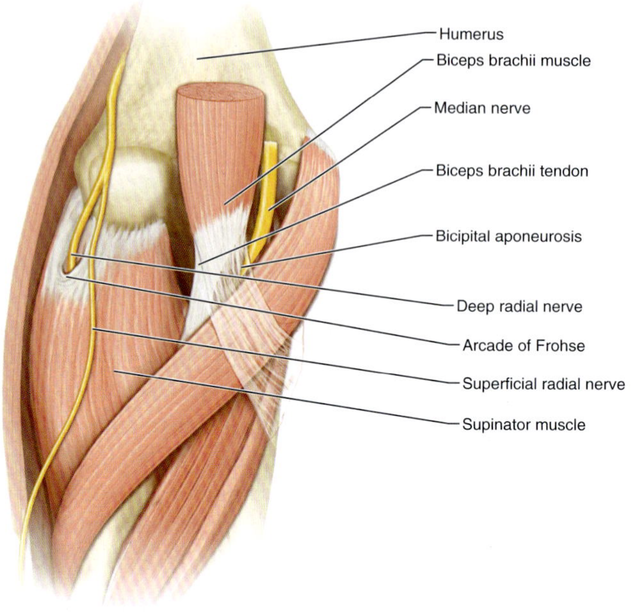


**FIGURE 6.29** Anterior aspect of right elbow. (From Tank PW, Gest TR. *Lippincott Williams & Wilkins Atlas of Anatomy*. Philadelphia, PA: Lippincott Williams & Wilkins, 2009.)

## EQUIPMENT

- 3-mL syringe
- 25-gauge, 1-in. needle
- 1 mL of 1% lidocaine without epinephrine
- 1 mL of the steroid solution (40 mg of triamcinolone acetonide)
- One alcohol prep pad
- Two povidone–iodine prep pads
- Sterile gauze pads
- Sterile adhesive bandage
- Nonsterile, clean chucks pad

## TECHNIQUE

1. Prep the insertion site with alcohol followed by the povidone–iodine pads.
2. Achieve good local anesthesia by using topical vapocoolant spray.
3. Position the needle and syringe perpendicular to the skin with the needle tip directed posteriorly.
4. Using the no-touch technique, introduce the needle at the insertion site (Fig. 6.30).
5. Slowly advance the needle until the needle tip is at the anticipated injection site at the radial nerve.
6. If any pain, paresthesias, or numbness is encountered, withdraw the needle slightly.
7. When the needle is placed along the radial nerve, slowly deposit the steroid solution as a bolus around that structure.
8. If increased resistance is encountered, advance or withdraw the needle slightly before attempting further injection.

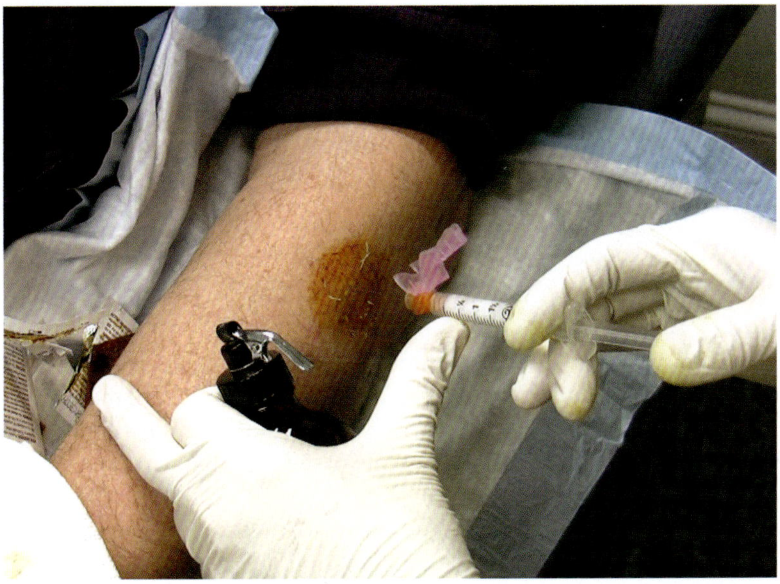

***FIGURE 6.30*** ● Left arm radial nerve entrapment injection.

9. Following injection of the corticosteroid solution, withdraw the needle.
10. Apply a sterile adhesive bandage.
11. Instruct the patient to move his or her wrist and elbow through their full range of motion.
12. Reexamine the proximal forearm in 5 min to confirm pain relief and the development of numbness in the distribution of the radial nerve from the local anesthetic.

## AFTERCARE

- Avoid excessive wrist extension and supination over the next 2 weeks.
- NSAIDs, ice, and/or physical therapy as indicated.
- Consider follow-up examination in 2 weeks.

**CPT code:** 64450—Injection, nerve block, therapeutic, other peripheral nerve or branch

## PEARLS

- Entrapment of branches of the radial nerve in the elbow and forearm can mimic the pain of lateral epicondylitis.

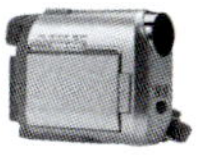

A video clip showing a radial nerve entrapment injection can be found in the companion eBook.

# Carpal Tunnel Syndrome—Preferred Flexor Carpi Radialis Approach

Carpal tunnel syndrome is a very common condition encountered in primary care. It represents a compressive injury to the median nerve as it traverses the carpal tunnel in the wrist. This usually occurs as a result of an overuse injury following repetitive handgrip movements or compression of the contents of the carpal tunnel from various disease processes. Predisposing factors may include previous injury, pregnancy, diabetes, hypothyroidism, rheumatoid arthritis, or amyloidosis. Corticosteroid injection of the carpal tunnel is an effective but underutilized treatment option by primary care providers.

In the traditional approach, the needle is inserted 1 cm proximal to the wrist crease and 1 cm ulnar to the palmaris longus tendon, then directed radially and distally at a 30-degree angle to the horizontal. With the preferred flexor carpi radialis (FCR) approach, the needle is inserted 1 cm proximal to the wrist crease, at the ulnar border of the FCR tendon, then in an ulnar direction and distally at a 30-degree angle to the horizontal. Anatomic studies of cadavers have demonstrated a higher risk of ulnar artery and median nerve injury due to the close proximity of those structures as well as median nerve swelling and/or flattening around the distal wrist crease when using the traditional approach.[1–3] The preferred FCR approach gives the highest accuracy rate and is also the safest injection site.[4] Ultrasound guidance further increases the safety and efficacy of this procedure.[1,5]

A single local injection of corticosteroid at or proximal to the carpal tunnel results in long-lasting improvement in approximately half of treated patients.[6–9] A second corticosteroid injection appears at least as effective as the first.[10] Favorable prognostic factors include patients with electrodiagnostically mild disease,[11] lower symptom severity scores, and lower median nerve ultrasonographic cross-sectional areas at the pisiform bone.[12]

Objective measurable changes following corticosteroid injections include improvement in distal motor latency of the median nerve,[13] improvement in sonoelasticity of the intracarpal tunnel contents,[14] decrease in the median nerve cross-sectional area, and decreased vascularity of the median nerve at the distal wrist crease.[15]

| Indication | ICD-9 Code | ICD-10 Code |
|---|---|---|
| Carpal tunnel syndrome | 354.0 | G56.00 |

**Relevant Anatomy:** (Figs. 6.31 and 6.32)

## PATIENT POSITION

- Supine on the examination table with the head of the bed elevated at an angle of 30 degrees.
- The elbow is slightly flexed with the wrist in supination.
- The wrist is then positioned in slight hyperextension with the placement of chucks pads or towels underneath the supinated wrist.
- Rotate the patient's head away from the side that is being injected. This minimizes anxiety and pain perception.

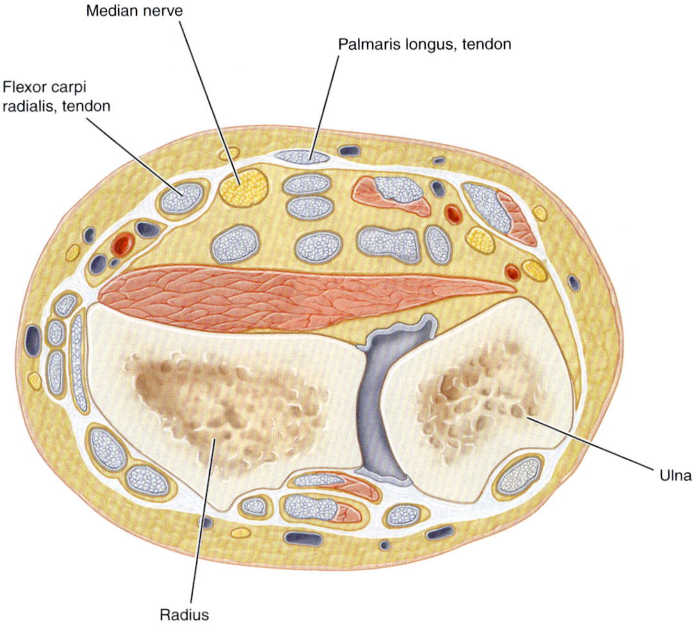


*FIGURE 6.31* • Right wrist cross-section at the level of the distal radioulnar joint. (From Tank PW, Gest TR. *Lippincott Williams & Wilkins Atlas of Anatomy*. Philadelphia, PA: Lippincott Williams & Wilkins, 2009.)

## LANDMARKS

1. With the patient supine on the examination table, the clinician stands lateral to the affected wrist.
2. Identify and mark the distal palmar crease as shown (Fig. 6.33).

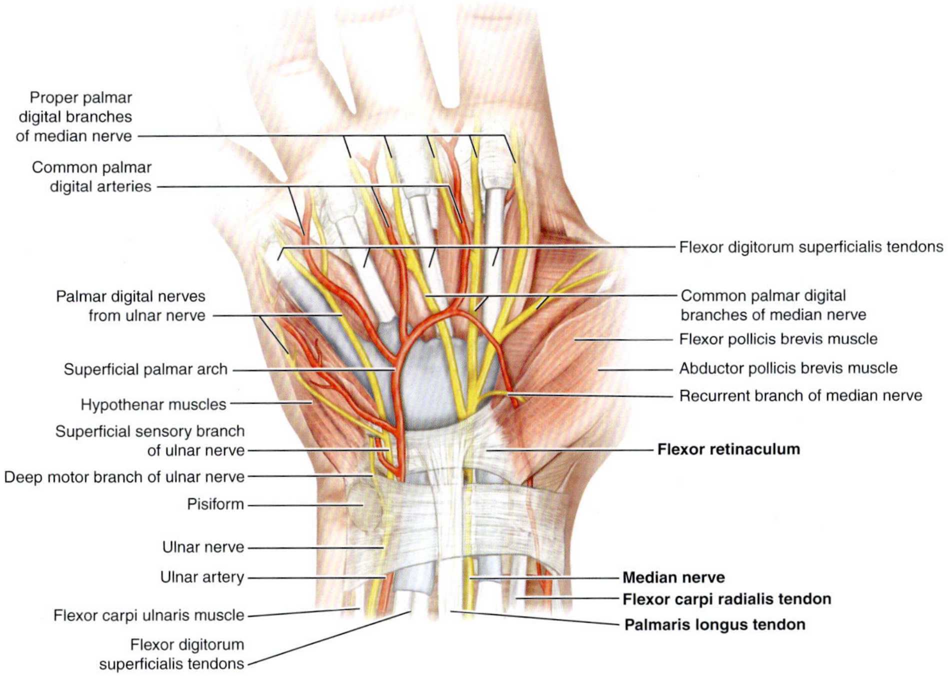


*FIGURE 6.32* • Right wrist—volar aspect.

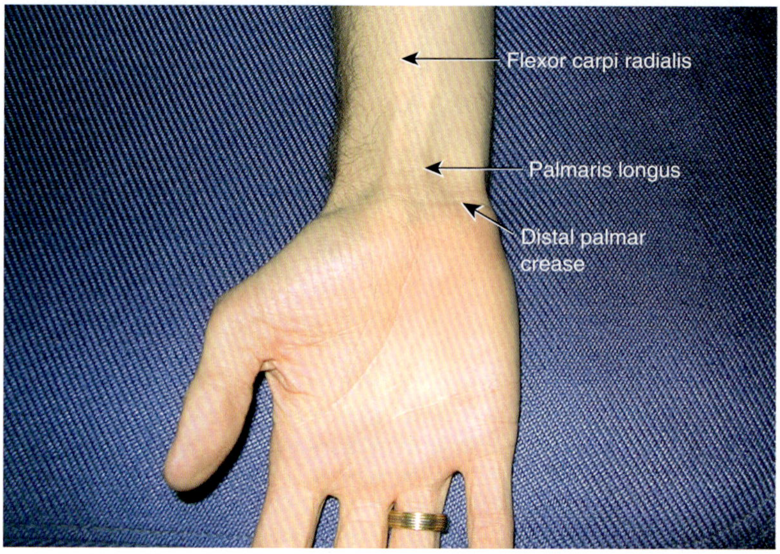


**FIGURE 6.33** Right carpal tunnel injection surface anatomy.

3. Identify and mark the course of the palmaris longus and FCR tendons (Fig. 6.34).
4. Mark a point 1 cm proximal to the distal palmar crease on the ulnar border of the FCR tendon. This is the entry point for the needle.
5. At both the entry point and target site, press firmly on the skin with the retracted tip of a ballpoint pen.
6. After the landmarks are identified, the patient should not move the wrist.

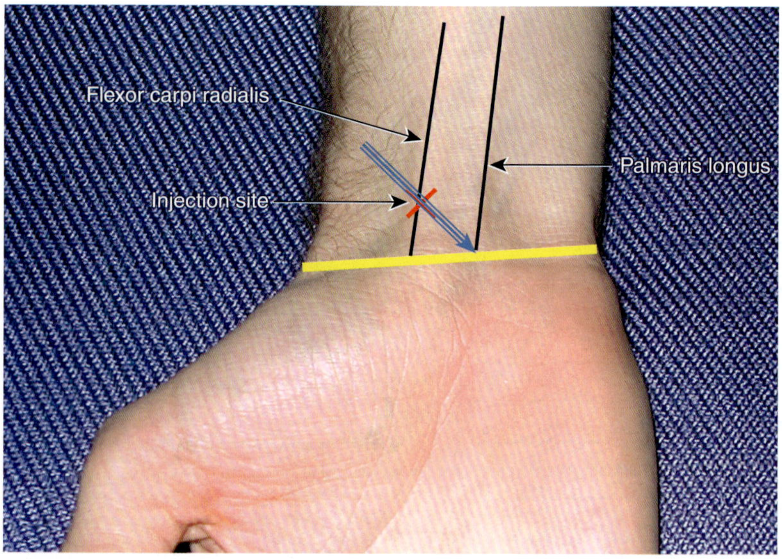


**FIGURE 6.34** Right carpal tunnel injection landmarks.

## ANESTHESIA

- Local anesthesia of the skin using topical vapocoolant spray.

## EQUIPMENT

- 3-mL syringe
- 25-gauge, 1-in. needle
- 1 mL of 1% lidocaine without epinephrine
- 1 mL of the steroid solution (40 mg of triamcinolone acetonide)
- One alcohol prep pad
- Two povidone–iodine prep pads
- Sterile gauze pads
- Sterile adhesive bandage
- Nonsterile, clean chucks pad

## TECHNIQUE

1. Prep the insertion site with alcohol followed by the povidone–iodine pads.
2. Achieve good local anesthesia by using topical vapocoolant spray.
3. Position the needle and syringe at a 30-degree angle to the skin with the needle tip directed in an ulnar and distal direction.
4. Using the no-touch technique, introduce the needle at the insertion site (Fig. 6.35).
5. Very slowly advance the needle approximately 1.5 cm.
6. If any pain, paresthesias, or numbness is encountered, withdraw the needle 1 to 2 mm.
7. Slowly inject the steroid solution as a bolus around the median nerve.
8. If increased resistance is encountered, withdraw the needle slightly before attempting further injection.
9. Following injection of the corticosteroid solution, withdraw the needle.
10. Apply a sterile adhesive bandage.
11. Reexamine the hand in 5 min to confirm pain relief and/or the development of numbness in the distribution of the medial nerve from the local anesthetic.

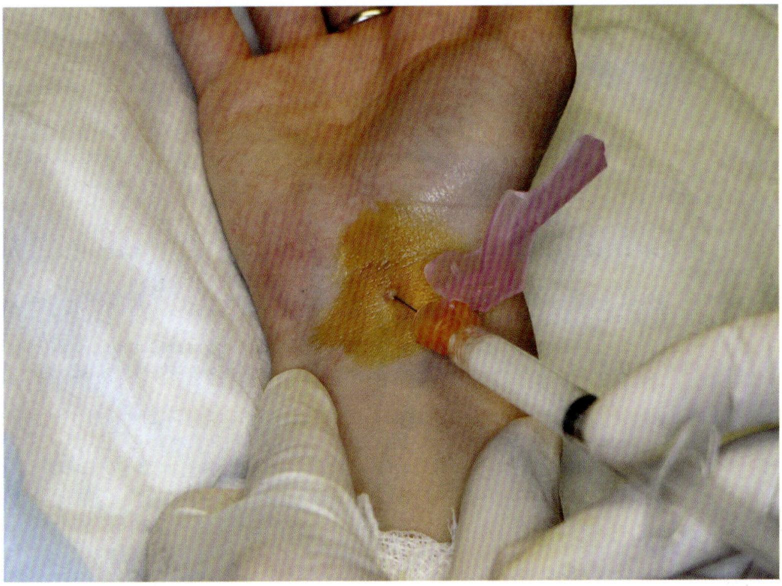

**FIGURE 6.35** • Right carpal tunnel injection - preferred FCR approach.

## AFTERCARE

- Avoid further overuse mechanisms of injury.
- Use a carpal tunnel wrist brace while sleeping to avoid wrist flexion and extension.
- NSAIDs, ice, and/or physical therapy as indicated.
- Consider follow-up examination in 2 weeks.

**CPT code:** 20526—Injection of carpal tunnel

## PEARLS

- The preferred FCR approach illustrated here is easy to perform and has few side effects.
- Steroid injections into the carpal tunnel may damage the median nerve.
- Warn the patients that the median nerve may be contacted when using this approach. Ask them to calmly report any pain or electrical shock sensation without jerking their arm away. If this occurs, simply withdraw the needle a few millimeters before injecting.

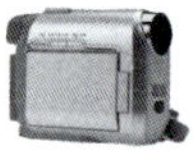

A video clip showing a carpal tunnel injection using the preferred FCR approach can be found in the companion eBook.

## REFERENCES


1. Kim DH, Jang JE, Park BK. Anatomical basis of ulnar approach in carpal tunnel injection. *Pain Physician*. 2013;16(3):E191–E198.
2. Dubert T, Racasan O. A reliable technique for avoiding the median nerve during carpal tunnel injections. *Joint Bone Spine*. 2006;73(1):77–79.
3. MacLennan A, Schimizzi A, Meier KM. Comparison of needle position proximity to the median nerve in 2 carpal tunnel injection methods: a cadaveric study. *J Hand Surg Am*. 2009;34(5):875–879.
4. Ozturk K, Esenyel CZ, Sonmez M, et al. Comparison of carpal tunnel injection techniques: a cadaver study. *Scand J Plast Reconstr Surg Hand Surg*. 2008;42(6):300–304.
5. Ustün N, Tok F, Yagz AE, et al. Ultrasound-guided vs. blind steroid injections in carpal tunnel syndrome: a single-blind randomized prospective study. *Am J Phys Med Rehabil*. 2013;92(11):999–1004.
6. Marshall S, Tardif G, Ashworth N. Local corticosteroid injection for carpal tunnel syndrome. *Cochrane Database Syst Rev*. 2007;(2):CD001554.
7. Ly-Pen D, Andréu JL, Millán I, et al. Comparison of surgical decompression and local steroid injection in the treatment of carpal tunnel syndrome: 2-year clinical results from a randomized trial. *Rheumatology (Oxford)*. 2012;51(8):1447–1454.
8. Peters-Veluthamaningal C, Winters JC, Groenier KH, et al. Randomised controlled trial of local corticosteroid injections for carpal tunnel syndrome in general practice. *BMC Fam Pract*. 2010;11:54.
9. Dammers JW, Roos Y, Veering MM, et al. Injection with methylprednisolone in patients with the carpal tunnel syndrome: a randomised double blind trial testing three different doses. *J Neurol*. 2006;253(5):574–577.
10. Ashworth NL, Bland JD. Effectiveness of second corticosteroid injections for carpal tunnel syndrome. *Muscle Nerve*. 2013;48(1):122–126.
11. Visser LH, Ngo Q, Groeneweg SJ, et al. Long term effect of local corticosteroid injection for carpal tunnel syndrome: a relation with electrodiagnostic severity. *Clin Neurophysiol*. 2012;123(4):838–841.
12. Meys V, Thissen S, Rozeman S, et al. Prognostic factors in carpal tunnel syndrome treated with a corticosteroid injection. *Muscle Nerve*. 2011;44(5):763–768.
13. Milo R, Kalichman L, Volchek L, et al. Local corticosteroid treatment for carpal tunnel syndrome: a 6-month clinical and electrophysiological follow-up study. *J Back Musculoskelet Rehabil*. 2009;22(2): 59–64.
14. Miyamoto H, Siedentopf C, Kastlunger M, et al. Intracarpal tunnel contents: evaluation of the effects of corticosteroid injection with sonoelastography. *Radiology*. 2014;270(3):809–815.
15. Cartwright MS, White DL, Demar S, et al. Median nerve changes following steroid injection for carpal tunnel syndrome. *Muscle Nerve*. 2011;44(1):25–29.

# Carpal Tunnel Syndrome—Traditional Approach

Carpal tunnel syndrome is a very common condition encountered in primary care. It represents a compressive injury to the median nerve as it traverses the carpal tunnel in the wrist. This usually occurs as a result of an overuse injury following repetitive hand-grip movements or compression of the contents of the carpal tunnel from various disease processes. Predisposing factors may include previous injury, pregnancy, diabetes, hypothyroidism, rheumatoid arthritis, or amyloidosis. Corticosteroid injection of the carpal tunnel is an effective but underutilized treatment option by primary care providers. This injection technique is the most commonly performed injection of the carpal tunnel. Although it is straightforward to perform, there is a higher risk for direct needle injury to the ulnar artery and median nerve compared to the alternative carpal tunnel injection approach described in the preceding chapter.

| Indication | ICD-9 Code | ICD-10 Code |
|---|---|---|
| Carpal tunnel syndrome | 354.0 | G56.00 |

**Relevant Anatomy:** (Figs. 6.36 and 6.37)

## PATIENT POSITION

- Supine on the examination table with the head of the bed elevated 30 degrees.
- The elbow is slightly flexed with the wrist in supination.
- The wrist is then positioned in slight hyperextension with the placement of chucks pads or towels underneath the supinated wrist.
- Rotate the patient's head away from the side that is being injected. This minimizes anxiety and pain perception.

## LANDMARKS

1. With the patient supine on the examination table, the clinician stands lateral to the affected wrist.
2. Identify and mark the distal palmar crease as shown (Fig. 6.38).
3. Identify and mark the intersection of the palmaris longus tendon with the distal palmar crease (Fig. 6.39).
4. Mark a spot 1 cm proximal and 1 cm ulnar to this intersection.
5. At that site, press firmly with the retracted tip of a ballpoint pen. This indention represents the entry point for the needle.
6. After the landmarks are identified, the patient should not move the wrist.

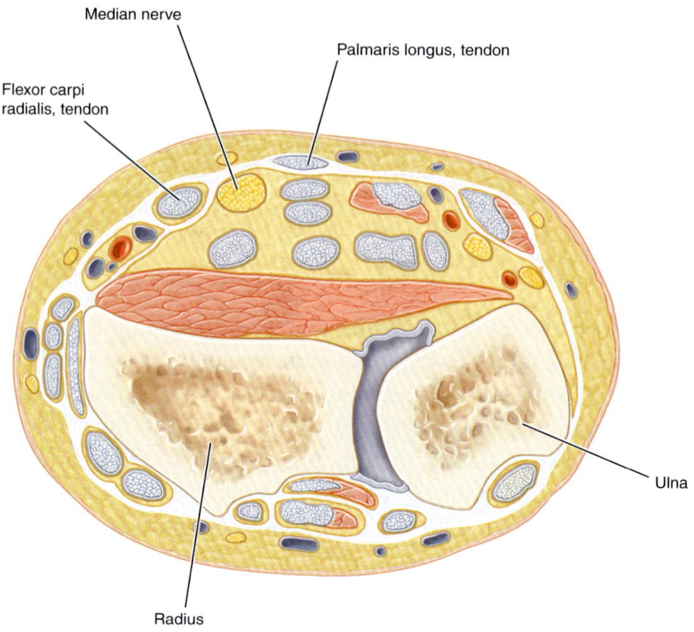


**FIGURE 6.36** Right wrist cross-section at the level of the distal radioulnar joint. (From Tank PW, Gest TR. *Lippincott Williams & Wilkins Atlas of Anatomy*. Philadelphia, PA: Lippincott Williams & Wilkins, 2009.)

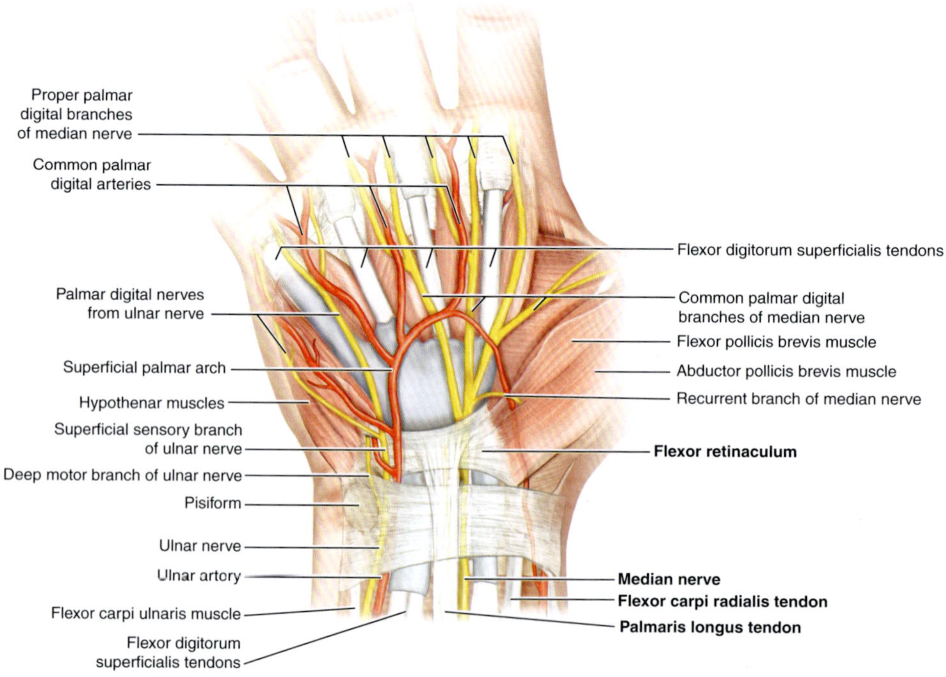


**FIGURE 6.37** Right wrist—volar aspect.

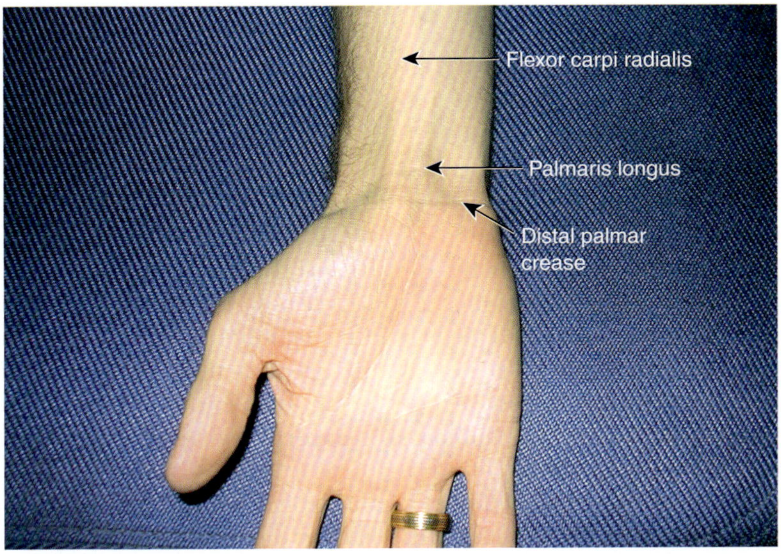


***FIGURE 6.38*** ● Right carpal tunnel injection surface anatomy.

## ANESTHESIA

- Local anesthesia of the skin using topical vapocoolant spray.

## EQUIPMENT

- 3-mL syringe
- 25-gauge, 1-in. needle
- 1 mL of 1% lidocaine without epinephrine
- 1 mL of the steroid solution (40 mg of triamcinolone acetonide)
- One alcohol prep pad

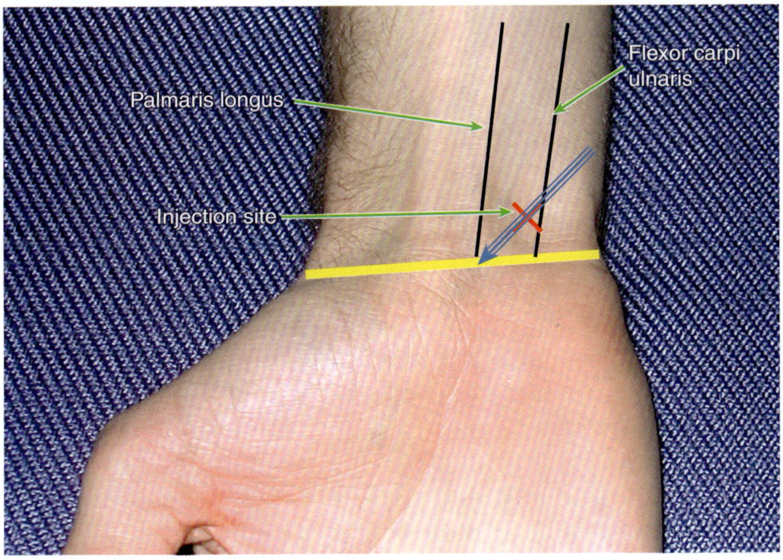


***FIGURE 6.39*** ● Right carpal tunnel injection landmarks.

- Two povidone–iodine prep pads
- Sterile gauze pads
- Sterile adhesive bandage
- Nonsterile, clean chucks pad

## TECHNIQUE

1. Prep the insertion site with alcohol followed by the povidone–iodine pads.
2. Achieve good local anesthesia by using topical vapocoolant spray.
3. Position the needle and syringe at a 30-degree angle to the skin of the wrist with the needle tip directed toward the base of the thumb.
4. Using the no-touch technique, introduce the needle at the insertion site (Fig. 6.40).
5. Very slowly advance the needle approximately 1 cm toward the base of the thumb.
6. If any pain, paresthesias, or numbness is encountered, withdraw the needle 1 to 2 mm.
7. Slowly inject the steroid solution as a bolus around the median nerve.
8. If increased resistance is encountered, withdraw the needle slightly before attempting further injection.
9. Following injection of the corticosteroid solution, withdraw the needle.
10. Apply a sterile adhesive bandage.
11. Reexamine the hand in 5 min to confirm pain relief or the development of numbness in the distribution of the medial nerve from the local anesthetic.

## AFTERCARE

- Avoid further overuse mechanisms of injury.
- Use a carpal tunnel wrist brace while sleeping to avoid wrist flexion and extension.
- NSAIDs, ice, and/or physical therapy as indicated.
- Consider follow-up examination in 2 weeks.

**CPT code:** 20526—Injection of carpal tunnel

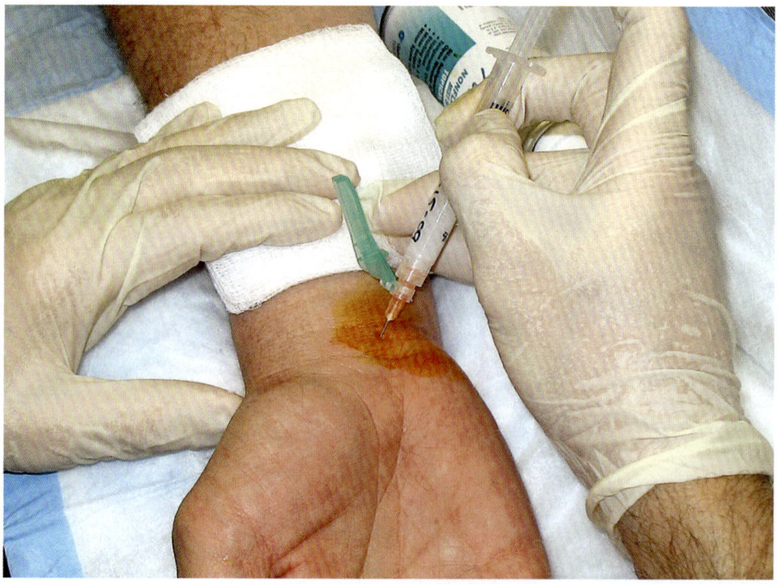

***FIGURE 6.40*** ● Right carpal tunnel injection - traditional approach.

## PEARLS

- The approach illustrated here is easy to perform and has few side effects.
- However, the possibility of direct needle injury to the median nerve is greater with the traditional technique because the nerve is "fixed" in position by the carpal tunnel.
- Warn the patients that the median nerve may be contacted when using this approach. Ask them to report any pain or electrical shock sensation. If this occurs, simply withdraw the needle a few millimeters before continuing to advance the needle using a slightly different path medially or laterally.

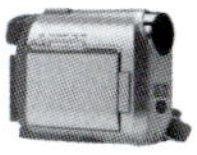

A video clip showing a carpal tunnel injection can be found in the companion eBook.

## REFERENCES

Please consult references listed in the preceding chapter.

# Wrist Joint

Injection of the wrist joint is a relatively uncommon procedure in primary care. Pain and swelling in the wrist may be the result of trauma, osteoarthritis, an infectious etiology, or an inflammatory disorder such as rheumatoid arthritis. Occasionally, there will be a small collection of synovial fluid to remove. The success rates of corticosteroid injections can be significantly improved with use of ultrasound guidance.[1–4] In the absence of a fluid collection, a small-diameter needle is used for corticosteroid injection.

| Indications | ICD-9 Code | ICD-10 Code |
|---|---|---|
| Wrist pain | 719.43 | M25.539 |
| Wrist sprain of unspecified site | 842.00 | S63.50 |
| Wrist joint arthritis, unspecified | 716.93 | M12.9 |
| Wrist joint osteoarthritis, primary | 715.13 | M19.039 |
| Wrist joint osteoarthritis, posttraumatic | 716.13 | M19.139 |
| Wrist joint osteoarthritis, secondary | 715.23 | M19.239 |

**Relevant Anatomy:** (Fig. 6.41)

## PATIENT POSITION

- Supine on the examination table with the head of the bed elevated 30 degrees.
- The elbow is slightly flexed with neutral positioning of the wrist in pronation.
- The wrist is supported with the placement of chucks pads or towels.
- Rotate the patient's head away from the side that is being injected. This minimizes anxiety and pain perception.

## LANDMARKS

1. With the patient supine on the examination table, the clinician stands lateral to the affected wrist.
2. Identify and mark the area of maximal tenderness and/or swelling over the dorsal aspect of the wrist joint.
3. At that site, press firmly on the skin with the retracted tip of a ballpoint pen. This indention represents the entry point for the needle.
4. After the landmarks are identified, the patient should not move the wrist.

## ANESTHESIA

- Local anesthesia of the skin using topical vapocoolant spray.

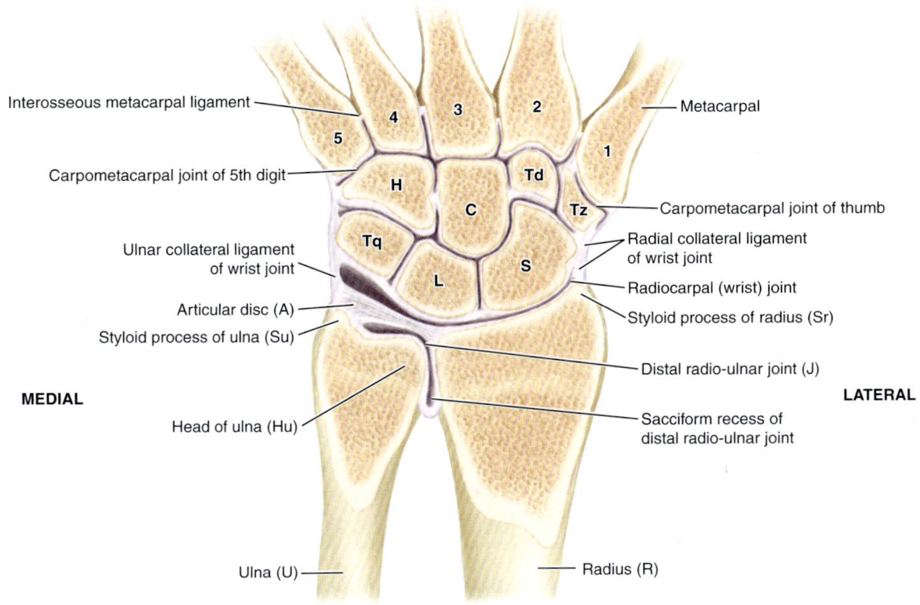


***FIGURE 6.41*** • Coronal section of the wrist. (From Tank PW, Gest TR. *Lippincott Williams & Wilkins Atlas of Anatomy*. Philadelphia, PA: Lippincott Williams & Wilkins, 2009.)

## EQUIPMENT

- 3-mL syringe
- 5-mL syringe—for optional aspiration
- 25-gauge, 1-in. needle—for injection
- 20-gauge, 1-in. needle—for optional aspiration
- 0.5 mL of 1% lidocaine without epinephrine
- 0.5 mL of the steroid solution (20 mg of triamcinolone acetonide)
- One alcohol prep pad
- Two povidone–iodine prep pads
- Sterile gauze pads
- Sterile adhesive bandage
- Nonsterile, clean chucks pad

## TECHNIQUE

1. Prep the insertion site with alcohol followed by the povidone–iodine pads.
2. Achieve good local anesthesia by using topical vapocoolant spray.
3. Position the needle and syringe perpendicular to the skin with the needle tip directed posteriorly.
4. Using the no-touch technique, introduce the needle at the insertion site (Fig. 6.42).
5. Advance the needle down into the wrist joint.
6. If aspirating, withdraw the fluid using a 20-gauge, 1-in. needle with the 5-mL syringe and then inject through the same syringe.
7. If only injecting, use a 25-gauge, 1-in. needle with the 3-mL syringe.
8. If injection following aspiration is elected, remove the large syringe from the 20-gauge needle and then attach the 3-mL syringe filled with the steroid solution.

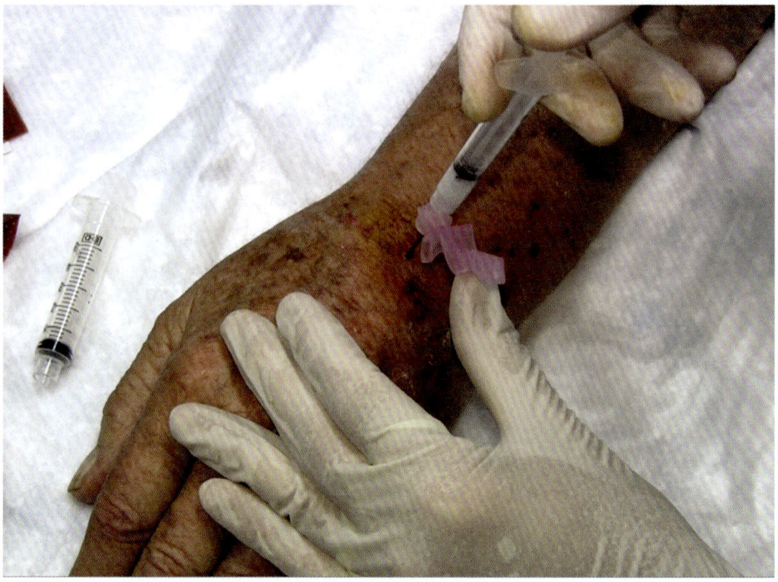

**FIGURE 6.42** ● Right dorsal wrist joint injection.

9. Inject the steroid solution as a bolus into the wrist joint. The injected solution should flow smoothly into the space. If increased resistance is encountered, advance or withdraw the needle slightly before attempting further injection.
10. Following injection of the corticosteroid solution, withdraw the needle.
11. Apply a sterile adhesive bandage.
12. Instruct the patient to move his or her wrist through its full range of motion. This movement distributes the steroid solution throughout the joint.
13. Reexamine the wrist in 5 min to confirm pain relief.

## AFTERCARE

- Consider the use of a wrist brace.
- Avoid excessive use of the wrist over the next 2 weeks.
- NSAIDs, ice, and/or physical therapy as indicated.
- Consider follow-up examination in 2 weeks.

**CPT code:** 20605—Arthrocentesis, aspiration, and/or injection of intermediate joint or bursa

## PEARLS

- There are many septa that create multiple partitions within the wrist joint complex. Increasing degrees of synovitis also inhibit flow to all wrist compartments. Therefore, a single injection into a standard injection site in the proximal part of the wrist cannot be assumed to distribute and treat the whole joint.[5] Successful administration of corticosteroid involves pinpoint precision and may require multiple injections during the same office visit.
- Ultrasound guidance will improve accuracy.
- Work on the dorsal aspect of the wrist. The volar aspect contains the radial artery, median nerve, and ulnar artery. These must all be avoided.

- If multiple injections are performed, do not give more than 1 mL (40 mg of triamcinolone) of the steroid solution to the patient at any single office visit.

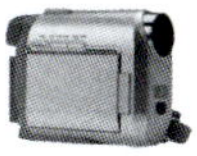

A video clip showing a wrist joint injection can be found in the companion eBook.

## REFERENCES


1. Dubreuil M, Greger S, LaValley M, et al. Improvement in wrist pain with ultrasound-guided glucocorticoid injections: a meta-analysis of individual patient data. *Semin Arthritis Rheum*. 2013;42(5):492–497.
2. Smith J, Brault JS, Rizzo M, et al. Accuracy of sonographically guided and palpation guided scaphotrapezio-trapezoid joint injections. *J Ultrasound Med*. 2011;30(11):1509–1515.
3. Cunnington J, Marshall N, Hide G, et al. A randomized, double-blind, controlled study of ultrasound-guided corticosteroid injection into the joint of patients with inflammatory arthritis. *Arthritis Rheum*. 2010;62(7):1862–1869.
4. Lohman M, Vasenius J, Nieminen O. Ultrasound guidance for puncture and injection in the radiocarpal joint. *Acta Radiol*. 2007;48(7):744–747.
5. Boesen M, Jensen KE, Torp-Pedersen S, et al. Intra-articular distribution pattern after ultrasound-guided injections in wrist joints of patients with rheumatoid arthritis. *Eur J Radiol*. 2009;69(2):331–338.

# de Quervain Tenosynovitis

Injection of corticosteroids for the treatment of de Quervain tenosynovitis is a fairly common procedure for primary care physicians. This condition represents a stenosing tenosynovitis of the first dorsal compartment over the radial aspect of the wrist. The extensor pollicis brevis and abductor pollicis longus tendons run alongside each other and share a common tendon sheath. Overuse movements that require repetitive extension and abduction of the thumb generally cause this condition.

Studies show that one or two local injections of corticosteroid leads to a high rate of improvement both in the short and long term with few side effects.[1] Ultrasound studies show a 28% to 52% incidence of a tendon sheath septum isolating the extensor pollicis brevis from the abductor pollicis longus.[2,3] The presence of these subcompartments plays a role in recurrence rates.[3] The use of ultrasound has been shown to detect the septum, improve injection accuracy by enabling injection into each subcompartment, and improve clinical outcomes.[4]

| Indication | ICD-9 Code | ICD-10 Code |
|---|---|---|
| de Quervain tenosynovitis | 727.04 | M65.4 |

**Relevant Anatomy:** (Fig. 6.43)

## PATIENT POSITION

- Supine on the examination table with the head of the bed elevated 30 degrees.
- The affected wrist is held in a neutral position. The thumb is directed superiorly midway between supination and pronation.
- The wrist is supported with the placement of chucks pads or towels.
- Rotate the patient's head away from the side that is being injected. This minimizes anxiety and pain perception.

## LANDMARKS

1. With the patient supine on the examination table, the clinician stands lateral to the affected wrist.
2. Identify tenderness located in the tendon sheath that contains the abductor pollicis longus and the extensor pollicis brevis.
3. The injection point is located directly between these two tendons. Mark this spot.
4. At that site, press firmly on the skin with the retracted tip of a ballpoint pen. This indention represents the entry point for the needle.
5. After the landmarks are identified, the patient should not move the wrist or thumb.

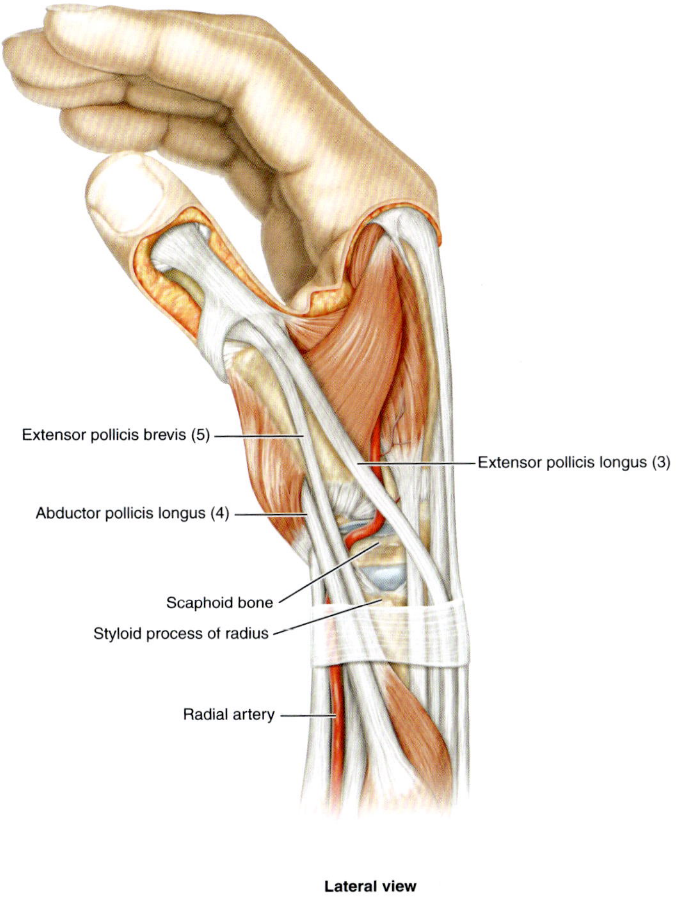


***FIGURE 6.43*** • Right hand anatomy. (From Tank PW, Gest TR. *Lippincott Williams & Wilkins Atlas of Anatomy*. Philadelphia, PA: Lippincott Williams & Wilkins, 2009.)

## ANESTHESIA

- Local anesthesia of the skin using topical vapocoolant spray.

## EQUIPMENT

- 3-mL syringe
- 25-gauge, 5/8-in. needle
- 0.5 mL of 1% lidocaine without epinephrine
- 0.25 mL of the steroid solution (10 mg of triamcinolone acetonide)
- One alcohol prep pad
- Two povidone–iodine prep pads
- Sterile gauze pads
- Sterile adhesive bandage
- Nonsterile, clean chucks pad

## TECHNIQUE

1. Prep the insertion site with alcohol followed by the povidone–iodine pads.
2. Achieve good local anesthesia by using topical vapocoolant spray.

3. Position the needle and syringe at a 45-degree angle to the skin with the needle tip directed proximally.
4. Using the no-touch technique, introduce the needle at the insertion site (Fig. 6.44).
5. Advance the needle toward the convergence of the abductor pollicis longus and the extensor pollicis brevis tendons until the needle tip is located between the tendons in the tendon sheath.
6. Slowly inject the steroid solution as a bolus into the tendon sheath. A small bulge in the shape of a sausage should develop in the tendon sheath.
7. Following injection of the corticosteroid solution, withdraw the needle.
8. Apply a sterile adhesive bandage.
9. Instruct the patient to move his or her thumb through its full range of motion. This movement distributes the steroid solution throughout the tenosynovial sheath.
10. Reexamine the hand and wrist in 5 min to confirm pain relief.

## AFTERCARE

- Ensure no excessive wrist flexion or pronation over the next 2 weeks by the application of a wrist thumb spica splint.
- NSAIDs, ice, heat, and/or physical therapy as indicated.
- Consider follow-up examination in 2 weeks.

**CPT code:** 20550—Injection of single tendon sheath

## PEARLS

- The de Quervain tenosynovitis injection is superficial—especially in thin persons. Depositing corticosteroid in the subcutaneous tissues can result in the complication of skin atrophy and hypopigmentation. de Quervain's injection is notorious for the development of this complication. Avoid the development of an intradermal wheal while performing all injections of corticosteroid solutions.

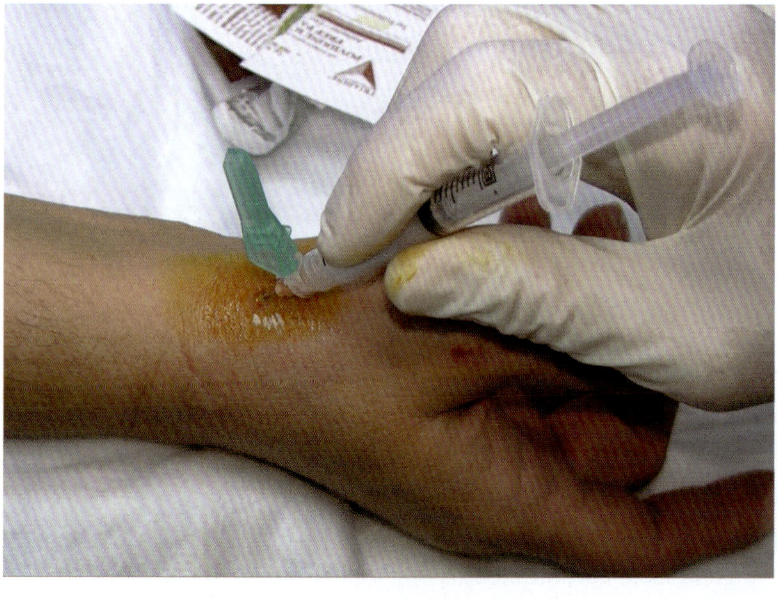

***FIGURE 6.44*** ● de Quervain's tenosynovitis injection.

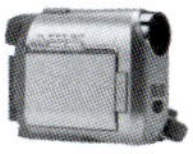

A video clip showing a de Quervain's injection can be found in the companion eBook.

## REFERENCES


1. Peters-Veluthamaningal C, Winters JC, Groenier KH, et al. Randomised controlled trial of local corticosteroid injections for de Quervain's tenosynovitis in general practice. *BMC Musculoskelet Disord.* 2009;10:131.
2. Mirzanli C, Ozturk K, Esenyel CZ, et al. Accuracy of intrasheath injection techniques for de Quervain's disease: a cadaveric study. *J Hand Surg Eur Vol.* 2012;37(2):155–160.
3. McDermott JD, Ilyas AM, Nazarian LN, et al. Ultrasound-guided injections for de Quervain's tenosynovitis. *Clin Orthop Relat Res.* 2012;470(7):1925–1931.
4. Kume K, Amano K, Yamada S, et al. In de Quervain's with a separate EPB compartment, ultrasound-guided steroid injection is more effective than a clinical injection technique: a prospective open-label study. *J Hand Surg Eur Vol.* 2012;37(6):523–527.

# Dorsal Wrist Ganglion Cyst

Aspiration of wrist ganglion cysts is a common procedure for primary care physicians. Ganglions are cysts containing clear mucinous fluid. They may originate from the wrist joint or tendon sheaths. A common site of occurrence is along the extensor carpi radialis brevis as it passes over the dorsum of the wrist joint. Although most prevalent found in the wrist, ganglion cysts may also occur in other joints. Ganglion cysts located over the dorsal surface of the wrist joint are generally treated with needle aspiration and rarely with corticosteroid.

The very few studies reported in the medical literature suggest a poor response rate to single aspiration attempts with 27% reported by Richman[1] and 42% by Dias.[2] Aspiration combined with corticosteroid injection gave only a 38.5% success rate.[3] In a study by Zubowicz,[4] up to three separate aspirations yielded 85% resolution.

The author suspects that the reason for the poor overall response rate is due to incomplete evacuation of the contents of the ganglion cyst. Therefore, he developed a technique that combines aspiration with a large-bore needle followed by firm compression of the cyst with the wrist in a flexed position. Corticosteroid is not injected. Since employing this technique for more than 10 years, he is aware of only two patients who have failed this conservative treatment. Both were young women with chronic, large dorsal wrist ganglion cysts greater than 1 cm in diameter (unpublished).

Ganglion cysts involving the volar surface of the wrist are intimately associated with the radial artery and best managed by surgical referral.

| Indication | ICD-9 Code | ICD-10 Code |
|---|---|---|
| Ganglion cyst of wrist | 727.41 | M67.439 |

**Relevant Anatomy:** (Fig. 6.45)

## PATIENT POSITION

- Supine on the examination table with the head of the bed elevated 30 degrees.
- For ganglion cysts over the dorsal aspect, the wrist is held in pronation and slight flexion.
- The wrist is supported with the placement of chucks pads or towels.
- Rotate the patient's head away from the side that is being injected. This minimizes anxiety and pain perception.

## LANDMARKS

1. With the patient supine on the examination table, the clinician stands lateral to the affected wrist.
2. Identify the cystic structure over the dorsal aspect of the wrist joint.

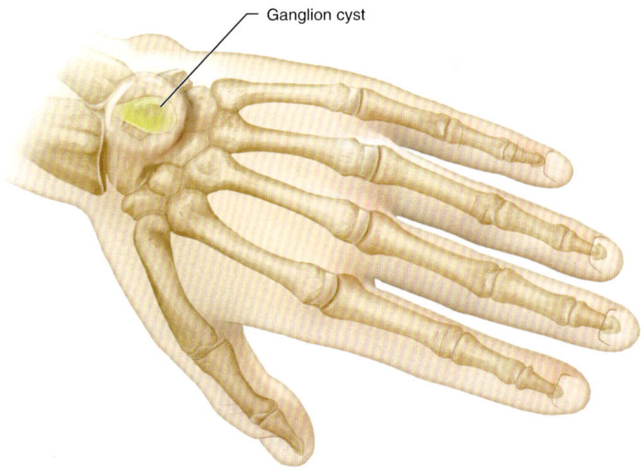


*FIGURE 6.45* • Dorsal wrist ganglion cyst.

3. The injection point is located directly over the cyst.
4. At that site, press firmly on the skin with the retracted tip of a ballpoint pen. This indention represents the entry point for the needle.
5. After the landmarks are identified, the patient should not move the wrist.

## ANESTHESIA

- Local anesthesia of the skin using topical vapocoolant spray.

## EQUIPMENT

- 3-mL syringe
- 18-gauge, 1½ in. needle
- One alcohol prep pad
- Two povidone–iodine prep pads
- Sterile gauze pads
- Sterile adhesive bandage
- Nonsterile, clean chucks pad

## TECHNIQUE

1. Prep the insertion site with alcohol followed by the povidone–iodine pads.
2. Achieve good local anesthesia by using topical vapocoolant spray.
3. Position the needle and syringe perpendicular to the skin with the needle tip directed posteriorly.
4. Using the no-touch technique, introduce the needle at the insertion site (Fig. 6.46).
5. Advance the needle quickly but carefully into the cyst.
6. Apply suction with the syringe and withdraw the expected small amount of a clear gel.
7. Withdraw the needle.
8. With gloved fingers, apply firm pressure to the tissues surrounding the punctured cyst. Do not contact the injection site with nonsterile gloves. Remove all extruded clear gel with sterile gauze pads (Fig. 6.47).
9. Apply a sterile adhesive bandage.

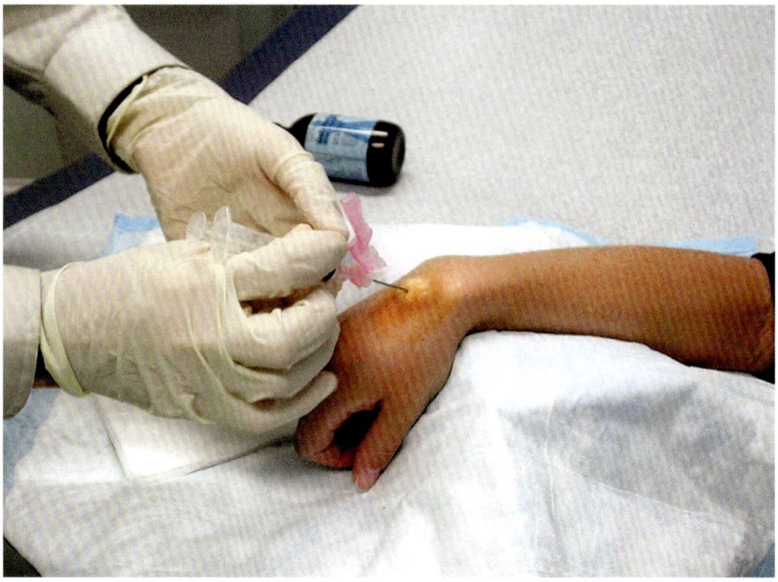

*FIGURE 6.46* Right wrist dorsal ganglion cyst aspiration.

## AFTERCARE

- Consider immobilizing the wrist with a splint for 2 weeks.
- Consider follow-up examination in 2 weeks.

**CPT code:** 20612—Aspiration and/or injection of ganglion cyst(s) any location. (To report multiple ganglion cyst aspirations/injections, use 20612 and append modifier 59.)

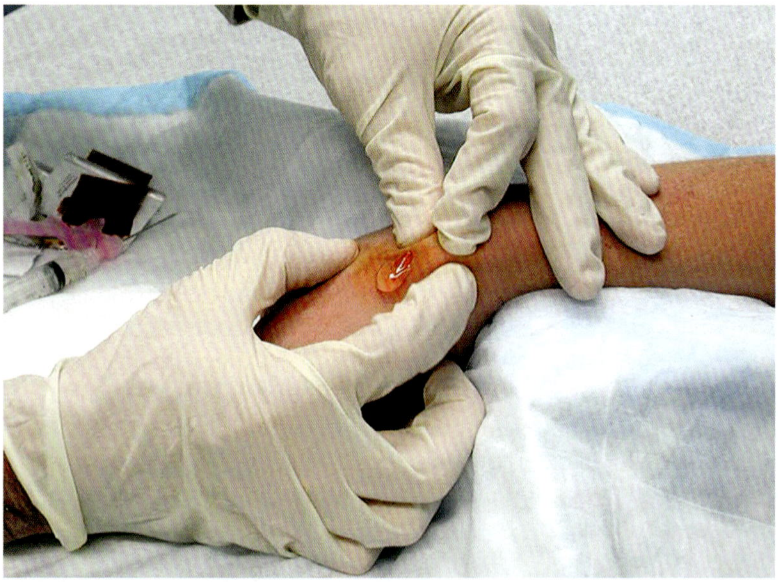

*FIGURE 6.47* Expression of fluid remaining following aspiration of a ganglion cyst with direct pressure to the surrounding tissues.

## PEARLS

- Use extreme caution when treating ganglion cysts over the volar aspect of the wrist. These commonly involve the area immediately next to the radial artery. An accidental injury of this artery with an 18-gauge needle can have disastrous results.
- Initial treatment of a symptomatic ganglion cyst usually requires only cyst aspiration with manual extrusion of remaining contents.
- Treatment success may improve with wrist immobilization for 3 weeks.[1]
- Even with proficient technique, ganglion cysts frequently recur and may require surgical referral for definitive management.

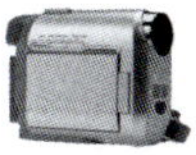

A video clip showing a dorsal wrist ganglion cyst aspiration can be found in the companion eBook.

## REFERENCES

1. Richman JA, Gelberman RH, Engber WD, et al. Ganglions of the wrist and digits: results of treatment by aspiration and cyst wall puncture. *J Hand Surg*. 1987;12:1041–1043.
2. Dias JJ, Dhukaram V, Kumar P. The natural history of untreated dorsal wrist ganglia and patient reported outcome 6 years after intervention. *J Hand Surg Eur Vol*. 2007;32(5):502–508.
3. Limpaphayom N, Wilairatana V. Randomized controlled trial between surgery and aspiration combined with methylprednisolone acetate injection plus wrist immobilization in the treatment of dorsal carpal ganglion. *J Med Assoc Thai*. 2004;87(12):1513–1517.
4. Zubowicz VN. Management of ganglion cysts of the hand by simple aspiration. *J Hand Surg Am*. 1987;12A(4):618.

# Thumb Carpometacarpal Joint

The carpometacarpal (CMC) joint of the thumb is a relatively common injection site for most primary care physicians. This joint articulates the trapezium and the first metacarpal bone of the thumb. It is the most common site of osteoarthritis in the hand. The diagnosis of thumb CMC osteoarthritis is based on symptoms of localized pain, tenderness, and instability on physical examination and radiographic findings.

Although there has been some inconsistency, a review of the medical literature supports the use of corticosteroid injections for short-term[1,2] and perhaps medium- and long-term treatment.[3,4] Improvements are noted in pain, grip strength, and overall hand function. The therapeutic effect may be more beneficial in mild rather than moderate or severe osteoarthritis.[5,6] Hyaluronic acid viscosupplements may play a future role in this condition.[7,8]

A small-diameter needle is appropriate as this technique is only used to inject steroid solution into the CMC joint. There is no joint effusion to remove.

| Indications | ICD-9 Code | ICD-10 Code |
|---|---|---|
| Pain of thumb CMC joint | 719.44 | M79.643 |
| CMC joint arthropathy, unspecified | 716.94 | M12.9 |
| CMC joint osteoarthritis, primary | 715.14 | M18.10 |
| CMC joint osteoarthritis, posttraumatic | 716.14 | M18.30 |
| CMC joint osteoarthritis, secondary | 715.24 | M18.50 |

**Relevant Anatomy:** (Fig. 6.48)

## PATIENT POSITION

- Supine on the examination table with the head of the bed elevated 30 degrees.
- The affected wrist is held in a neutral position between supination and pronation.
- The wrist is supported with the placement of chucks pads or towels.
- Rotate the patient's head away from the side that is being injected. This minimizes anxiety and pain perception.

## LANDMARKS

1. With the patient supine on the examination table, the clinician stands lateral to the affected hand.
2. Locate the CMC joint by palpating the thumb metacarpal bone in a distal-to-proximal direction. At the proximal aspect of the first metacarpal, there will be tenderness as the examiner's finger passes over, then drops into the CMC joint. This is located between the first metacarpal and the trapezium bone. The patient will report tenderness in this joint.
3. Mark the injection point directly over the CMC joint.

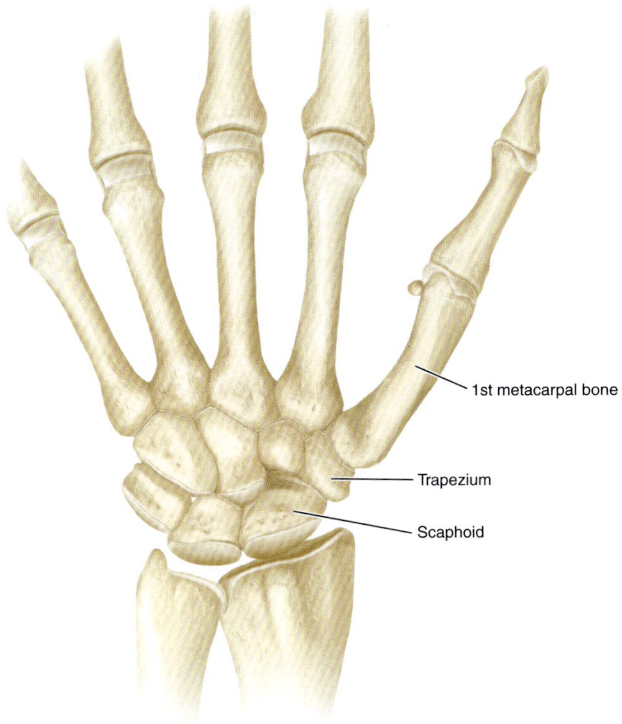


**FIGURE 6.48** ● Dorsal aspect of the right hand. (From Tank PW, Gest TR. *Lippincott Williams & Wilkins Atlas of Anatomy*. Philadelphia, PA: Lippincott Williams & Wilkins, 2009.)

4. At that site, press firmly on the skin with the retracted tip of a ballpoint pen. This indention represents the entry point for the needle.
5. After the landmarks are identified, the patient should not move the hand or thumb.

## ANESTHESIA

- Local anesthesia of the skin using topical vapocoolant spray.

## EQUIPMENT

- 3-mL syringe
- 25-gauge, 5/8 in. needle
- 0.25 mL of 1% lidocaine without epinephrine
- 0.25 mL of the steroid solution (10 mg of triamcinolone acetonide)
- One alcohol prep pad
- Two povidone–iodine prep pads
- Sterile gauze pads
- Sterile adhesive bandage
- Nonsterile, clean chucks pad

## TECHNIQUE

1. Prep the insertion site with alcohol followed by the povidone–iodine pads.
2. Achieve good local anesthesia by using topical vapocoolant spray.

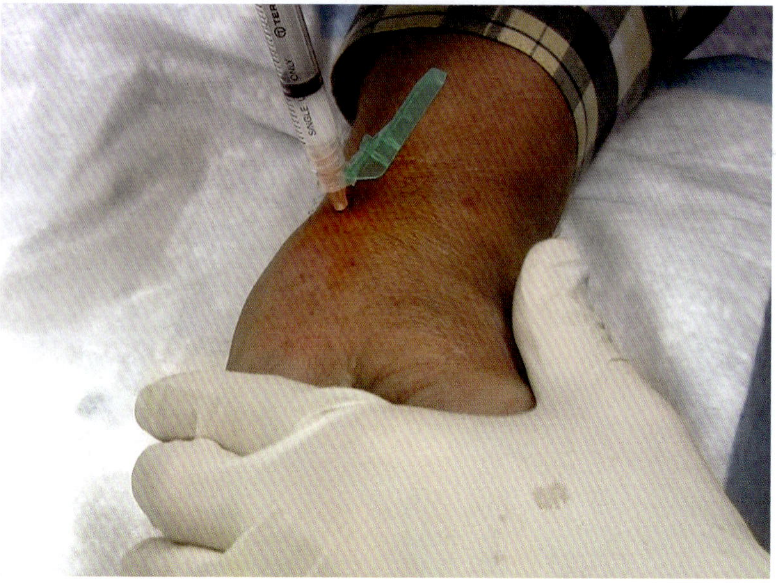

*FIGURE 6.49* Left hand—thumb CMC joint injection.

3. Position the needle and syringe perpendicular to the skin with the needle tip directed posteriorly toward the first CMC joint.
4. Using the no-touch technique, introduce the needle at the insertion site (Fig. 6.49).
5. Advance the needle down into the joint.
6. Inject the steroid solution as a bolus into the joint. The injected solution should flow smoothly into the space. If increased resistance is encountered, advance or withdraw the needle slightly before attempting further injection.
7. Following injection of the corticosteroid solution, withdraw the needle.
8. Apply a sterile adhesive bandage.
9. Instruct the patient to move his or her thumb through its full range of motion. This movement distributes the steroid solution throughout the CMC joint.
10. Reexamine the CMC joint in 5 min to confirm pain relief.

## AFTERCARE

- Avoid excessive use of the thumb over the next 2 weeks.
- Consider the use of a thumb spica splint.
- NSAIDs, ice, and/or physical therapy as indicated.
- Consider follow-up examination in 2 weeks.

**CPT code:** 20600—Injection of small joint

## PEARLS

- Applying traction to the thumb in a distal direction as shown in the photo will help open up the joint to accommodate the needle.

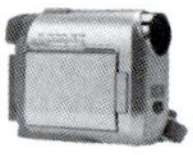

A video clip of thumb CMC joint injection can be found in the companion eBook.

## REFERENCES

1. Maarse W, Watts AC, Bain GI. Medium-term outcome following intra-articular corticosteroid injection in first CMC joint arthritis using fluoroscopy. *Hand Surg*. 2009;14(2–3):99–104.
2. Joshi R. Intraarticular corticosteroid injection for first carpometacarpal osteoarthritis. *J Rheumatol*. 2005;32(7):1305–1306.
3. Swindells MG, Logan AJ, Armstrong DJ, et al. The benefit of radiologically-guided steroid injections for trapeziometacarpal osteoarthritis. *Ann R Coll Surg Engl*. 2010;92(8):680–684.
4. Bahadir C, Onal B, Dayan VY, et al. Comparison of therapeutic effects of sodium hyaluronate and corticosteroid injections on trapeziometacarpal joint osteoarthritis. *Clin Rheumatol*. 2009;28(5):529–533.
5. Meenagh GK, Patton J, Kynes C, et al. A randomised controlled trial of intra-articular corticosteroid injection of the carpometacarpal joint of the thumb in osteoarthritis. *Ann Rheum Dis*. 2004;63(10):1260–1263.
6. Day CS, Gelberman R, Patel AA, et al. Basal joint osteoarthritis of the thumb: a prospective trial of steroid injection and splinting. *J Hand Surg Am*. 2004;29(2):247–251.
7. Bahadir C, Onal B, Dayan VY, et al. Comparison of therapeutic effects of sodium hyaluronate and corticosteroid injections on trapeziometacarpal joint osteoarthritis. *Clin Rheumatol*. 2009;28(5):529–533.
8. Stahl S, Kaufman T. The efficacy of an injection of steroids for medial epicondylitis: a prospective study of sixty elbows. *J Bone Joint Surg Am*. 1997;79(11):1648–1652.

# Metacarpophalangeal Joint

Metacarpophalangeal (MCP) joints of the hand are uncommon injection sites for most primary care clinicians. An MCP joint may become inflamed with osteoarthritis, inflammatory arthritis, or septic arthritis.

A small-diameter needle is appropriate as this technique is only used to inject steroid solution into the MCP joint. There should not be a significant joint effusion to remove in the absence of infection.

| Indications | ICD-9 Code | ICD-10 Code |
|---|---|---|
| Pain of MCP joint | 719.44 | M79.643 |
| Sprain of MCP joint | 842.12 | S63.64 |
| MCP joint arthritis, unspecified | 716.94 | M12.9 |
| MCP joint osteoarthritis, primary | 715.14 | M19.049 |
| MCP joint osteoarthritis, posttraumatic | 716.14 | M19.149 |
| MCP joint osteoarthritis, secondary | 715.24 | M19.249 |

**Relevant Anatomy:** (Fig. 6.50)

## PATIENT POSITION

- Supine on the examination table with the head of the bed elevated 30 degrees.
- The affected wrist is held in a neutral position. The wrist is pronated, and the patient is asked to make a loose fist.
- The hand is supported with the placement of chucks pads or towels.
- Rotate the patient's head away from the side that is being injected. This minimizes anxiety and pain perception.

## LANDMARKS

1. With the patient supine on the examination table, the clinician stands anterior to the affected hand.
2. Locate the affected MCP joint.
3. The point of entry is located directly over the MCP joint, just radial or ulnar to the extensor tendon.
4. At that site, press firmly on the skin with the retracted tip of a ballpoint pen. This indention represents the entry point for the needle.
5. After the landmarks are identified, the patient should not move the hand or fingers.

## ANESTHESIA

- Local anesthesia of the skin using topical vapocoolant spray.

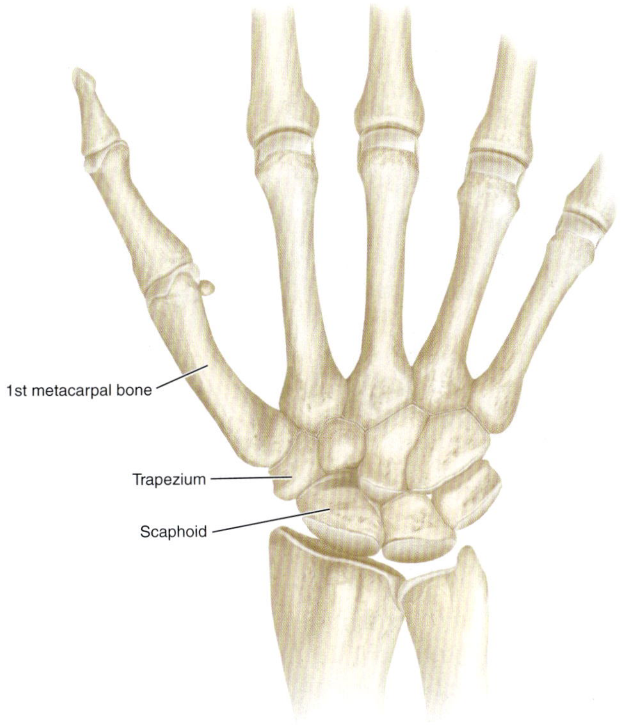


**FIGURE 6.50** • Dorsal aspect of the right hand. (From Tank PW, Gest TR. *Lippincott Williams & Wilkins Atlas of Anatomy*. Philadelphia, PA: Lippincott Williams & Wilkins, 2009.)

## EQUIPMENT

- 3-mL syringe
- 25-gauge, 5/8-in. needle
- 0.25 mL of 1% lidocaine without epinephrine
- 0.25 mL of the steroid solution (10 mg of triamcinolone acetonide)
- One alcohol prep pad
- Two povidone–iodine prep pads
- Sterile gauze pads
- Sterile adhesive bandage
- Nonsterile, clean chucks pad

## TECHNIQUE

1. Prep the insertion site with alcohol followed by the povidone–iodine pads.
2. Achieve good local anesthesia by using topical vapocoolant spray.
3. Position the needle and syringe perpendicular to the skin with the needle tip directed posteriorly toward the first MCP joint.
4. Using the no-touch technique, introduce the needle at the insertion site (Fig. 6.51).
5. Advance the needle down into the joint.
6. Inject the steroid solution as a bolus into the joint. The injected solution should flow smoothly into the space. If increased resistance is encountered, advance or withdraw the needle slightly before attempting further injection.

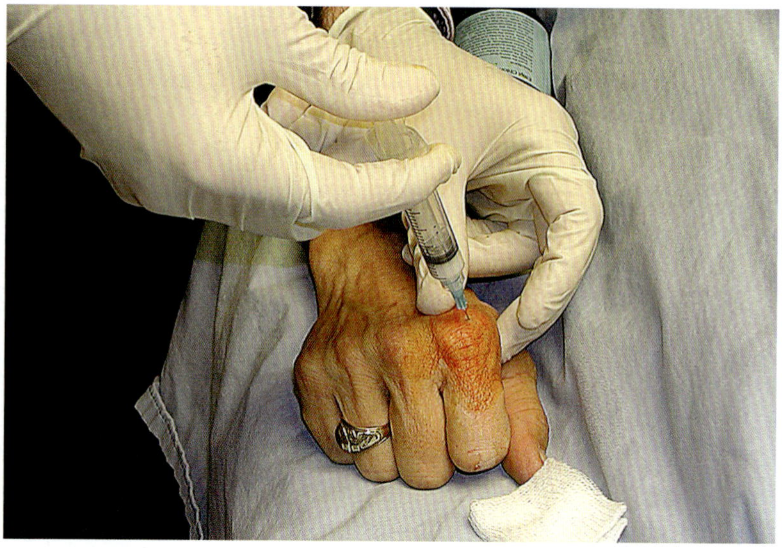

*FIGURE 6.51* ● Metacarpophalangeal joint injection.

7. Following injection of the corticosteroid solution, withdraw the needle.
8. Apply a sterile adhesive bandage.
9. Instruct the patient to move his or her MCP joint through its full range of motion. This movement distributes the steroid solution throughout the joint.
10. Reexamine the MCP joint in 5 min to confirm pain relief.

## AFTERCARE

- Avoid excessive use of the affected hand and finger over the next 2 weeks.
- Consider the use of a volar wrist splint.
- NSAIDs, ice, and/or physical therapy as indicated.
- Consider follow-up examination in 2 weeks.

**CPT code:** 20600—Injection of small joint

## PEARLS

- Approach the MCP joint dorsally, but avoid inserting the needle through the extensor tendon.
- Avoid the development of a subdermal wheal during injection. This indicates the deposition of steroid solution that may cause localized skin atrophy and hypopigmentation.

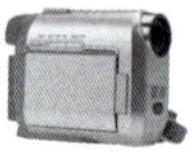

A video clip showing a MCP joint injection can be found in the companion eBook.

# Trigger Finger

Stenosing tenosynovitis, or trigger finger, is the term given for tendinosis of the flexor tendons of the digits. This tendinopathy with nodule formation usually occurs as a result of repetitive compression injury. It is more common in patients with diabetes and rheumatoid arthritis. In this disorder, the nodule forms where the flexor tendon passes over the metacarpal head of a finger or, less commonly, the CMC joint of the thumb. With flexion of the digit, the nodule passes over the proximal edge of the first annular (A-1) pulley of the tendon sheath and becomes entrapped. This is a fairly common procedure performed by primary care providers. A discrete injection of corticosteroid at the site of the palpable, painful nodule offers an effective nonsurgical treatment of this condition.

Injection of corticosteroid is a useful first-line treatment for trigger finger.[1] A recent study by Dala-Ali[2] and colleagues showed a 66% success rate. Prognostic indicators for recurrence include younger age, insulin-dependent diabetes mellitus, involvement of multiple digits, and a history of other tendinopathies of the upper extremity.[3] Alternative injection techniques may be useful and include extrasynovial[4] (subcutaneous) and injections in the mid proximal phalanx.[5] Recently, the NSAID, diclofenac, has been shown to be a treatment option with 53% response compared to 70% in the corticosteroid group.[6]

| Indications | ICD-9 Code | ICD-10 Code |
|---|---|---|
| Trigger finger | 727.03 | M65.309 |
| Trigger thumb | 727.03 | M65.319 |

**Relevant Anatomy:** (Fig. 6.52)

## PATIENT POSITION

- Supine on the examination table with the head of the bed elevated 30 degrees.
- The affected wrist is held in a neutral position.
- The wrist is fully supinated.
- The hand is supported with the placement of chucks pads or towels.
- Rotate the patient's head away from the side that is being injected. This minimizes anxiety and pain perception.

## LANDMARKS

1. With the patient supine on the examination table, the clinician stands anterior to the affected hand.
2. Identify and mark the tender nodule located in the finger's flexor tendon and its sheath. This should be located over the metatarsal heads.

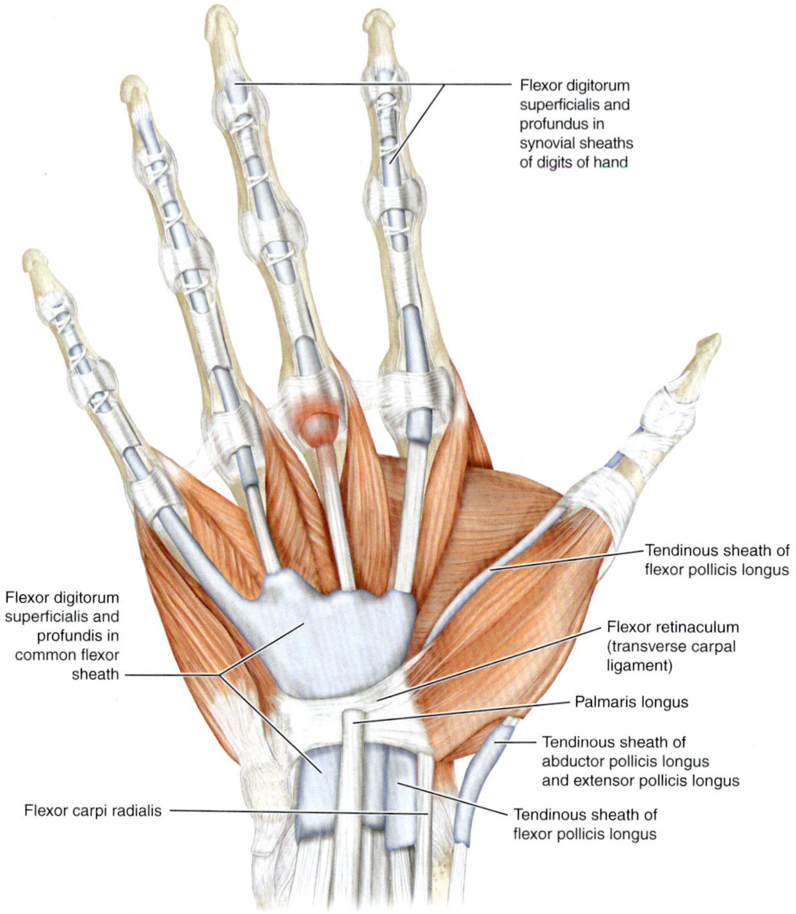


***FIGURE 6.52*** Tendinous (synovial) sheaths of long flexor tendons of the digits. An inflamed nodule is shown in the flexor tendon of the long finger. (From Tank PW, Gest TR. *Lippincott Williams & Wilkins Atlas of Anatomy*. Philadelphia, PA: Lippincott Williams & Wilkins, 2009.)

3. Mark a point 1 cm distal to the nodule.
4. At that site, press firmly on the skin with the retracted tip of a ballpoint pen. This indention represents the entry point for the needle.
5. After the landmarks are identified, the patient should not move the hand or the fingers.

## ANESTHESIA

- Local anesthesia of the skin using topical vapocoolant spray.

## EQUIPMENT

- 3-mL syringe
- 25-gauge, 5/8-in. needle
- 0.5 mL of 1% lidocaine without epinephrine
- 0.5 mL of the steroid solution (20 mg of triamcinolone acetonide)
- One alcohol prep pad
- Two povidone–iodine prep pads

- Sterile gauze pads
- Sterile adhesive bandage
- Nonsterile, clean chucks pad

## TECHNIQUE

1. Prep the insertion site with alcohol followed by the povidone–iodine pads.
2. Achieve good local anesthesia by using topical vapocoolant spray.
3. Position the needle and syringe at a 45-degree angle to the skin with the needle tip directed proximally.
4. Using the no-touch technique, introduce the needle at the insertion site (Fig. 6.53).
5. Advance the needle until the needle tip is located at the tendon nodule. Back up the needle 1 to 2 mm.
6. Slowly inject the steroid solution around the nodule into the tendon sheath. A subtle bulge in the shape of a sausage may develop in the tendon sheath.
7. If increased resistance is encountered, advance or withdraw the needle slightly before attempting further injection.
8. Following injection of the corticosteroid solution, withdraw the needle.
9. Apply a sterile adhesive bandage.
10. Instruct the patient to move his or her finger through its full range of motion. This movement distributes the steroid solution throughout the tenosynovial sheath.
11. Reexamine the hand in 5 min to confirm pain relief.

## AFTERCARE

- Avoid excessive repetitive handgrip activities over the next 2 weeks.
- NSAIDs, ice, heat, and/or physical therapy as indicated.
- Consider follow-up examination in 2 weeks.

**CPT code:** 20550—Injection of single tendon sheath

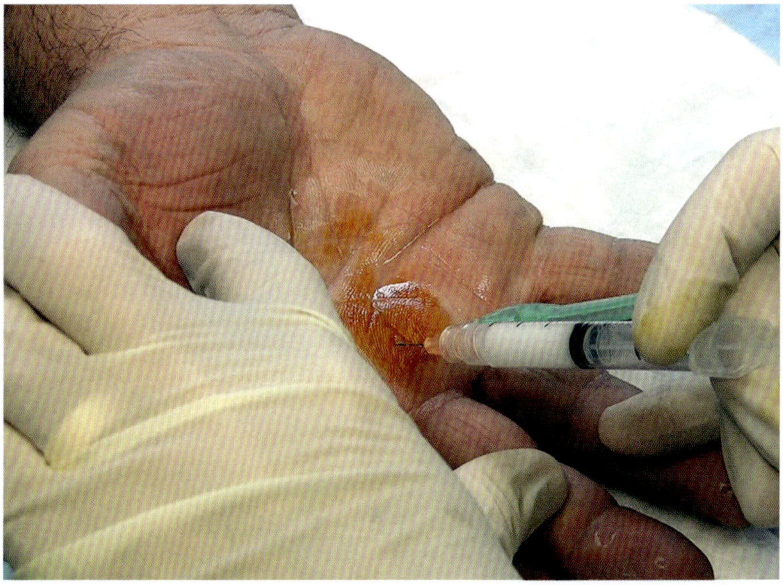

***FIGURE 6.53*** ● Trigger finger injection.

## PEARLS

- The flexor tendon nodule may be approached from either a distal or a proximal direction. It however is easier to perform this injection in a distal-to-proximal direction.

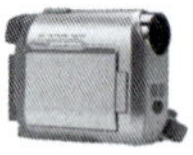

A video clip showing a trigger finger injection can be found in the companion eBook.

## REFERENCES


1. Peters-Veluthamaningal C, van der Windt DA, Winters JC, et al. Corticosteroid injection for trigger finger in adults. *Cochrane Database Syst Rev*. 2009;(1):CD005617.
2. Dala-Ali BM, Nakhdjevani A, Lloyd MA, et al. The efficacy of steroid injection in the treatment of trigger finger. *Clin Orthop Surg*. 2012;4(4):263–268.
3. Rozental TD, Zurakowski D, Blazar PE. Trigger finger: prognostic indicators of recurrence following corticosteroid injection. *J Bone Joint Surg Am*. 2008;90(8):1665–1672.
4. Kazuki K, Egi T, Okada M, et al. Clinical outcome of extrasynovial steroid injection for trigger finger. *Hand Surg*. 2006;11(1–2):1–4.
5. Pataradool K, Buranapuntaruk T. Proximal phalanx injection for trigger finger: randomized controlled trial. *Hand Surg*. 2011;16(3):313–317.
6. Shakeel H, Ahmad TS. Steroid injection versus NSAID injection for trigger finger: a comparative study of early outcomes. *J Hand Surg Am*. 2012;37(7):1319–1323.

# Digital Mucous Cyst

Patients frequently present to their primary care providers with digital mucous cysts (a.k.a. digital myxoid cysts). These cysts, which have either a ganglion or myxomatous origin,[1] are located over the dorsal aspect of terminal digits adjacent to the fingernail. They contain clear mucinous fluid. Typically, there is underlying osteoarthritis of the DIP joint. It is believed that a dorsal osteophyte weakens the joint capsule and allows the fluid to track distally. This pedicle terminates at the proximal nailfold where the fluid accumulates in a cystic structure. Over time, the cyst enlarges, applies pressure on the nail matrix, and produces an indention in the fingernail.[1] Digital mucous cysts are commonly treated with recurrent aspiration or needling, but the recurrence rate is high.[2] Corticosteroid injection is not beneficial.[3] If recurrent, they are best managed with surgical excision of the cyst that includes a rotation advancement skin flap.[4,5]

| Indication | ICD-9 Code | ICD-10 Code |
|---|---|---|
| Digital mucous cyst | 727.40 | M71.30 |

**Relevant Anatomy:** (Figs. 6.54 and 6.55)

## PATIENT POSITION

- Supine on the examination table with the head of the bed elevated 30 degrees.
- The wrist is held in pronation.
- The hand is supported with the placement of chucks pads or towels.
- Rotate the patient's head away from the side that is being injected. This minimizes anxiety and pain perception.

## LANDMARKS

1. With the patient supine on the examination table, the clinician stands lateral to the affected hand.
2. Identify the cystic structure over the dorsal aspect of the finger, just proximal to the nailfold.
3. The injection point is located directly over the cyst.
4. The patient should not move the hand.

## ANESTHESIA

- Digital block anesthesia of the finger using injected 1% lidocaine.

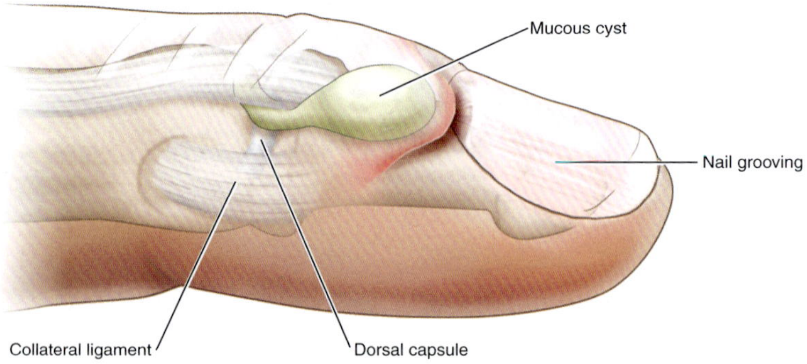


**FIGURE 6.54** Digital mucous cyst.

## EQUIPMENT

- 3-mL syringe
- 18-gauge, 1½ in. needle
- One alcohol prep pad
- Two povidone–iodine prep pads
- Sterile gauze pads
- Sterile adhesive bandage
- Nonsterile, clean chucks pad

## TECHNIQUE

1. Achieve good digital block anesthesia.
2. Prep the insertion site with alcohol followed by the povidone–iodine pads.

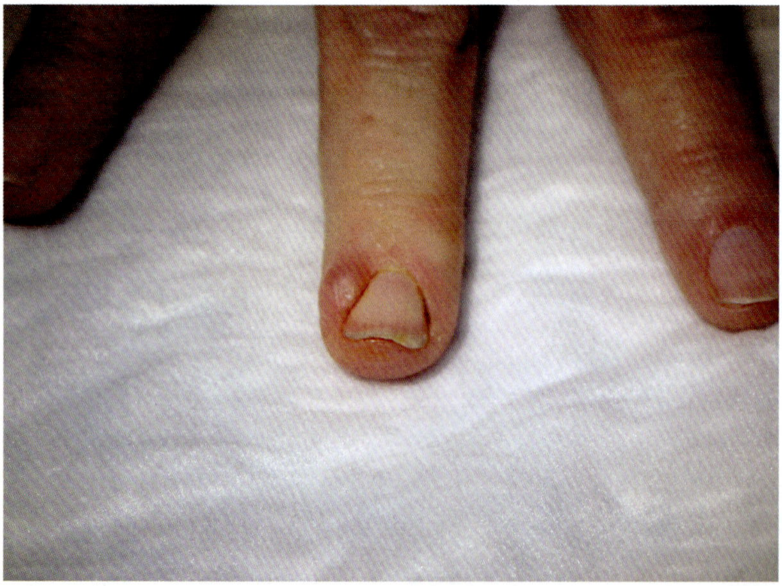

**FIGURE 6.55** Digital mucous cyst.

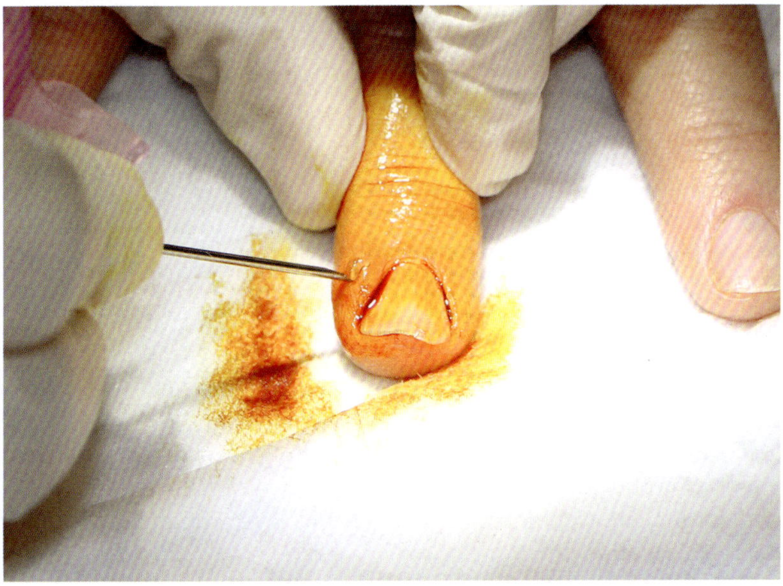

***FIGURE 6.56*** • Digital mucous cyst aspiration.

3. Position the needle and syringe perpendicular to the skin with the needle tip directed to the center of the cyst.
4. Using the no-touch technique, introduce the needle at the insertion site (Fig. 6.56).
5. Advance the needle quickly but carefully into the cyst.
6. Apply suction with the syringe and withdraw the expected small amount of a clear gel.
7. Withdraw the needle.
8. With either the shaft of the needle or gloved fingers, apply firm pressure to the tissues surrounding the punctured cyst. Remove all extruded clear gel with sterile gauze pads (Fig. 6.57).

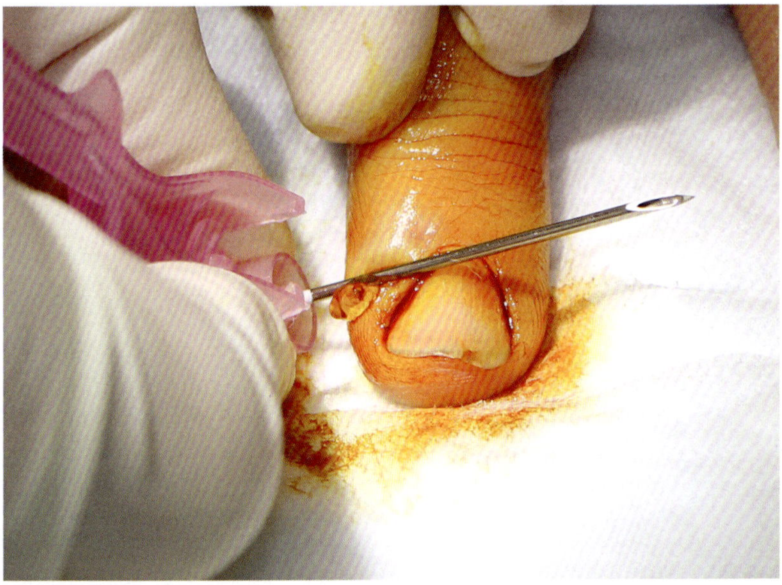

***FIGURE 6.57*** • Expression of fluid remaining following aspiration of a ganglion cyst with direct pressure to the surrounding tissues.

9. Injection of steroid solution is not indicated.
10. Apply a sterile adhesive bandage.

## AFTERCARE

- Consider follow-up examination in 2 weeks.

**CPT code:** 26160—Aspiration and/or injection of mucoid DIP cyst

## PEARLS

- Initial treatment of a symptomatic digital mucous cyst usually requires only cyst aspiration with manual extrusion of remaining contents.
- Cysts that recur despite repeated aspirations/needling have not been found to respond to injections of corticosteroid.
- Even with proficient technique, digital mucous cysts frequently recur and may require surgical treatment.

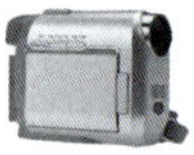

A video clip showing a digital mucous cyst aspiration can be found in the companion eBook.

## REFERENCES

1. Lin YC, Wu YH, Scher RK. Nail changes and association of osteoarthritis in digital myxoid cyst. *Dermatol Surg*. 2008;34(3):364–369.
2. Epstein E. A simple technique for managing digital mucous cysts. *Arch Dermatol*. 1979;115(11):1315–1316.
3. Epstein E. Steroid injection of myxoid finger cysts. *JAMA*. 1965;194:98–99.
4. Zuber TJ. Office management of digital mucous cysts. *Am Fam Physician*. 2001;64(12):1987–1991.
5. Johnson SM, et al. A reliable surgical treatment for digital mucous cysts. *J Hand Surg Eur* Vol. 2013 Oct 25. [Epub ahead of print]

# 7 Myofascial Trigger Points

Myofascial pain syndrome is a common condition that arises from muscles or related fascia and is associated with painful trigger points. Each point is a highly localized, hyperirritable focal area in a palpable, taut band of skeletal muscle fibers (Fig. 7.1). Patients present frequently to primary care physicians with this condition. Although the trigger points may be injected with corticosteroids or local anesthetics, the nodules are also commonly treated with multiple needle piercings without the introduction of medication. This practice of "dry needling" is attributed to Travell and Simons[1] who empirically developed techniques involving the passage of needles into isolated trigger points. This therapeutic modality, also known as intramuscular stimulation, is based on theories similar, but not exclusive, to traditional acupuncture. However, dry needling targets discrete trigger points, which are the direct and palpable source of pain, rather than traditional meridians.

Dry needling is an invasive procedure in which a standard hollow hypodermic needle or a solid core acupuncture needle is inserted through the skin and directly into a myofascial trigger point. Proper dry needling of a myofascial trigger point will elicit both referred pain and a local twitch response. This is an involuntary spinal cord reflex in which the muscle fibers in the taut band of muscle quickly contract. The local twitch response indicates the proper placement of the needle in a trigger point. At the site of an active trigger point, there are elevated levels of inflammatory mediators, known to be associated with persistent pain states and myofascial tenderness. This local milieu positively changes with the occurrence of a local twitch response.[2] Lewit[3] demonstrated that the therapeutic effect from passage of a needle is distinct from that of the injected substance.

Several adverse effects associated specifically with dry needling have been reported. These include pain, hematoma, syncopal episodes, and pneumothorax.[4] Overall, the rate of complications is low, and dry needling/acupuncture provided by experienced physicians is considered a safe treatment.[5]

An examination of the peer-reviewed literature regarding the benefit of dry needling is inconclusive. There are randomized clinical trials indicating both positive effect[6] and no difference.[7–9] The use of ultrasound may improve the accuracy, clinical response, and safety of the procedure.[10] A systematic review[11] indicated no difference in outcomes in patients treated with dry needling for the treatment of myofascial pain syndrome. Another comprehensive review[12] yielded insufficient evidence to make any recommendations about acupuncture or dry needling for acute low back pain. But, for chronic low back pain, results show that acupuncture is more effective for pain relief and improving function than is no treatment or sham treatment in the short term. The technique has a small incremental effect when added to other conventional therapies, but is not more effective than are other conventional and "alternative" treatments.

Several other percutaneous treatments for tendinopathy that include corticosteroid injection, prolotherapy, autologous whole blood injection, and autologous platelet-rich

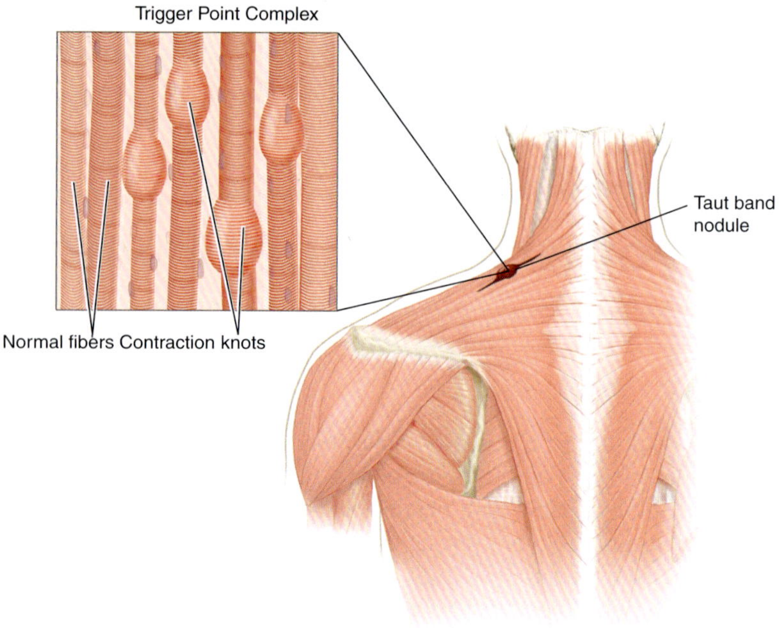


**FIGURE 7.1** ● Myofascial trigger point.

plasma injection are often performed in conjunction with fenestration. It is currently unknown if these other percutaneous procedures have any benefit over dry needling alone.

Most reported studies suffer from significant methodologic limitations and may not be generalizable.[12,13] Furthermore, rigorous evidence regarding the potential physiologic mechanisms of actions and effects of this modality is sparse and incomplete. Studies performed in an acupuncture setting do not necessarily apply to dry needling.[14] Since it appears that significant symptomatic improvement occurs in some patients who are treated with injection of myofascial trigger points, further high-quality research is required to determine the proper place of this intervention in the treatment of myofascial pain syndrome. Areas that need to be addressed include proper study design that include blinding, randomization, use of controls, and sufficient numbers of patients.

| Indications | ICD-9 Code | ICD-10 Code |
|---|---|---|
| Fibromyalgia/Fibromyositis | 729.1 | M79.7 |
| Spinal enthesopathy | 720.1 | M46.0 |
| Cervicalgia | 723.1 | M54.2 |
| Tension headache | 307.81 | G44.2 |

## PATIENT POSITION

- Lying prone on the examination table.

## LANDMARKS

1. With the patient lying prone on the examination table, the clinician stands lateral to the affected myofascial trigger point(s).
2. Identify tender nodules that are commonly located in the sternocleidomastoid, scalene, levator scapulae, upper trapezius, quadratus lumborum, gluteus maximus, gluteus medius, quadriceps, and calf muscles.

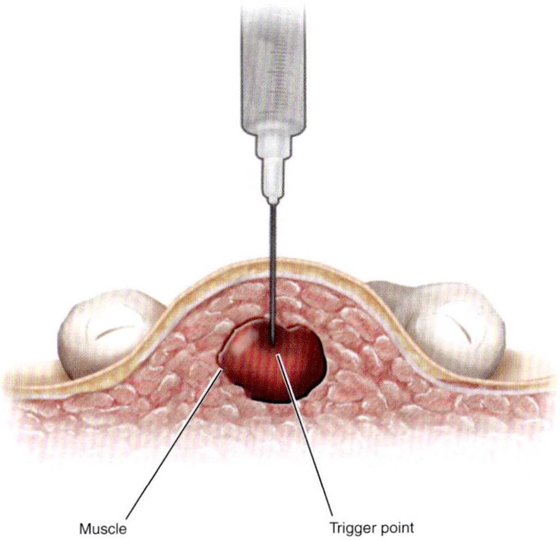


*FIGURE 7.2* • Trigger point in the trapezius muscle.

3. The injection point is located directly over the nodule(s) (Fig. 7.2).
4. At that site, press firmly on the skin with the retracted tip of a ballpoint pen. This indention represents the entry point for the needle.
5. After the landmarks are identified, the patient should not move.

## ANESTHESIA

- Skin distraction or local anesthesia of the skin using topical vapocoolant spray.

## EQUIPMENT

- 3-mL syringe
- 25- to 30-gauge, 1- to 2-in. needle
- (Optional) 0.5 to 1 mL of 1% lidocaine without epinephrine per trigger point
- One alcohol prep pad
- Two povidone–iodine prep pads
- Sterile gauze pads
- Sterile adhesive bandage

## TECHNIQUE

1. Prep the insertion site with alcohol followed by the povidone–iodine pads.
2. Achieve good local anesthesia by using topical vapocoolant spray.
3. With the nondominant hand, firmly press on either side of the nodule with the index and long fingers in order to "fix" the position of the muscular nodule.
4. Position the needle and syringe at a 30- to 45-degree angle to the skin with the tip of the needle directed toward the trigger point.
5. Using the no-touch technique, introduce the needle at the insertion site (Fig. 7.3).
6. Advance the needle carefully into the nodule until the needle tip is located in the center of the trigger point. Successful entry into the nodule will be accompanied by a quick muscle contraction known as the local twitch response. There may also be increased pain at the site of the trigger point or referred pain. Leave the needle in place until the muscle twitch (spasm) relaxes.

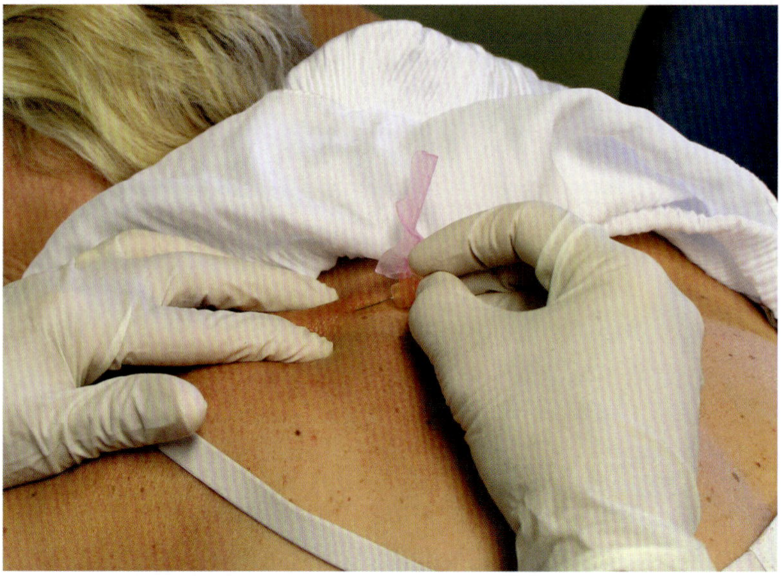

**FIGURE 7.3** ● Myofascial trigger point injection using the dry-needling technique.

7. If performing dry needling, withdraw the needle from the nodule and back to the subcutaneous fat before advancing again into the trigger point. Repeat the process 5 to 10 times or until the twitch response is extinguished.
8. If desired, 0.5 to 1 mL of 1% lidocaine without epinephrine may be injected slowly into the nodule during the final entry of the needle.
9. Finally, withdraw the needle through the skin.
10. Apply a sterile adhesive bandage.
11. Massage and stretch each of the injection sites.
12. Reexamine the area of involvement in 5 min to confirm pain relief and observe for any complications.

## AFTERCARE

- Ice, heat, stretching, and/or physical therapy as indicated.
- Treatment of the underlying condition.
- Consider follow-up examination in 2 weeks.

### CPT codes

20552—Injection of trigger point(s) in one to two muscle groups
20553—Injection of trigger point(s) in three+ muscle groups.

These codes are used only once in each session, regardless of the number of injections performed.

## PEARLS

- The key objective with this procedure is to elicit the local twitch response when directing a needle into a myofascial trigger point.
- Avoid advancing the needle so deeply as to risk complications including pneumothorax.

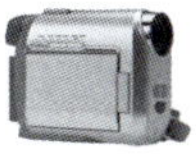

A video clip showing a muscular trigger point injection can be found in the companion eBook.

## REFERENCES


1. Simons DG, Travell JG, Simons LS. *Travell and Simons' Myofascial Pain and Dysfunction: The Trigger Point Manual,* 2nd Ed, Vol. 1. Baltimore, MD: Williams & Wilkins, 1999.
2. Vulfsons S, Ratmansky M, Kalichman L. Trigger point needling: techniques and outcome. *Curr Pain Headache Rep*. 2012;16(5):407–412.
3. Lewit K. The needle effect in the relief of myofascial pain. *Pain*. 1979;6:83–90.
4. Witt CM, Pach D, Brinkhaus B, et al. Safety of acupuncture: results of a prospective observational study with 229,230 patients and introduction of a medical information and consent form. *Forsch Komplementmed*. 2009;16:91–97.
5. White A, Hayhoe S, Hart A, et al. Adverse events following acupuncture: prospective survey of 32,000 consultations with doctors and physiotherapists. *BMJ*. 2001;323:485–486.
6. Tekin L, Akarsu S, Durmuş O, et al. The effect of dry needling in the treatment of myofascial pain syndrome: a randomized double-blinded placebo-controlled trial. *Clin Rheumatol*. 2013;32(3):309–315.
7. Ga H, Choi JH, Park CH, et al. Acupuncture needling versus lidocaine injection of trigger points in myofascial pain syndrome in elderly patients–a randomised trial. *Acupunct Med*. 2007;25:130–136.
8. Barbagli P, Bollettin R, Ceccherelli F. Acupuncture (dry needle) versus neural therapy (local anesthesia) in the treatment of benign back pain. Immediate and long-term results. *Minerva Med*. 2003;94:17–25.
9. Hong CZ. Lidocaine injection versus dry needling to myofascial trigger point. The importance of the local twitch response. *Am J Phys Med Rehabil*. 1994;73:256–263.
10. Chiavaras MM, Jacobson JA. Ultrasound-guided tendon fenestration. *Semin Musculoskelet Radiol*. 2013;17(1):85–90.
11. Cummings TM, White AR. Needling therapies in the management of myofascial trigger point pain: a systematic review. *Arch Phys Med Rehabil*. 2001;82:986–992.
12. Furlan AD, van Tulder MW, Cherkin DC, et al. Acupuncture and dry-needling for low back pain. *Cochrane Database Syst Rev*. 2005;(1):CD001351.
13. Tough EA, White AR, Cummings TM, et al. Acupuncture and dry needling in the management of myofascial trigger point pain: a systematic review and meta-analysis of randomised controlled trials. *Eur J Pain*. 2009;13:3–10.
14. Cagnie B, Dewitte V, Barbe T, et al. Physiologic effects of dry needling. *Curr Pain Headache Rep*. 2013;17(8):348.

# Suprascapular Neuropathy

Patients uncommonly present to the primary care office for evaluation of suprascapular neuropathy. It is an underdiagnosed disorder that is the result of nerve entrapment. The suprascapular nerve is vulnerable as it passes through the suprascapular notch and again at the spinoglenoid notch. Entrapment at the former leads to weakness of the supraspinatus and infraspinatus muscles as well as vague posterior unilateral shoulder pain that is described as a deep, dull, aching discomfort that is exacerbated with overhead throwing motions. Entrapment at the latter causes weakness of the infraspinatus muscle and is generally painless. The most common causes of suprascapular neuropathy are acute trauma, inflammatory processes (i.e., brachial neuritis), a spinoglenoid notch cyst, and rotator cuff tears and overuse.[1] Spinoglenoid notch cysts and suprascapular notch entrapment respond best to surgical decompression, while overuse and viral etiologies respond best to conservative measures.[2] A nerve block at the suprascapular notch can be used in the conservative management of this condition as well as to treat shoulder pain following surgery,[3] pain following strokes,[4] and that associated with adhesive capsulitis.[5]

| Indication | ICD-9 Code | ICD-10 Code |
|---|---|---|
| Neuritis, unspecified | 729.2 | M79.2 |

**Relevant Anatomy:** (Fig. 7.4)

## PATIENT POSITION

- Sitting on an exam stool, with arms resting on the exam table and neck in a neutral position.

## LANDMARKS

1. With the patient sitting on an exam stool, the clinician stands posterior to the affected scapula.
2. Find the midpoint between the tip of the acromion and the medial aspect of the spine of the scapula, and mark it with an ink pen.
3. Find the coracoid process, and mark it with an ink pen.
4. Draw a line between these two points, and mark the midposition of this line.
5. At that site, press firmly on the skin with the retracted tip of a ballpoint pen. This indention represents the entry point for the needle.
6. After the landmarks are identified, the patient should not move.

## ANESTHESIA

- Local anesthesia of the skin using topical vapocoolant spray.

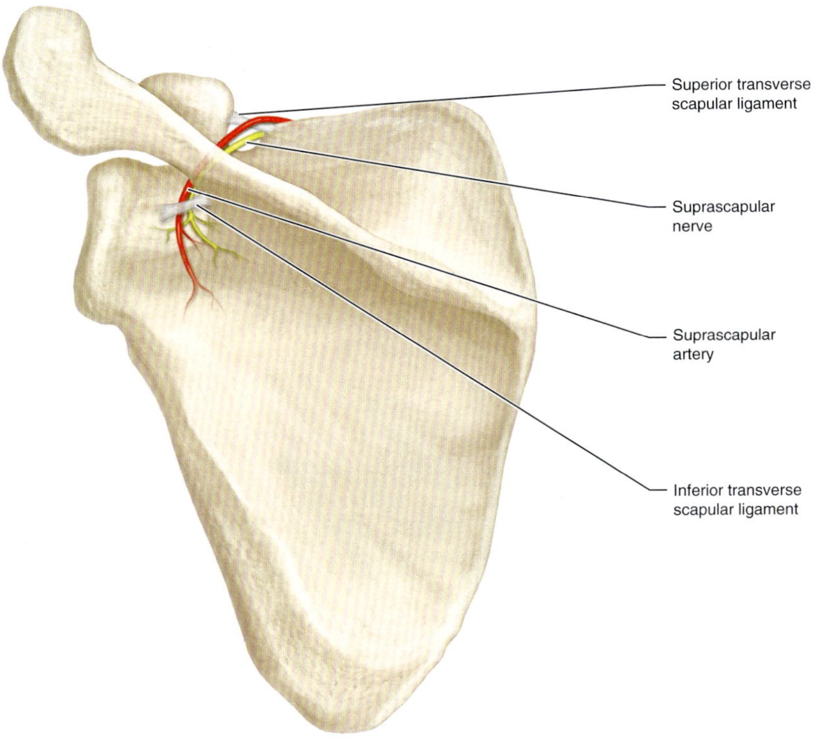


**FIGURE 7.4** ● Nerves and vessels of left posterior scapular region. (From Tank PW, Gest TR. *Lippincott Williams & Wilkins Atlas of Anatomy*. Philadelphia, PA: Lippincott Williams & Wilkins, 2009.)

## EQUIPMENT

- 3-mL syringe
- 25-gauge, 1½ in. needle
- 1 mL of 1% lidocaine without epinephrine
- 1 mL of the steroid solution (40 mg of triamcinolone acetonide)
- One alcohol prep pad
- Two povidone–iodine prep pads
- Sterile gauze pads
- Sterile, adhesive bandage

## TECHNIQUE

1. Prep the insertion site with alcohol followed by the povidone–iodine pads.
2. Achieve good local anesthesia by using topical vapocoolant spray.
3. Position the needle and syringe perpendicular to the skin with the tip of the needle directed toward the suprascapular notch.
4. Using the no-touch technique, introduce the needle at the insertion site (Fig. 7.5).
5. Advance the needle completely through the supraspinatus muscle and touch the bone of the suprascapular fossa. Back up the needle 1 to 2 mm.
6. Aspirate to make sure that the needle tip is not in the suprascapular artery. If there is no blood return, then inject the steroid solution as a bolus into the muscle around the suprascapular nerve. The injected solution should flow smoothly into this area. If increased resistance is encountered, advance or withdraw the needle slightly before attempting further injection.

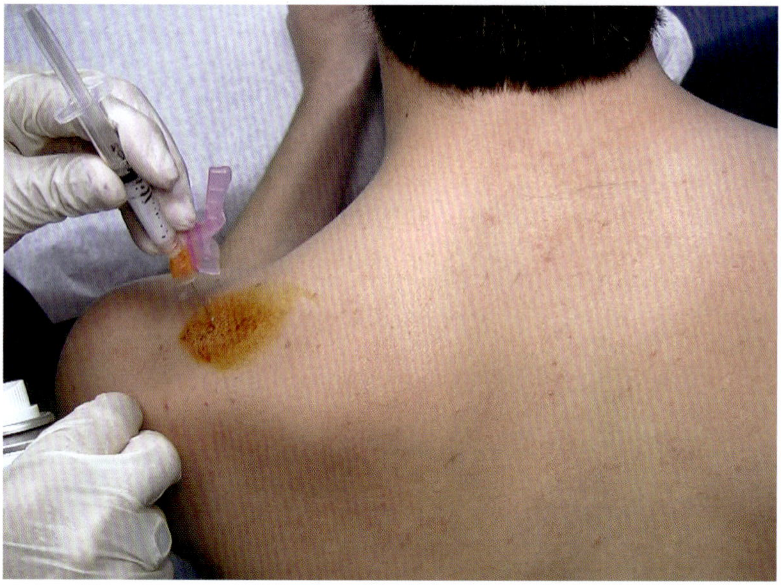

**FIGURE 7.5** ● Suprascapular neuritis injection.

7. Following injection of the corticosteroid solution, withdraw the needle.
8. Apply a sterile adhesive bandage.
9. Instruct the patient to move his or her shoulder through its full range of motion in external rotation and abduction. This movement distributes the steroid solution throughout the suprascapular fossa.
10. Reexamine the shoulder and scapula in 5 min to confirm pain relief.

## AFTERCARE

- Avoid excessive abduction, external rotation, and overhead throwing motions of the shoulder over the next 2 weeks.
- Nonsteroidal anti-inflammatory drugs (NSAIDs), ice, and/or physical therapy as indicated.
- Consider follow-up examination in 2 weeks.

**CPT code:** 64418—Injection, suprascapular nerve

## PEARLS

- Always aspirate before injecting to make sure that the needle tip is not in the suprascapular artery.
- If there is no significant improvement in pain or weakness and the diagnosis has been confirmed by EMG, then refer the patient for surgical decompression of the superior or inferior transverse scapular ligaments.

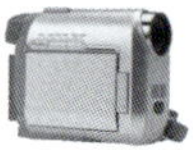

A video clip showing a suprascapular neuritis injection can be found in the companion eBook.

## REFERENCES

1. Hill LJ, Jelsing EJ, Terry MJ, et al. Evaluation, Treatment, and outcomes of suprascapular neuropathy: a 5-year review. *PM R*. 2014;pii:S1934-1482(14)00071-9.
2. Antoniou J, Tae SK, Williams GR, et al. Suprascapular neuropathy. Variability in the diagnosis, treatment, and outcome. *Clin Orthop Relat Res*. 2001;(386):131–138.
3. Jerosch J, Saad M, Greig M, et al. Suprascapular nerve block as a method of preemptive pain control in shoulder surgery. *Knee Surg Sports Traumatol Arthrosc*. 2008;16(6):602–607.
4. Adey-Wakeling Z, Crotty M, Shanahan EM. Suprascapular nerve block for shoulder pain in the first year after stroke: a randomized controlled trial. *Stroke*. 2013;44(11):3136–3141.
5. Jones DS, Chattopadhyay C. Suprascapular nerve block for the treatment of frozen shoulder in primary care: a randomized trial. *Br J Gen Pract*. 1999;49(438):39–41.

# Scapulothoracic Syndrome

Scapulothoracic syndrome is a relatively uncommon problem. It primarily affects middle-aged persons whose occupations require them to extend their arms for prolonged periods of time. This can also occur as a complication from preexisting shoulder lesions or in disabled patients who are unable to control the scapulothoracic relationship. The abnormal positioning causes a bursitis because of abnormal biomechanics of the scapula and the underlying posterior chest wall. Scapulothoracic syndrome is characterized by pain that may be localized to the medial superior border of the scapula or may radiate to the neck and shoulder. Nonsurgical therapy utilizing scapular stabilization, postural exercises, and/or injections is the initial treatment of choice but is less successful than is surgical management in patients with anatomic abnormalities.[1] In patients with normal anatomy, this condition can be successfully treated with a local corticosteroid injection at site of maximum tenderness at the medial superior scapular border.[2]

| Indications | ICD-9 Code | ICD-10 Code |
|---|---|---|
| Bursitis of shoulder | 727.3 | M75.50 |
| Specified injury to scapula | 719.48 | S49.80 |
| Unspecified injury to scapula | 959.2 | S49.90 |
| Other specified arthropathy of scapula | 716.81 | M12.819 |
| Unspecified arthropathy of scapula | 716.91 | M12.9 |

**Relevant Anatomy:** (Fig. 7.6)

## PATIENT POSITION

- Sitting erect on an exam stool, with ipsilateral hand on the contralateral shoulder.

## LANDMARKS

1. With the patient seated on the exam stool, the clinician stands or sits behind the affected scapula.
2. Palpate to determine the area of most intense pain. This is usually along the medial superior scapular border of the scapula. Mark this site with an ink pen.
3. At that site, press firmly on the skin with the retracted tip of a ballpoint pen. This indention represents the entry point for the needle.
4. After the landmarks are identified, the patient should not move.

## ANESTHESIA

- Local anesthesia of the skin using topical vapocoolant spray.

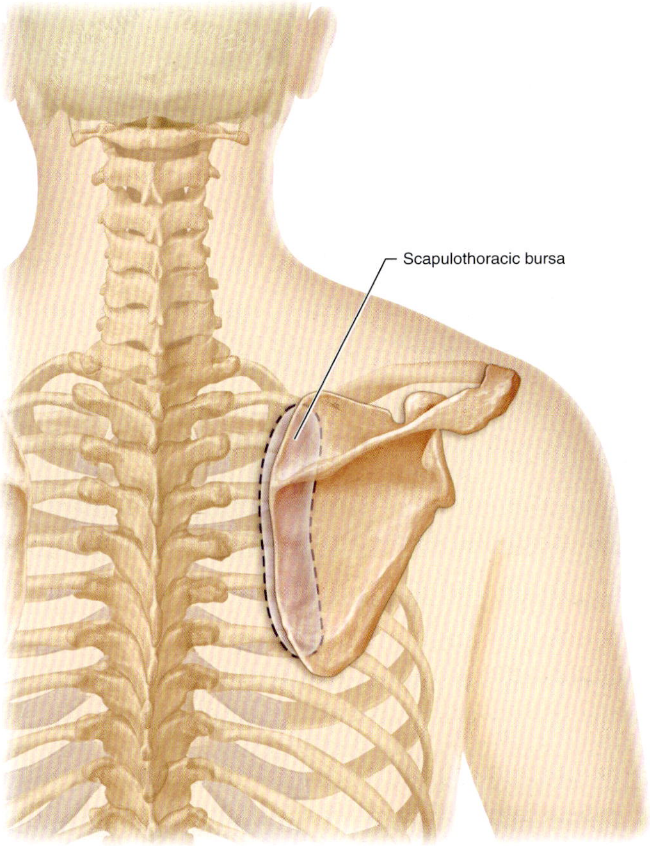


*FIGURE 7.6* • Scapulothoracic bursitis. (From Tank PW, Gest TR. *Lippincott Williams & Wilkins Atlas of Anatomy*. Philadelphia, PA: Lippincott Williams & Wilkins, 2009.)

## EQUIPMENT

- 3-mL syringe
- 25-gauge, 1½ in. needle
- 1 mL of 1% lidocaine without epinephrine
- 1 mL of the steroid solution (40 mg of triamcinolone acetonide)
- One alcohol prep pad
- Two povidone–iodine prep pads
- Sterile gauze pads
- Sterile adhesive bandage

## TECHNIQUE

1. Prep the insertion site with alcohol followed by the povidone–iodine pads.
2. Achieve good local anesthesia by using topical vapocoolant spray.
3. Position the needle and syringe at a 20-degree angle to the skin with the tip of the needle directed toward the area of tenderness in the scapulothoracic space.
4. Using the no-touch technique, introduce the needle at the insertion site (Fig. 7.7).
5. Advance the needle into the point of maximal tenderness in a plane parallel to the undersurface of the scapula, not toward the chest wall.
6. Inject half of the steroid solution as a bolus at the point of maximal tenderness and the remainder in the scapulothoracic space. The injected solution should flow

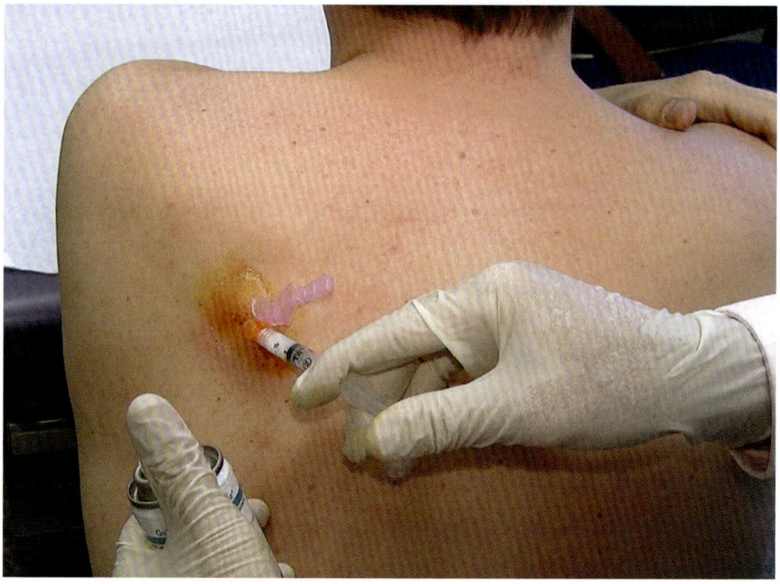

**FIGURE 7.7** ● Scapulothoracic bursitis injection.

smoothly into the space. If increased resistance is encountered, advance or withdraw the needle slightly before attempting further injection.

7. Following injection of the corticosteroid solution, withdraw the needle.
8. Apply a sterile adhesive bandage.
9. Instruct the patient to move his or her shoulder through its full range of motion. This movement distributes the steroid solution throughout the area.
10. Reexamine the scapula in 5 min to confirm pain relief.

## AFTERCARE

- Avoid excessive shoulder abduction, reaching in front, pushing, pulling, and overhead throwing motions over the next 2 weeks.
- NSAIDs, ice, and/or physical therapy as indicated.
- Consider follow-up examination in 2 weeks.

**CPT code:** 20610—Injection of major joint or bursa

## PEARLS

- Avoid advancing the needle so deeply as to risk the complication of pneumothorax.

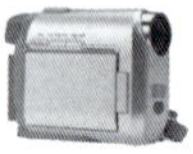

A video clip showing a scapulothoracic injection can be found in the companion eBook.

## REFERENCES


1. Gaskill T, Millett PJ. Snapping scapula syndrome: diagnosis and management. *J Am Acad Orthop Surg*. 2013;21(4):214–224.
2. Boneti C, Arentz C, Klimberg VS. Scapulothoracic bursitis as a significant cause of breast and chest wall pain: underrecognized and undertreated. *Ann Surg Oncol*. 2010;17(Suppl 3):321–324.

# Sacroiliac Joint

Pain involving the sacroiliac joint(s) is a common condition seen by primary care physicians. Sacroiliitis may be caused by acute or repetitive trauma, spondyloarthropathies, degenerative arthritis, pregnancy, and rarely by an infection of the joint. Corticosteroid injections are an effective conservative treatment option for this condition.[1] Furthermore, these can be safely and effectively performed using landmark-guided techniques with similar outcomes compared to the use of imaging.[2] In fact, equal and even improved outcomes may be seen in patients who receive periarticular injections because significant extra-articular sources of sacroiliac region pain exist.[3,4] Botulinum toxin injections[5] and prolotherapy[6] utilizing dextrose show promise for the treatment of sacroiliac joint pain.

| Indications | ICD-9 Code | ICD-10 Code |
|---|---|---|
| SI pain | 724.6 | M53.3 |
| SI sprain | 846.1 | S33.6 |
| Sacroiliitis | 720.2 | M46.1 |
| SI joint arthritis—unspecified | 716.95 | M12.9 |
| SI joint osteoarthrosis—primary | 715.95 | M19.91 |

**Relevant Anatomy:** (Fig. 7.8)

## PATIENT POSITION

- Standing with back in 45 degrees of forward flexion and hands/arms supported by the examination table.

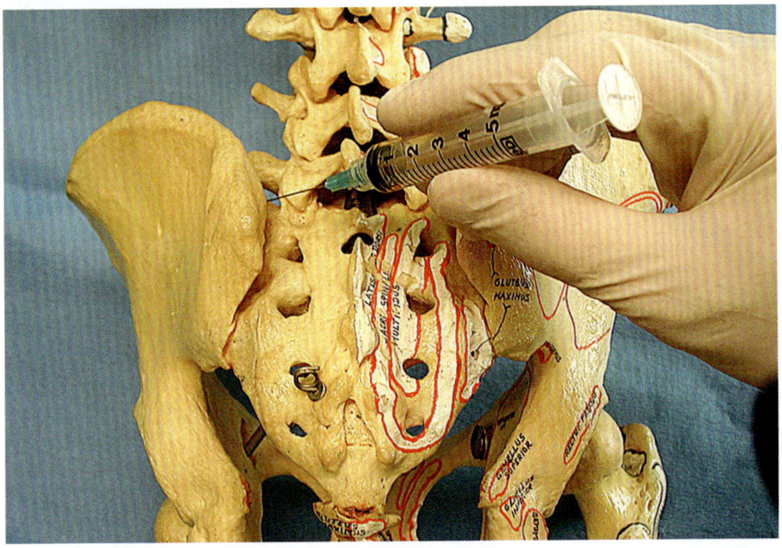

***FIGURE 7.8*** ● Sacroiliac anatomy—note the angle of insertion.

## LANDMARKS

- With the patient standing up with back in forward flexion, the clinician stands directly behind the patient.
- Identify tenderness over the sacroiliac joint. Mark it with ink.
- At that site, press firmly on the skin with the retracted tip of a ballpoint pen. This indention represents the entry point for the needle.

## ANESTHESIA

- Local anesthesia of the skin using topical vapocoolant spray.

## EQUIPMENT

- 5-mL syringe
- 25-gauge, 1½ or 2 in. needle
- 3 mL of 1% lidocaine without epinephrine
- 1 mL of the steroid solution (40 mg of triamcinolone acetonide)
- One alcohol prep pad
- Two povidone–iodine prep pads
- Sterile gauze pads
- Sterile adhesive bandage

## TECHNIQUE

1. Prep the insertion site with alcohol followed by the povidone–iodine pads.
2. Achieve good local anesthesia by using topical vapocoolant spray.
3. Position the needle at a 30-degree angle laterally, relative to the sagittal plane, and 15 degrees inferiorly, relative to the transverse plane, with the tip of the needle directed toward the sacroiliac joint.
4. Using the no-touch technique, introduce the needle at the insertion site (Fig. 7.9).

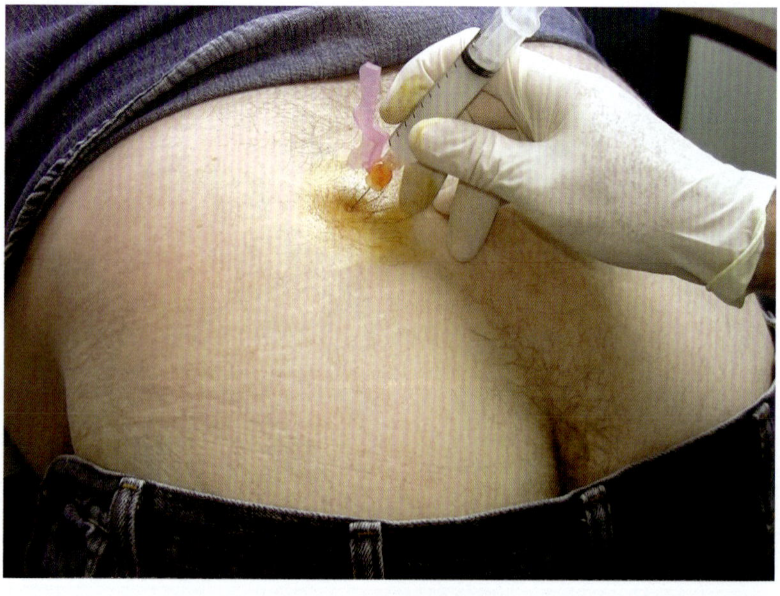

***FIGURE 7.9*** ● Sacroiliac joint injection.

5. Advance the needle slowly and carefully into the SI joint.
6. Inject the steroid solution as a bolus into the sacroiliac joint. The injected solution should flow smoothly into the space. If increased resistance is encountered, advance or withdraw the needle slightly before attempting further injection.
7. Following injection of the corticosteroid solution, withdraw the needle.
8. Apply a sterile adhesive bandage.
9. Reexamine the sacroiliac joint in 5 min to confirm pain relief.

## AFTERCARE

- NSAIDs, ice, and/or physical therapy as indicated.
- Treatment of the underlying condition.
- Consider follow-up examination in 2 weeks.

**CPT code:** 20610—Arthrocentesis, aspiration, and/or injection of major joint or bursa

## PEARLS

- The successful placement of this injection may need ultrasound or fluoroscopic guidance.
- Use Pain Ease mist spray to provide a topical vapocoolant anesthetic effect. Both Ethyl Chloride and Pain Ease stream spray run down the skin. In this location, the product will follow gravity and accumulate in the patients' groin, thus turning this injection into a very uncomfortable experience!

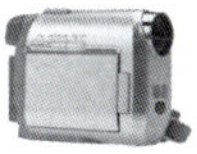

A video clip showing a sacroiliac joint injection can be found in the companion eBook.

## REFERENCES

1. Hawkins J, Schofferman J. Serial therapeutic sacroiliac joint injections: a practice audit. *Pain Med.* 2009;10(5):850–853.
2. Sadreddini S, Noshad H, Molaeefard M, et al. Unguided sacroiliac injection: effect on refractory buttock pain in patients with spondyloarthropathies. *Presse Med.* 2009;38(5):710–716.
3. Borowsky CD, Fagen G. Sources of sacroiliac region pain: insights gained from a study comparing standard intra-articular injection with a technique combining intra- and peri-articular injection. *Arch Phys Med Rehabil.* 2008;89(11):2048–2056.
4. Hartung W, Ross CJ, Straub R, et al. Ultrasound-guided sacroiliac joint injection in patients with established sacroiliitis: precise IA injection verified by MRI scanning does not predict clinical outcome. *Rheumatology (Oxford).* 2010;49(8):1479–1482.
5. Lee JH, Lee SH, Song SH. Clinical effectiveness of botulinum toxin A compared to a mixture of steroid and local anesthetics as a treatment for sacroiliac joint pain. *Pain Med.* 2010;11(5):692–700.
6. Kim WM, Lee HG, Jeong CW, et al. A randomized controlled trial of intra-articular prolotherapy versus steroid injection for sacroiliac joint pain. *J Altern Complement Med.* 2010;16(12):1285–1290.

# 8 Hip Joint—Preferred Lateral Approach

Hip joint pain from arthritis or capsulitis is a common condition seen in primary care medical practice. This often occurs as a result of osteoarthrosis, posttraumatic arthritis, and rheumatoid arthritis. Patients typically represent the middle-aged and older population. Septic arthritis in children is fortunately now a rare occurrence since the development of the *Haemophilus influenzae* and pneumococcal vaccines. Because of the joint's perceived inaccessibility, fear of vascular puncture, and the remote risk of avascular necrosis of the head of the femur, primary care physicians rarely perform aspiration and corticosteroid injections of the hip joint. In fact, access to this joint is straightforward. Anterior and lateral approaches have been described. The landmark-guided anterior approach has success rates of 60% to 93%.[1,2] The lateral approach also has good success rates of about 80%.[1,3] However, the anterior approach is associated with significantly more risk to the femoral artery and femoral nerve than the lateral approach.[1,3] For this reason, the lateral approach is preferred in the setting where image guidance is not available. In both cases, the use of ultrasound to guide needle placement significantly improves the safety and success rates of hip injections.[4,5] Guidance is particularly important in obese patients, patients with advanced osteoarthritis with no joint space, and those with flexion deformity.[6]

| Indications | ICD-9 Code | ICD-10 Code |
|---|---|---|
| Hip pain | 719.45 | M25.559 |
| Hip capsulitis | 726.5 | M70.70 |
| Hip arthritis, unspecified | 716.95 | M12.9 |
| Hip osteoarthritis, primary | 715.15 | M16.10 |
| Hip osteoarthritis, posttraumatic | 716.15 | M12.559 |
| Hip osteoarthritis, secondary | 715.25 | M16.7 |

**Relevant Anatomy:** (Fig. 8.1)

## PATIENT POSITION

- Lying on the examination table in the lateral decubitus position on the unaffected hip.

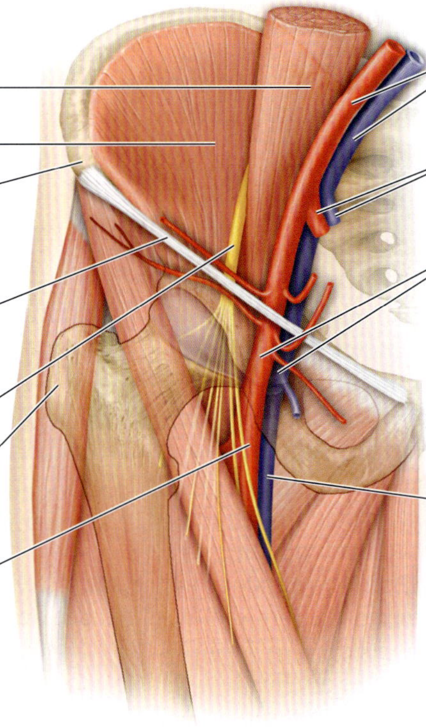


***FIGURE 8.1*** • Right lateral hip and femoral triangle. (From Tank PW, Gest TR. *Lippincott Williams & Wilkins Atlas of Anatomy*. Philadelphia, PA: Lippincott Williams & Wilkins, 2009.)

## LANDMARKS

1. With the patient lying on the examination table in the lateral decubitus position on the unaffected hip, the clinician stands posterior to the affected hip.
2. Identify the trochanter of the femur.
3. Mark a point 1 cm proximal to the tip of the greater trochanter.
4. (Optional) Use ultrasound to image the hip joint.
5. At that site, press firmly on the skin with the retracted tip of a ballpoint pen. This indention represents the entry point for the needle.
6. After the landmarks are identified, the patient should not move the hip.

## ANESTHESIA

- Local anesthesia of the skin using topical vapocoolant spray

## EQUIPMENT

- 20-mL syringe—for aspiration
- 3-mL syringe—for the injection of corticosteroid/local anesthetic mixture
- 25-gauge, 2 in. needle in thin individuals. Otherwise, use a 25-gauge, 3½ in. needle (for injections only)
- 20-gauge, 2 in. needle in thin individuals. Otherwise, use a 20-gauge, 3½ in. needle (for aspirations and injections)

- 3 mL of 1% lidocaine without epinephrine
- 1 mL of the steroid solution (40 mg of triamcinolone acetonide)
- One alcohol prep pad
- Two povidone–iodine prep pads
- Sterile gauze pads
- Sterile adhesive bandage
- Nonsterile, clean chucks pad

## TECHNIQUE

1. (Optional) Use an ultrasound to image the hip joint using an adjacent but separate acoustic window. This allows imaging separate from the injection site so that there is no contamination from the ultrasound gel. Alternatively, the entire site may be prepped in an aseptic manner and sterile ultrasound gel utilized.
2. Prep the insertion site with alcohol followed by the povidone–iodine pads.
3. Achieve good local anesthesia by using topical vapocoolant spray.
4. Position the needle and syringe perpendicular to the skin with the tip of the needle directed medially toward the hip joint.
5. Using the no-touch technique, introduce the needle at the insertion site (Fig. 8.2).
6. Advance the needle toward the hip joint until the needle tip contacts the femoral neck/head. Back up the needle 1 to 2 mm.
7. Inject the steroid solution as a bolus into the hip joint capsule. The injected solution should flow smoothly into the space. If increased resistance is encountered, advance or withdraw the needle slightly before attempting further injection.
8. Following injection of the corticosteroid solution, withdraw the needle.
9. Apply a sterile adhesive bandage.
10. Instruct the patient to move his or her hip through its full range of motion. This movement distributes the steroid solution throughout the hip joint capsule.
11. Reexamine the hip in 5 min to confirm pain relief.

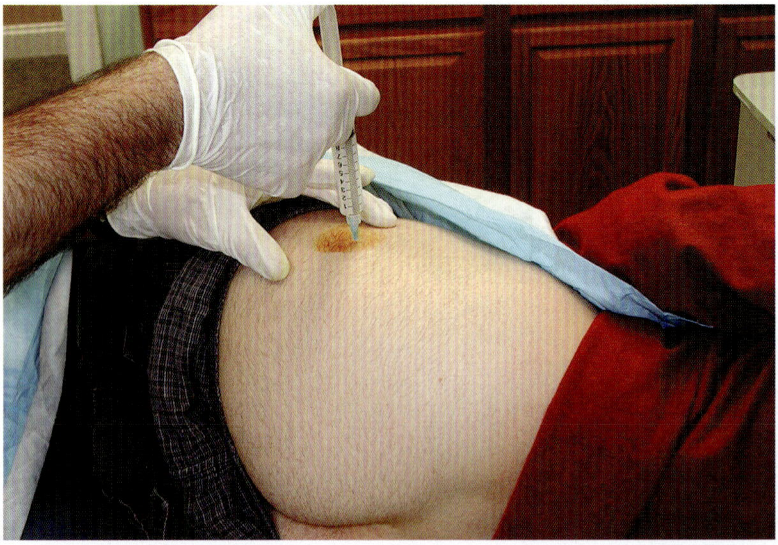

**FIGURE 8.2** Hip joint injection—preferred lateral approach.

## AFTERCARE

- Avoid excessive weight bearing and hip movement over the next 2 weeks.
- Nonsteroidal anti-inflammatory drugs (NSAIDs), and/or physical therapy as indicated.
- Consider follow-up examination in 2 weeks.

**CPT code:** 20610—Arthrocentesis, aspiration, and/or injection of the major joint or bursa

## PEARLS

- Guidance is particularly important in obese patients, patients with advanced osteoarthritis with no joint space, and those with flexion deformity.[6]

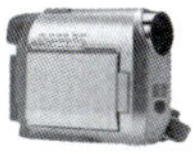

A video clip showing a hip joint injection can be found in the companion eBook.

## REFERENCES


1. Leopold SS, Battista V, Oliverio JA. Safety and efficacy of intraarticular hip injection using anatomic landmarks. *Clin Orthop Relat Res*. 2001;(391):192–197.
2. Mei-Dan O, McConkey MO, Petersen B, et al. The anterior approach for a non-image-guided intra-articular hip injection. *Arthroscopy*. 2013;29(6):1025–1033.
3. Ziv YB, Kardosh R, Debi R, et al. An inexpensive and accurate method for hip injections without the use of imaging. *J Clin Rheumatol*. 2009;15(3):103–105.
4. Gilliland CA, Salazar LD, Borchers JR. Ultrasound versus anatomic guidance for intra-articular and periarticular injection: a systematic review. *Phys Sportsmed*. 2011;39(3):121–131.
5. Migliore A, Tormenta S, Martin Martin LS, et al. Safety profile of 185 ultrasound-guided intra-articular injections for treatment of rheumatic diseases of the hip. *Reumatismo*. 2004;56(2):104–109.
6. Kurup H, Ward P. Do we need radiological guidance for hip joint injections? *Acta Orthop Belg*. 2010;76(2): 205–207.

# Hip Joint—Anterior Approach

Hip joint pain from arthritis or capsulitis is a common condition seen in primary care medical practice. This often occurs as a result of osteoarthrosis, posttraumatic arthritis, and rheumatoid arthritis. Patients typically represent the middle-aged and older population. Septic arthritis in children is fortunately now a rare occurrence since the development of the *H. influenzae* and pneumococcal vaccines. Because of the joint's perceived inaccessibility, fear of vascular puncture, and the remote risk of avascular necrosis of the head of the femur, primary care physicians rarely perform aspiration and corticosteroid injections of the hip joint. In fact, access to this joint is straightforward. Anterior and lateral approaches have been described. The landmark-guided anterior approach has success rates of 60% to 93%.[1,2] The lateral approach also has good success rates of about 80%.[1,3] However, the anterior approach is associated with significantly more risk to the femoral artery and femoral nerve than the lateral approach.[1,3] For this reason, the anterior approach is not recommended and the lateral approach is preferred in the setting where image guidance is not available. In both cases, the use of ultrasound to guide needle placement significantly improves the safety and success rates of hip injections.[4,5] Guidance is particularly important in obese patients, patients with advanced osteoarthritis with no joint space, and those with flexion deformity.[6]

| Indications | ICD-9 Code | ICD-10 Code |
|---|---|---|
| Hip pain | 719.45 | M25.559 |
| Hip capsulitis | 726.5 | M70.70 |
| Hip arthritis, unspecified | 716.95 | M12.9 |
| Hip osteoarthritis, primary | 715.15 | M16.10 |
| Hip osteoarthritis, posttraumatic | 716.15 | M12.559 |
| Hip osteoarthritis, secondary | 715.25 | M16.7 |

**Relevant Anatomy:** (Fig. 8.3)

## PATIENT POSITION

- Supine on the examination table with the head of the bed slightly elevated.

## LANDMARKS

1. With the patient supine on the examination table, the clinician stands lateral to the affected hip.
2. Over the anterior aspect of the hip, identify the point at the intersection of two perpendicular lines. The first is distal and sagittal from the anterior superior iliac spine,

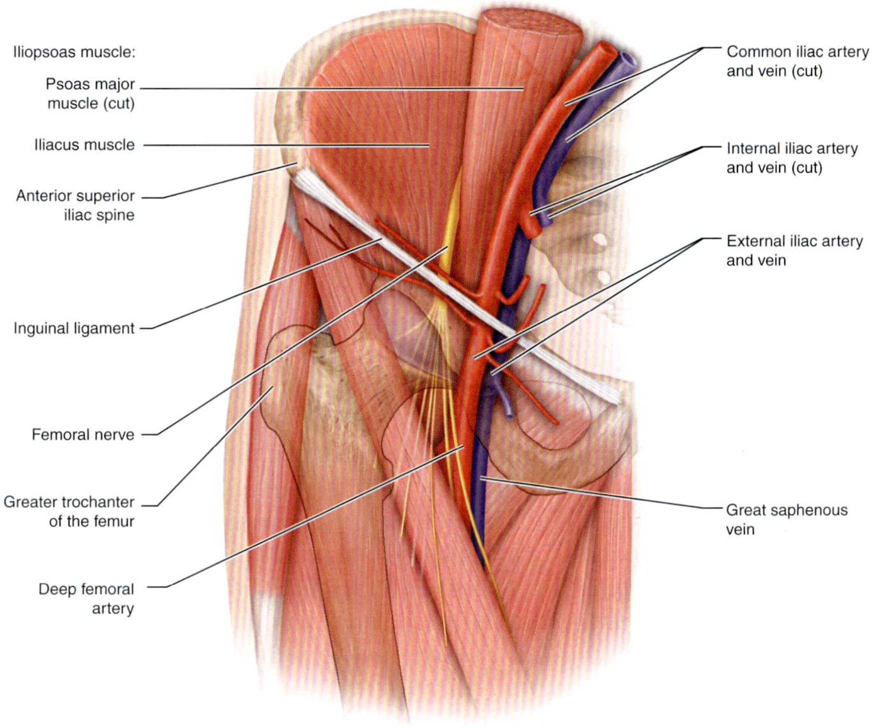


***FIGURE 8.3*** • Right anterior hip and femoral triangle. (From Tank PW, Gest TR. *Lippincott Williams & Wilkins Atlas of Anatomy*. Philadelphia, PA: Lippincott Williams & Wilkins, 2009.)

and the second line is transverse from the proximal tip of the greater trochanter. This point will be located about 3 cm lateral to the femoral artery. Mark that spot, which is directly over the hip joint.

3. (Optional) Use ultrasound to image the hip joint.
4. At that site, press firmly on the skin with the retracted tip of a ballpoint pen. This indention represents the entry point for the needle.
5. After the landmarks are identified, the patient should not move the hip.

## ANESTHESIA

- Local anesthesia of the skin using topical vapocoolant spray.

## EQUIPMENT

- 20-mL syringe—for aspiration
- 3-mL syringe—for the injection of corticosteroid/local anesthetic mixture
- 25-gauge, 1½ in. needle in thin individuals. Otherwise, use a 25-gauge, 3½ in. needle (for injections only)
- 20-gauge, 1½ in. needle in thin individuals. Otherwise, use a 20-gauge, 3½ in. needle (for aspirations and injections)
- 3 mL of 1% lidocaine without epinephrine
- 1 mL of the steroid solution (40 mg of triamcinolone acetonide)
- One alcohol prep pad
- Two povidone–iodine prep pads

- Sterile gauze pads
- Sterile adhesive bandage
- Nonsterile, clean chucks pad

## TECHNIQUE

1. (Optional) Use an ultrasound to image the hip joint using an adjacent but separate acoustic window. This allows imaging separate from the injection site so that there is no contamination from the ultrasound gel. Alternatively, the entire site may be prepped in an aseptic manner and sterile ultrasound gel utilized.
2. Prep the insertion site with alcohol followed by the povidone–iodine pads.
3. Achieve good local anesthesia by using topical vapocoolant spray.
4. Position the needle and syringe perpendicular to the skin with the tip of the needle directed posteriorly toward the hip joint.
5. Using the no-touch technique, introduce the needle at the insertion site (Fig. 8.4).
6. Advance the needle toward the hip joint until the needle tip contacts the junction of the femoral neck and femoral head. Back up the needle 1 to 2 mm.
7. Inject the steroid solution as a bolus into the hip joint capsule. The injected solution should flow smoothly into the space. If increased resistance is encountered, advance or withdraw the needle slightly before attempting further injection.
8. Following injection of the corticosteroid solution, withdraw the needle.
9. Apply a sterile adhesive bandage.
10. Instruct the patient to move his or her hip through its full range of motion. This movement distributes the steroid solution throughout the hip joint capsule.
11. Reexamine the hip in 5 min to confirm pain relief.

## AFTERCARE

- Avoid excessive weight bearing and hip movement over the next 2 weeks.
- NSAIDs and/or physical therapy as indicated.
- Consider follow-up examination in 2 weeks.

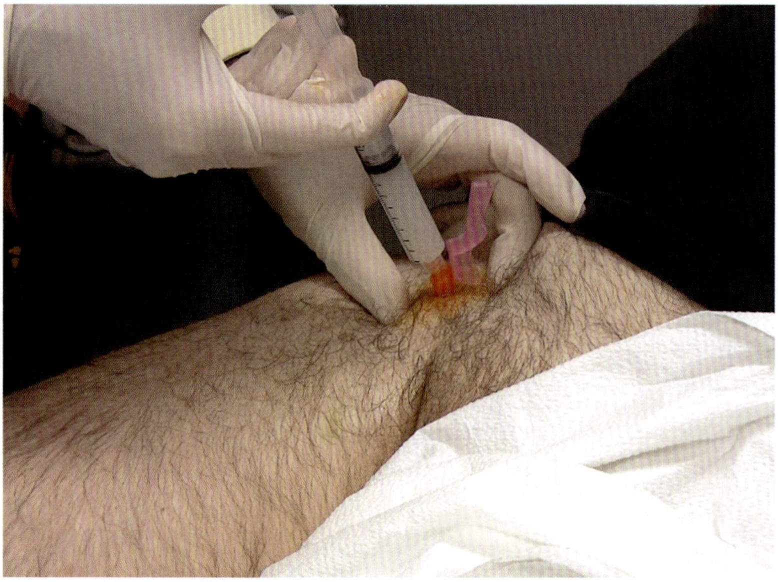

**FIGURE 8.4** ● Hip joint injection—anterior approach.

**CPT code:** 20610—Arthrocentesis, aspiration, and/or injection of the major joint or bursa

## PEARLS

- Guidance is particularly important in obese patients, patients with advanced osteoarthritis with no joint space, and those with flexion deformity.[6]

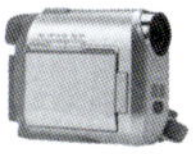

A video clip showing a hip joint injection can be found in the companion eBook.

## REFERENCES

1. Leopold SS, Battista V, Oliverio JA. Safety and efficacy of intraarticular hip injection using anatomic landmarks. *Clin Orthop Relat Res*. 2001;(391):192–197.
2. Mei-Dan O, McConkey MO, Petersen B, et al. The anterior approach for a non-image-guided intra-articular hip injection. *Arthroscopy*. 2013;29(6):1025–1033.
3. Ziv YB, Kardosh R, Debi R, et al. An inexpensive and accurate method for hip injections without the use of imaging. *J Clin Rheumatol*. 2009;15(3):103–105.
4. Gilliland CA, Salazar LD, Borchers JR. Ultrasound versus anatomic guidance for intra-articular and periarticular injection: a systematic review. *Phys Sportsmed*. 2011;39(3):121–131.
5. Migliore A, Tormenta S, Martin Martin LS, et al. Safety profile of 185 ultrasound-guided intra-articular injections for treatment of rheumatic diseases of the hip. *Reumatism*. 2004;56(2):104–109.
6. Kurup H, Ward P. Do we need radiological guidance for hip joint injections? *Acta Orthop Belg*. 2010;76(2): 205–207.

# Piriformis Syndrome

Patients uncommonly present to the primary care office for the evaluation of piriformis syndrome. This is an often overlooked disorder attributed to 6% to 8% of patients presenting with low back and leg pain. It is presumed to be a compression neuropathy that occurs when an abnormally tight piriformis muscle compresses the sciatic nerve. It may occur following trauma, vigorous physical activity, developmental abnormalities, or cerebral palsy or after total hip arthroplasty. The diagnosis may be made by excluding other causes of sciatica, palpating an abnormally tight and tender piriformis muscle, and the demonstration of a positive figure-four test. Treatment consists of stretching, physical therapy, local corticosteroid injection,[1] botulinum toxin injection,[2,3] and, rarely, surgery. Image guidance improves injection success rates.[1,4]

| Indication | ICD-9 Code | ICD-10 Code |
|---|---|---|
| Injury to the sciatic nerve at the thigh/hip | 956.0 | S74.00XA |

**Relevant Anatomy:** (Fig. 8.5)

## PATIENT POSITION

- Standing up with the back in forward flexion and hands/arms supported by the examination table.
- Alternatively, this injection may be performed with the patient lying in the lateral decubitus position on the examination table.

## LANDMARKS

1. With the patient standing up with the back in forward flexion and hands/arms supported by the examination table, the clinician stands directly behind the patient.
2. Locate the S2 median sacral crest and the lateral aspect of the femoral trochanter.
3. Identify the point of maximal tenderness over the piriformis muscle. This will be one-third to one-half of the distance from the sacral crest.
4. At that site, press firmly on the skin with the retracted tip of a ballpoint pen. This indention represents the entry point for the needle.
5. After the landmarks are identified, the patient should not move.

## ANESTHESIA

- Local anesthesia of the skin with a topical vapocoolant spray may be used, but it is not necessary in most patients.

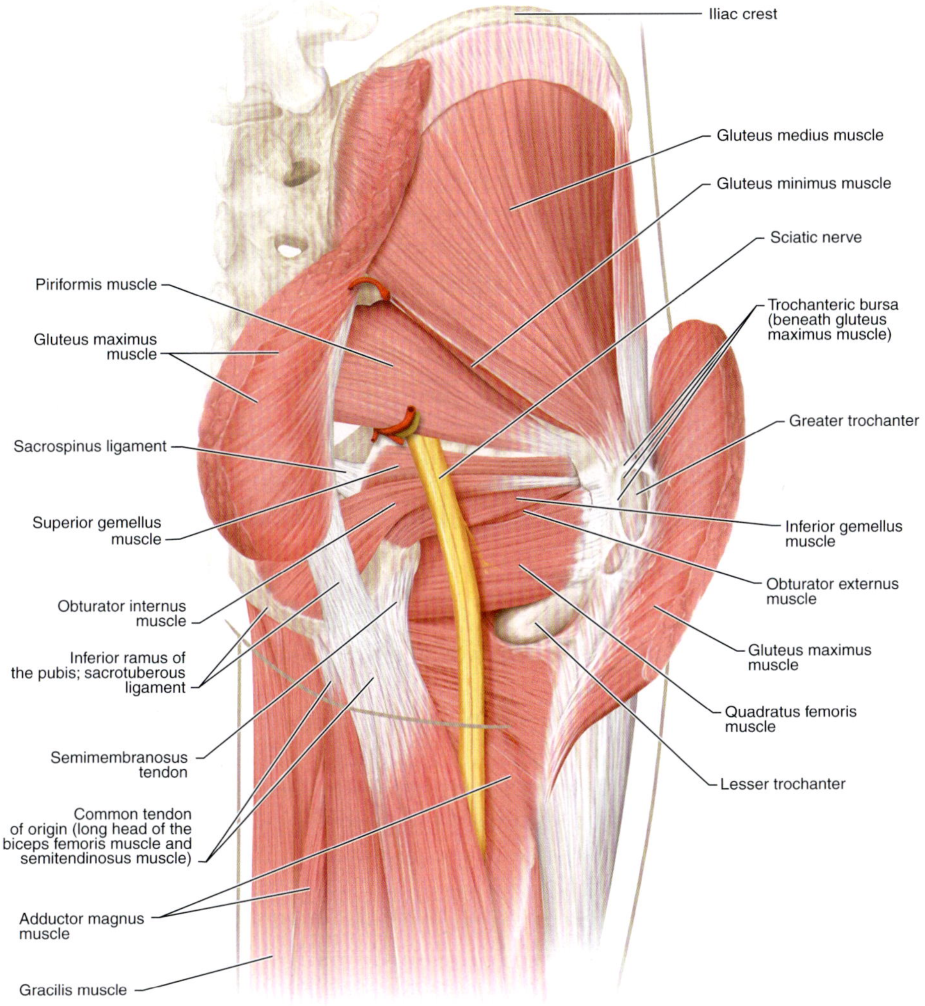


***FIGURE 8.5*** • Middle and deep gluteal muscles and sciatic nerve. (From Tank PW, Gest TR. *Lippincott Williams & Wilkins Atlas of Anatomy*. Philadelphia, PA: Lippincott Williams & Wilkins, 2009.)

## EQUIPMENT

- 3-mL syringe
- 25-gauge, 1½ to 2 in. needle
- 1 mL of 1% lidocaine without epinephrine
- 1 mL of the steroid solution (40 mg of triamcinolone acetonide)
- One alcohol prep pad
- Two povidone–iodine prep pads
- Sterile gauze pads
- Sterile adhesive bandage

## TECHNIQUE

1. Prep the insertion site with alcohol followed by the povidone–iodine pads.
2. Achieve good local anesthesia by using a topical vapocoolant spray.

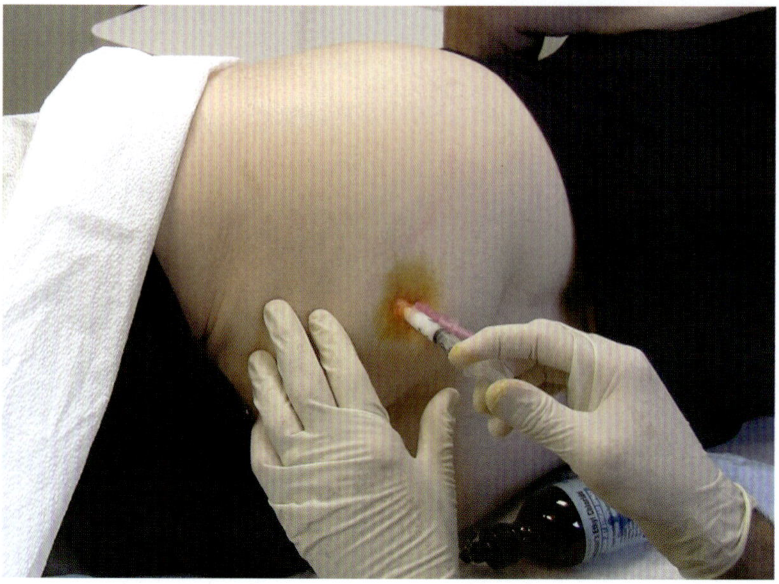

***FIGURE 8.6*** ● Piriformis muscle injection.

3. Position the needle and syringe perpendicular to the skin with the tip of the needle directed anteriorly.
4. Using the no-touch technique, introduce the needle at the insertion site (Fig. 8.6).
5. Advance the needle until you feel that there is an increase in resistance in the muscle due to spasm and/or fibrosis. If the patient experiences sudden shooting pain down the leg, the sciatic nerve has been contacted. Withdraw the needle a few millimeter until there is no pain.
6. Aspirate to ensure no blood return and inject the volume of the syringe into the soft tissues. The injected solution should flow smoothly. If increased resistance is encountered, advance or withdraw the needle slightly before attempting further injection.
7. Following injection of the corticosteroid solution, withdraw the needle.
8. Apply a sterile adhesive bandage.
9. Instruct the patient to move his or her hip through its full range of motion. This movement distributes the steroid solution throughout the course of the piriformis muscle.
10. Reexamine the piriformis muscle in 5 min to confirm pain relief.

## AFTERCARE

- Avoid excessive use of the affected hip over the next 2 weeks.
- NSAIDs, ice, and/or physical therapy as indicated.
- Consider follow-up examination in 2 weeks.

**CPT code:** 20552—Injection of trigger point(s) in one to two muscle groups

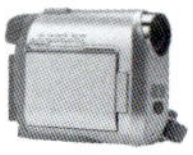

A video clip showing a piriformis injection can be found in the companion eBook.

## REFERENCES

1. Masala S, Crusco S, Meschini A, et al. Piriformis syndrome: long-term follow-up in patients treated with percutaneous injection of anesthetic and corticosteroid under CT guidance. *Cardiovasc Intervent Radiol.* 2012;35(2):375–382.
2. Waseem Z, Boulias C, Gordon A, et al. Botulinum toxin injections for low-back pain and sciatica. *Cochrane Database Syst Rev*. 2011;(1):CD008257.
3. Yoon SJ, Ho J, Kang HY, et al. Low-dose botulinum toxin type A for the treatment of refractory piriformis syndrome. *Pharmacotherapy*. 2007;27(5):657–665.
4. Clendenen SR, Candler SA, Osborne MD, et al. Needle placement for piriformis injection using 3-D imaging. *Pain Physician*. 2013;16(3):E301–E310.

# Meralgia Paresthetica

Patients occasionally present to their primary care provider with burning pain, numbness, or paresthesias over the lateral aspect of the thigh. Meralgia paresthetica is most commonly caused by a compression neuropathy of the lateral femoral cutaneous nerve of the thigh as it passes through a tunnel formed by the lateral attachment of the inguinal ligament and the anterior superior iliac spine. It is more common in patients with diabetes. Percussion of the nerve over this tunnel just anterior to the anterior iliac spine or extending the thigh posteriorly may reproduce or worsen the symptoms. Conservative management includes relieving chronic pressure over the nerve, weight loss, and antineuropathic medications. Corticosteroid injections at the site of nerve compression demonstrate high success rates when guided by ultrasound.[1] Other treatment options include ultrasound-guided hydrodissection of the nerve,[2] and surgical decompression[3] or nerve transection.

| Indication | ICD-9 Code | ICD-10 Code |
|---|---|---|
| Neuritis, unspecified | 729.2 | G57.10 |

**Relevant Anatomy:** (Figs. 8.7 and 8.8)

## PATIENT POSITION

- Lying supine on the examination table.
- Rotate the patient's head away from the side that is being injected. This minimizes anxiety and pain perception.

## LANDMARKS

1. With the patient supine on the examination table, the clinician stands lateral to the affected hip.
2. Find the anterior superior iliac spine and the pubic bone.
3. Firmly palpate the inguinal ligament that connects these two structures.
4. The lateral femoral cutaneous nerve of the thigh traverses the inguinal ligament about 2 cm inferior and medial to the anterior superior iliac spine under the inguinal ligament. Tap over this area or press firmly until discomfort is elicited. Mark that spot with ink.
5. At that site, press firmly on the skin with the retracted tip of a ballpoint pen. This indention represents the entry point for the needle.
6. After the landmarks are identified, the patient should not move the hip or leg.

## ANESTHESIA

- Local anesthesia of the skin with a topical vapocoolant spray may be used, but it is not necessary in most patients.

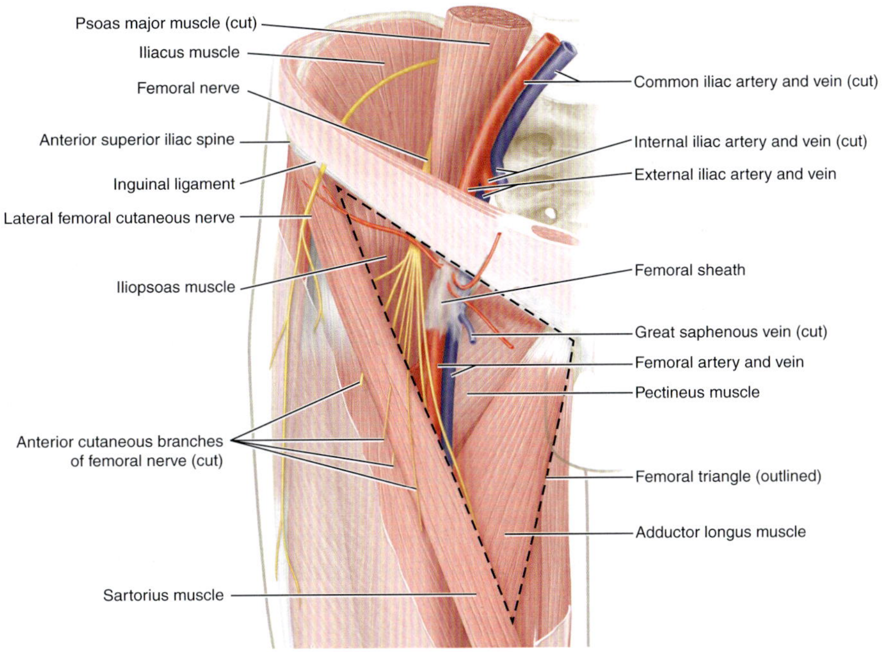


***FIGURE 8.7*** ● Anterior right hip neurovascular structures. (Adapted from Tank PW, Gest TR. *Lippincott Williams & Wilkins Atlas of Anatomy*. Philadelphia, PA: Lippincott Williams & Wilkins, 2009.)

## EQUIPMENT

- 3-mL syringe
- 25-gauge, 1½ in. needle
- 8 mL[1] of 1% lidocaine without epinephrine
- 1 mL of the steroid solution (40 mg of triamcinolone acetonide)
- One alcohol prep pad
- Two povidone–iodine prep pads
- Sterile gauze pads
- Sterile adhesive bandage

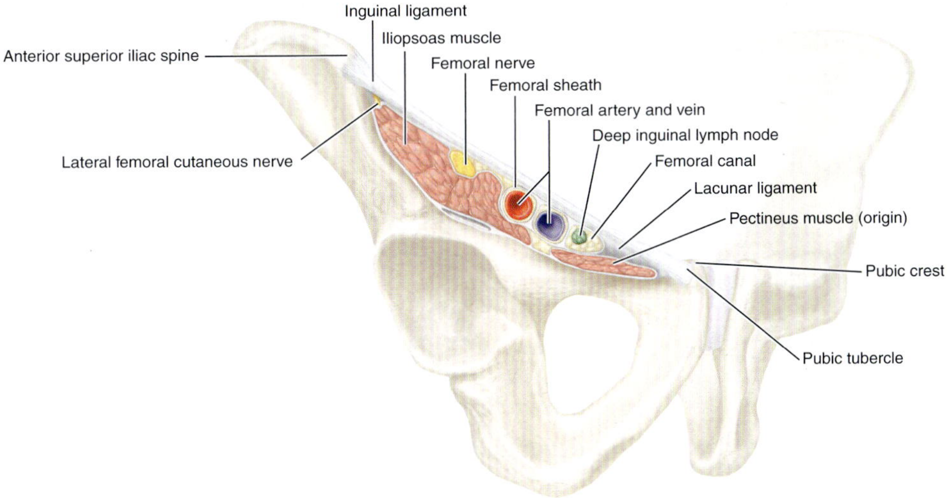


***FIGURE 8.8*** ● Section through the right femoral sheath. (Adapted from Tank PW, Gest TR. *Lippincott Williams & Wilkins Atlas of Anatomy*. Philadelphia, PA: Lippincott Williams & Wilkins, 2009.)

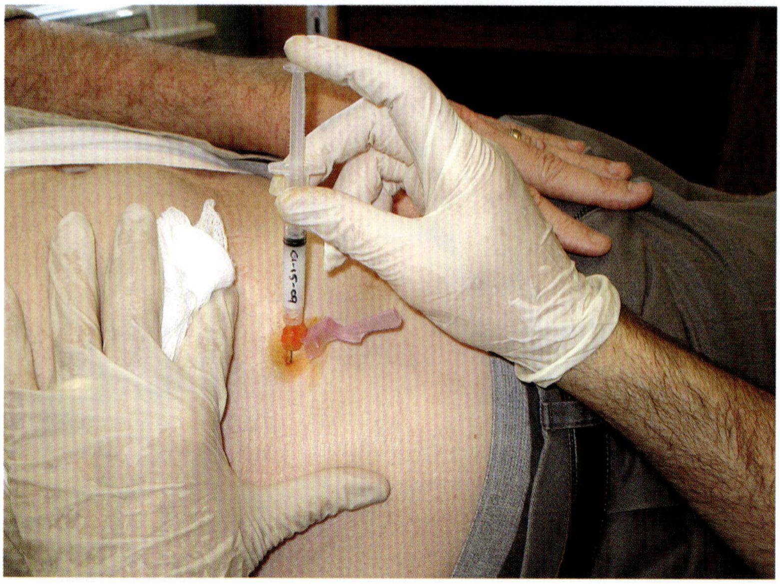

***FIGURE 8.9*** Meralgia paresthetica injection.

## TECHNIQUE

1. Prep the insertion site with alcohol followed by the povidone–iodine pads.
2. Achieve good local anesthesia by using a topical vapocoolant spray.
3. Position the needle and syringe perpendicular to the skin with the tip of the needle directed posteriorly.
4. Using the no-touch technique, introduce the needle at the insertion site (Fig. 8.9).
5. Advance the needle 2 to 3 cm until the needle tip is located under the inguinal ligament.
6. Inject the steroid solution as a bolus into the area. The injected solution should flow smoothly into the space. If increased resistance is encountered, advance or withdraw the needle slightly before attempting further injection.
7. Following injection of the corticosteroid solution, withdraw the needle.
8. Apply a sterile adhesive bandage.
9. Instruct the patient to move his or her hip through its full range of motion. This movement distributes the steroid solution throughout the area.

## AFTERCARE

- Treatment is directed at relieving the compression and usually consists of wearing looser clothing or losing weight.
- Consider follow-up examination in 2 weeks.

**CPT code:** 64450—Injection, nerve block, therapeutic, other peripheral nerve or branch

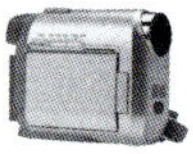

A video clip showing a meralgia paresthetica injection can be found in the companion eBook.

## REFERENCES

1. Tagliafico A, Serafini G, Lacelli F, et al. Ultrasound-guided treatment of meralgia paresthetica (lateral femoral cutaneous neuropathy): technical description and results of treatment in 20 consecutive patients. *J Ultrasound Med*. 2011;30(10):1341–1346.
2. Mulvaney SW. Ultrasound-guided percutaneous neuroplasty of the lateral femoral cutaneous nerve for the treatment of meralgia paresthetica: a case report and description of a new ultrasound-guided technique. *Curr Sports Med Rep*. 2011;10(2):99–104.
3. Siu TL, Chandran KN. Neurolysis for meralgia paresthetica: an operative series of 45 cases. *Surg Neurol*. 2005;63(1):19–23.

# Greater Trochanteric Pain Syndrome

Greater trochanteric pain syndrome is a term used to describe pain involving the lateral aspect of the hip. This regional pain syndrome includes pain from trochanteric bursitis but also often mimics pain from other sources including myofascial pain, degenerative joint disease, and spinal pathology. The prevalence is higher in women, and patients with coexisting low back pain, osteoarthritis, iliotibial band tenderness, and obesity. Symptoms include persistent pain over the lateral hip that may radiate along the lateral aspect of the thigh to the knee and occasionally to the buttock. Physical examination reveals point tenderness in the posterolateral area of the greater trochanter.[1] Conservative therapy includes stretching, therapeutic exercise, and physical modalities focused on the low back/pelvic core and sacroiliac joints. Local corticosteroid injection into the area of maximal tenderness has demonstrated effectiveness.[2,3] Recalcitrant cases may be treated with low-energy shock wave therapy, iliotibial band release, subgluteal bursectomy, and trochanteric reduction osteotomy.

| **Indication** | **ICD-9 Code** | **ICD-10 Code** |
|---|---|---|
| Trochanteric bursitis | 726.5 | M70.70 |

**Relevant Anatomy:** (Fig. 8.10)

## PATIENT POSITION

- Lying on the examination table in the lateral decubitus position on the unaffected hip.

## LANDMARKS

1. With the patient lying on the examination table in the lateral decubitus position on the unaffected hip, the clinician stands behind the patient.
2. Identify and mark the area(s) of maximal tenderness over the greater trochanter.
3. At that area, press firmly on the skin with the retracted tip of a ballpoint pen. This indention represents the entry point(s) for the needle.
4. After the landmarks are identified, the patient should not move the hip.

## ANESTHESIA

- Local anesthesia of the skin with topical vapocoolant spray may be used.

## EQUIPMENT

- 5-mL syringe
- 25-gauge, 1½ in. needle

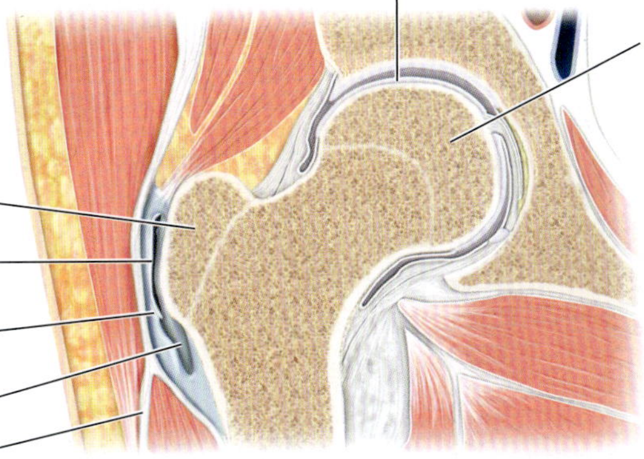


***FIGURE 8.10*** • Right anterior hip joint and trochanteric structures. (Adapted from Tank PW, Gest TR. *Lippincott Williams & Wilkins Atlas of Anatomy*. Philadelphia, PA: Lippincott Williams & Wilkins, 2009.)

- 3 mL of 1% lidocaine without epinephrine
- 1 mL of the steroid solution (40 mg of triamcinolone acetonide)
- One alcohol prep pad
- Two povidone–iodine prep pads
- Sterile gauze pads
- Sterile adhesive bandage

## TECHNIQUE

1. Prep the insertion site(s) with alcohol followed by the povidone–iodine pads.
2. Achieve good local anesthesia by using topical vapocoolant spray.
3. Position the needle and syringe perpendicular to the skin with the tip of the needle directed medially.
4. Using the no-touch technique, introduce the needle at the insertion site(s).
5. Advance the needle toward the femoral trochanter until the needle tip touches the bone. Back up the needle 1 to 2 mm.
6. Inject the steroid solution as a bolus steadily in the area of the trochanteric bursa. The injected solution should flow smoothly into the space. If increased resistance is encountered, advance or withdraw the needle slightly before attempting further injection.
7. Repeat the injection at other adjacent painful areas if needed.
8. Following injection(s) of the corticosteroid solution, withdraw the needle.
9. Apply a sterile adhesive bandage(s).
10. Instruct the patient to massage the area and move his or her hip through its full range of motion. This movement distributes the steroid solution throughout the trochanteric bursa.
11. Reexamine the area of the trochanteric bursa in 5 min to confirm pain relief (Fig. 8.11).

## AFTERCARE

- Avoid excessive hip movement over the next 2 weeks.
- NSAIDs, ice, heat, and/or physical therapy as indicated.
- Consider follow-up examination in 2 weeks.

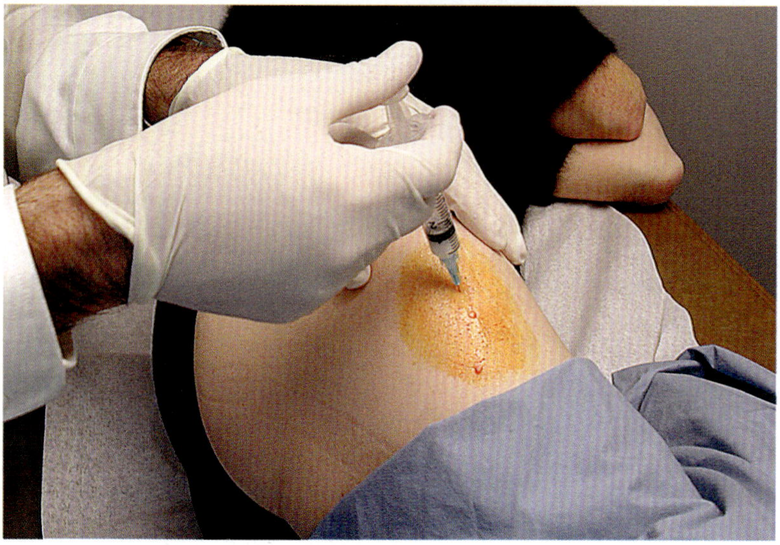

**FIGURE 8.11** Greater trochanteric pain syndrome injection.

**CPT code:** 20551—Injection of tendon origin or insertion

## PEARLS

- Consider fanning this injection to disperse the corticosteroid solution over a wider area.

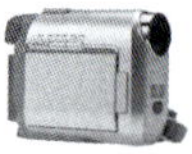

A video clip showing a trochanteric bursitis injection can be found in the companion eBook.

## REFERENCES


1. Williams BS, Cohen SP. Greater trochanteric pain syndrome: a review of anatomy, diagnosis and treatment. *Anesth Analg*. 2009;108(5):1662–1670.
2. Brinks A, van Rijn RM, Willemsen SP, et al. Corticosteroid injections for greater trochanteric pain syndrome: a randomized controlled trial in primary care. *Ann Fam Med*. 2011;9(3):226–234.
3. McEvoy JR, Lee KS, Blankenbaker DG, et al. Ultrasound-guided corticosteroid injections for treatment of greater trochanteric pain syndrome: greater trochanter bursa versus subgluteus medius bursa. *AJR Am J Roentgenol*. 2013;201(2):W313–W317.

# Hip Adductor Tendonitis

Patients occasionally present to the primary care office for the evaluation and treatment of pain upon adduction of the hip. The pectineus, adductor longus, magnus, and medius muscles connect the medial aspect of the femur to the pubic bone. Acute injury or chronic overuse may cause tendonitis or tendinopathy of the hip adductors. The adductor longus is most commonly injured, and patients classically present with pain upon palpation of the muscle belly and insertion, passive stretching, and resistance to contraction. In chronic tendonitis, treatment is often lengthy and difficult. Physical therapy is the cornerstone of treatment. It may be facilitated by the judicious use of corticosteroid injections given around the affected tendon(s).

| Indication | ICD-9 Code | ICD-10 Code |
|---|---|---|
| Enthesopathy of the hip | 726.5 | M76.819 |

**Relevant Anatomy:** (Fig. 8.12)

## PATIENT POSITION

- Lying supine on the examination table.
- Place the hip in a position of combined flexion abduction and external rotation.
- Rotate the patient's head away from the side that is being injected. This minimizes anxiety and pain perception.

## LANDMARKS

1. With the patient lying supine on the examination table, the clinician stands lateral and posterior to the affected hip.
2. Locate the symphysis pubis and trace the pubic bone laterally until the origin of the hip adductor muscles.
3. Determine the site of maximal tenderness over the tendons, and mark it with an ink pen.
4. At that site, press firmly on the skin with the retracted tip of a ballpoint pen. This indention represents the entry point for the needle.
5. After the landmarks are identified, the patient should not move the hip.

## ANESTHESIA

- Local anesthesia of the skin using a topical vapocoolant spray

## EQUIPMENT

- 3-mL syringe
- 25-gauge, 1½ in. needle

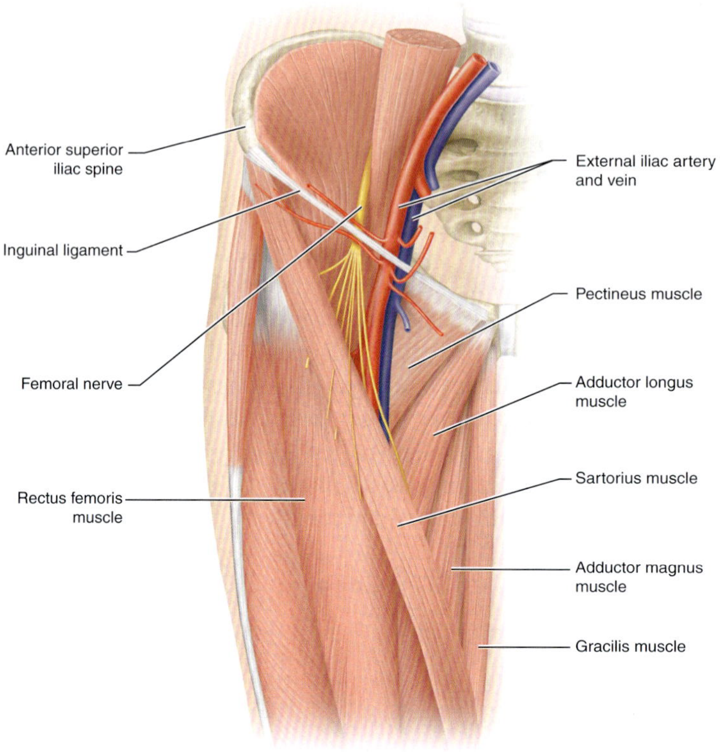


**FIGURE 8.12** Right thigh and femoral triangle structures. (From Tank PW, Gest TR. *Lippincott Williams & Wilkins Atlas of Anatomy*. Philadelphia, PA: Lippincott Williams & Wilkins, 2009.)

- 1 mL of 1% lidocaine without epinephrine
- 1 mL of the steroid solution (40 mg of triamcinolone acetonide)
- One alcohol prep pad
- Two povidone–iodine prep pads
- Sterile gauze pads
- Sterile adhesive bandage

## TECHNIQUE

1. Prep the insertion site with alcohol followed by the povidone–iodine pads.
2. Achieve good local anesthesia by using a topical vapocoolant spray.
3. Position the needle and syringe at an angle of 30 degrees to the skin with the tip of the needle directed proximally toward the pubic bone.
4. Using the no-touch technique, introduce the needle at the insertion site (Fig. 8.13).
5. Advance the needle so that it is positioned around the affected tendon, but not in the substance of the tendon.
6. Inject the steroid solution as a bolus around the adductor tendon(s). The injected solution should flow smoothly into the space. If increased resistance is encountered, advance or withdraw the needle slightly before attempting further injection.
7. Following injection of the corticosteroid solution, withdraw the needle.
8. Apply a sterile adhesive bandage.

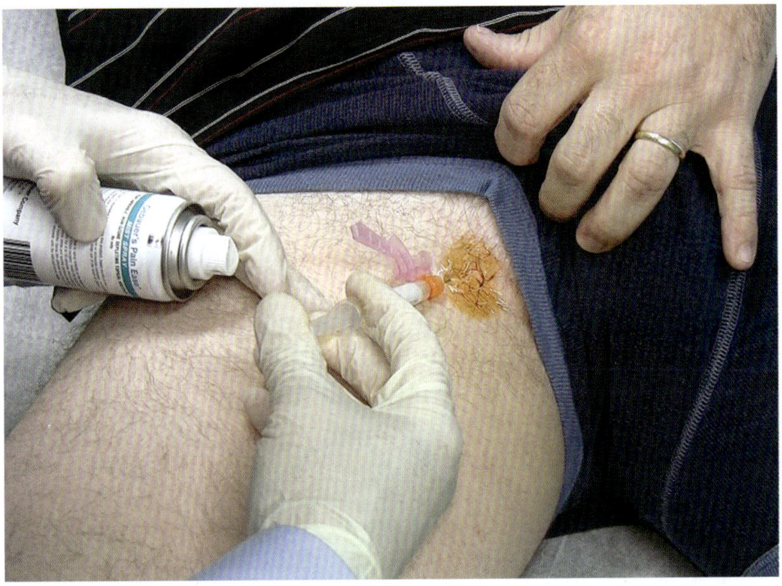

***FIGURE 8.13*** ● Hip adductor tendonitis injection.

9. Instruct the patient to massage the area and move his or her hip through its full range of motion. This movement distributes the steroid solution along the adductor tendon(s).
10. Reexamine the medial aspect of the hip in 5 min to confirm pain relief.

## AFTERCARE

- Avoid excessive use of the hip—especially hip abduction and adduction over the next 2 weeks.
- Begin a program of physical therapy.
- NSAIDs, ice, and heat as indicated.
- Consider follow-up examination in 2 weeks.

**CPT code:** 20551—Injection of tendon origin or insertion

## PEARLS

- This injection can be superficial—especially in thin persons. Depositing corticosteroid in the subcutaneous tissues can result in the complication of skin atrophy and hypopigmentation. Avoid the development of a subdermal wheal while performing all injections of corticosteroid solutions.

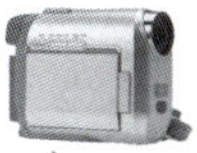

A video clip showing a hip adductor tendonitis injection can be found in the companion eBook.

# Knee Joint Injections

The need for aspiration and injection of the knee joint is commonly encountered by primary care physicians. The most common indications for this procedure include evaluation and treatment of monoarthritis, osteoarthritis, and inflammatory arthritis; to rule out septic arthritis; and removal of blood or reactive fluid following trauma. Arthrocentesis (aspiration) is employed to remove fluid from a joint for diagnostic synovial fluid analysis, to enhance comfort, to improve proprioception,[1] and to minimize dilution of injected substances. Injections of various products are also employed including corticosteroids,[2] hyaluronic acid viscosupplements,[3,4] platelet-rich plasma,[5] dextrose (prolotherapy),[6] etaneracept,[7] botulinum toxin,[8] and others.

Most practitioners use one of four palpation-based, anatomic landmark-guided approaches to perform aspirations and injections of the knee joint. Figure 8.14A and B shows the most common knee joint approaches—the extended-knee lateral suprapatellar, extended-knee lateral midpatellar, flexed-knee anteromedial, and flexed-knee anterolateral portals. The author avoids the medial suprapatellar and medial midpatellar approaches because of the limited operating space on the medial aspect of the knee/leg, to preserve patient modesty, and due to the lack of demonstrated accuracy and effectiveness in the medical literature. There is a general lack of consensus among experts regarding the best technique for knee joint injection and aspiration. An examination of the current medical literature (below), however, gives us some guidance. Although it appears that the lateral suprapatellar and lateral midpatellar approaches have an advantage over the others, the individual provider will ultimately determine the desired portal based on the scientific data, their expertise, history of success, and other patient-specific factors.

A review of literature however does give us some guidance in selecting the most successful approach and technique. A comprehensive review of injection accuracy was published in 2013 by Maricar et al.[9] Data from 23 publications were pooled and examined. Intra-articular knee injections at the lateral suprapatellar portal were most accurate (87%), while medial midpatellar (64%) and anterolateral joint line sites (70%) were least accurate. Furthermore, lateral suprapatellar, medial midpatellar, and medial suprapatellar sites were more accurate when using image guidance than when using anatomic landmarks.[9] Another systematic review of nine studies through July 2010 was done looking at the accuracy rates of various intra-articular injection approaches. Hermans[10] and associates found the extended-leg lateral suprapatellar approach (91%) to be the most accurate, as compared with the lateral midpatellar (85%), anteromedial (72%), and anterolateral (67%) approaches.[10] This success makes sense when the location of synovial fluid in the knee joint is considered. Hirsch[11] and colleagues demonstrated that small effusions were more commonly detected in the lateral suprapatellar pouch than elsewhere. In patients with painful knee arthritis, fluid distributes maximally to the lateral suprapatellar pouch in the extended knee.[11] Furthermore, Zhang et al.[12] found a "dry tap" rate of 10% in the extended leg supine position and 25% in the sitting position. This is a relatively easy procedure to perform, easily lends itself to ultrasound

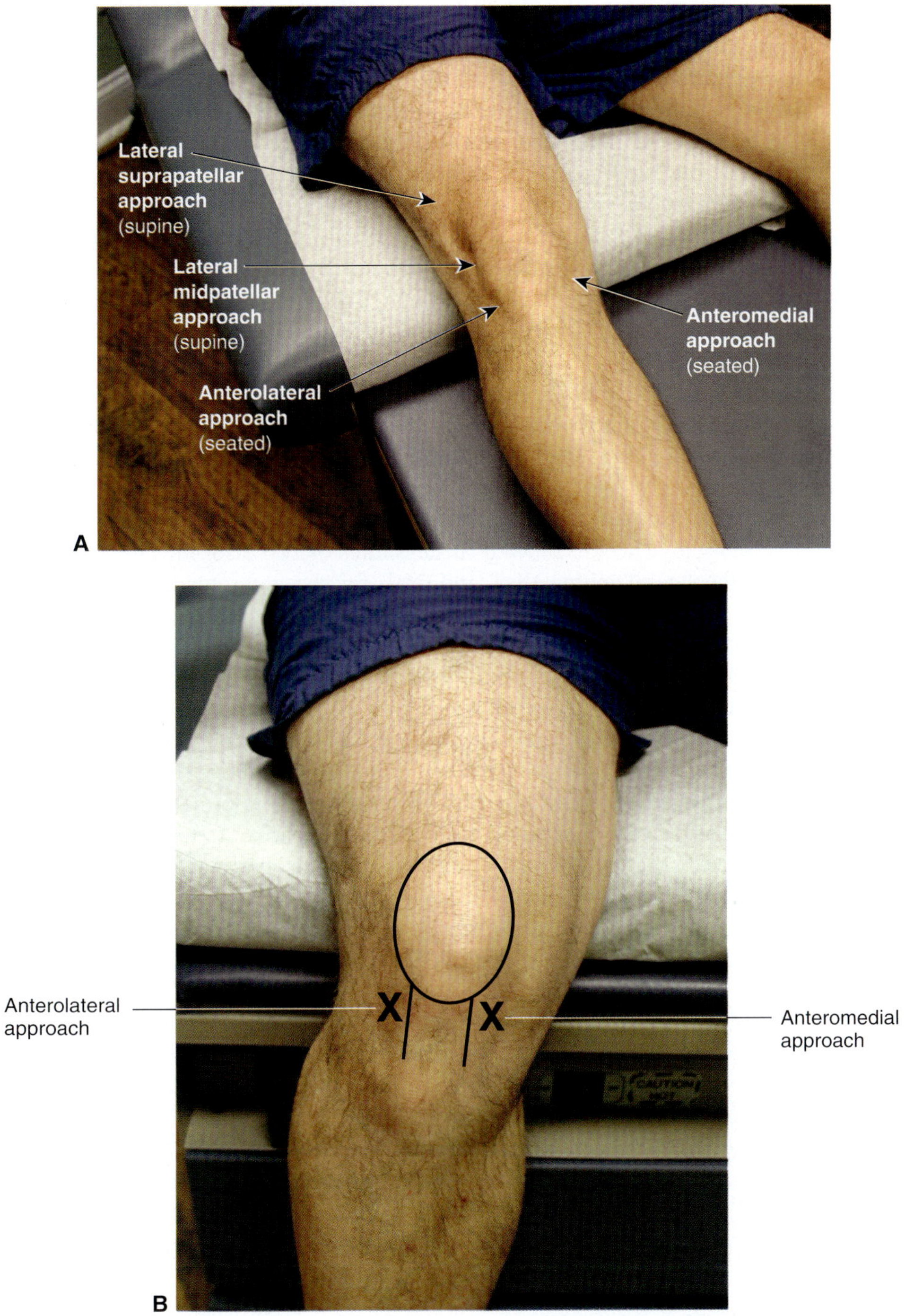


***FIGURE 8.14*** ● **A:** Right knee—the most common knee joint approaches. **B:** Flexed knee showing landmarks.

guidance without bony obstruction, and is well accepted by patients. Additionally, because of supine positioning, patients do not see the approaching needle and anxiety is diminished. For these reasons and based on the research, the extended-leg suprapatellar approach is the author's preferred technique and is highly recommended to others.

In an individual study by Jackson and colleagues using a 1½ in., 21-gauge needle, the lateral midpatellar approach was significantly more accurate (93%) than were the anteromedial (75%) and anterolateral (71%) approaches.[13] Toda and Tsukimura[14] reported that a modified 30-degree flexed-knee approach incorporating distal knee traction was significantly more accurate (86%) than were seated anteromedial (62%) and extended-leg lateral suprapatellar (70%) approaches using a 1½ in., 25-gauge needle. Accuracy rates increased with the presence of severe osteoarthritis.[14] In another investigation by Chavez-Chiang,[15] an anterolateral knee portal with 90-degree flexion targeting the synovial membrane of the medial femoral condyle with a 2-in., 21-gauge needle yielded an accuracy rate of 97%. This approach might be useful for patients who cannot lie down, transfer to an examination table, or extend the knee or those with flexion contractures.[15]

The use of musculoskeletal ultrasound dramatically increases the accuracy of knee injections. A number of studies now demonstrate significantly increased accuracy rates of injections when using ultrasound-guided techniques. The use of ultrasound increases the success rate to nearly 100%, even when performed by less experienced practitioners.[16] A study of ultrasound-guided injections in patients with moderate osteoarthritis using a 1½ in., 25-gauge needle showed success rates of 100% for the lateral suprapatellar, 95% for the lateral midpatellar, and 75% for the anteromedial approaches.[17] A review of 13 studies of the knee showed that imaging guidance with ultrasound improved the accuracy of intra-articular injections of the knee to 95.8% versus 77.8%, $P < 0.001$.[18] Employing a joint cupping maneuver from an inferior approach also improves the detection and removal of knee joint effusion by improving ultrasound visualization of the effusion.[19] The use of image-guided techniques is particularly important in patients without joint effusion and especially when injecting intra-articular viscosupplements to treat osteoarthritis of the knee.[20] Most importantly, there is statistically significant improvement in short-term (2 weeks) patient outcomes of pain and function with a reduction in adverse events when ultrasound-guided injections are compared to those guided by palpation of landmarks. These image-guided techniques also cause significantly less procedural pain, take no additional time to perform, lead to greater provider confidence with the procedure, and improve cost-effectiveness.[18,21,22]

## REFERENCES

1. Cho YR, Hong BY, Lim SH, et al. Effects of joint effusion on proprioception in patients with knee osteoarthritis: a single-blind, randomized controlled clinical trial. *Osteoarthritis Cartilage*. 2011;19(1):22–28.
2. Leung A, Liew D, Lim J, et al. The effect of joint aspiration and corticosteroid injections in osteoarthritis of the knee. *Int J Rheum Dis*. 2011;14(4):384–389.
3. Saito S, Kotake S. Is there evidence in support of the use of intra-articular hyaluronate in treating rheumatoid arthritis of the knee? A meta-analysis of the published literature. *Mod Rheumatol*. 2009;19(5):493–501.
4. Foti C, Cisari C, Carda S, et al. A prospective observational study of the clinical efficacy and safety of intra-articular sodium hyaluronate in synovial joints with osteoarthritis. *Eur J Phys Rehabil Med*. 2011;47(3):407–415.
5. Spaková T, Rosocha J, Lacko M, et al. Treatment of knee joint osteoarthritis with autologous platelet-rich plasma in comparison with hyaluronic acid. *Am J Phys Med Rehabil*. 2012;91(5):411–417.
6. Rabago D, Patterson JJ, Mundt M, et al. Dextrose prolotherapy for knee osteoarthritis: a randomized controlled trial. *Ann Fam Med*. 2013;11(3):229–237.
7. Liang DF, Huang F, Zhang JL, et al. A randomized, single-blind, parallel, controlled clinical study on single intra-articular injection of etanercept in treatment of inflammatory knee arthritis. *Zhonghua Nei Ke Za Zhi*. 2010;49(11):930–934.
8. Chou CL, Lee SH, Lu SY, et al. Therapeutic effects of intra-articular botulinum neurotoxin in advanced knee osteoarthritis. *J Chin Med Assoc*. 2010;73(11):573–580.
9. Maricar N, Parkes MJ, Callaghan MJ, et al. Where and how to inject the knee—a systematic review. *Semin Arthritis Rheum*. 2013;43(2):195–203.
10. Hermans J, Bierma-Zeinstra SM, Bos PK, et al. The most accurate approach for intra-articular needle placement in the knee joint: a systematic review. *Semin Arthritis Rheum*. 2011;41(2):106–115.

11. Hirsch G, O'Neill T, Kitas G, et al. Distribution of effusion in knee arthritis as measured by high-resolution ultrasound. *Clin Rheumatol.* 2012;31(8):1243–1246.
12. Zhang Q, Zhang T, Lv H, et al. Comparison of two positions of knee arthrocentesis: how to obtain complete drainage. *Am J Phys Med Rehabil.* 2012;91(7):611–615.
13. Jackson DW, Evans NA, Thomas BM. Accuracy of needle placement into the intra-articular space of the knee. *J Bone Joint Surg Am.* 2002;84-A(9):1522–1527.
14. Toda Y, Tsukimura N. A comparison of intra-articular hyaluronan injection accuracy rates between three approaches based on radiographic severity of knee osteoarthritis. *Osteoarthritis Cartilage.* 2008;16(9): 980–985.
15. Chavez-Chiang CE, Sibbitt WL Jr, Band PA, et al. The highly accurate anteriolateral portal for injecting the knee. *Sports Med Arthrosc Rehabil Ther Technol.* 2011;3(1):6.
16. Curtiss HM, Finnoff JT, Peck E, et al. Accuracy of ultrasound-guided and palpation-guided knee injections by an experienced and less-experienced injector using a superolateral approach: a cadaveric study. *PM R.* 2011;3(6):507–515.
17. Park Y, Lee SC, Nam HS, et al. Comparison of sonographically guided intra-articular injections at 3 different sites of the knee. *J Ultrasound Med.* 2011;30(12):1669–1676.
18. Berkoff DJ, Miller LE, Block JE. Clinical utility of ultrasound guidance for intra-articular knee injections: a review. *Clin Interv Aging.* 2012;7:89–95.
19. Uryasev O, Joseph OC, McNamara JP, et al. Novel joint cupping clinical maneuver for ultrasonographic detection of knee joint effusions. *Am J Emerg Med.* 2013;31(11):1598–1600.
20. Punzi L, Oliviero F. Arthrocentesis and synovial fluid analysis in clinical practice: value of sonography in difficult cases. *Ann N Y Acad Sci.* 2009;1154:152–158.
21. Wiler JL, Costantino TG, et al. Comparison of ultrasound-guided and standard landmark techniques for knee arthrocentesis. *J Emerg Med.* 2010;39(1):76–82.
22. Sibbitt WL Jr, Kettwich LG, Band PA, et al. Does ultrasound guidance improve the outcomes of arthrocentesis and corticosteroid injection of the knee? *Scand J Rheumatol.* 2012;41(1):66–72.

# Knee Joint—Preferred Lateral Suprapatellar Approach

The supine, extended-leg lateral suprapatellar approach to the knee joint is relatively easy to perform and is well accepted by patients. Because of supine positioning, patients do not see the approaching needle and anxiety is diminished. This approach is considered a safe procedure since there are no major arteries or nerves in the immediate path of the needle. Also, since the injection is done using the suprapatellar approach, it is extra-articular, but still within the joint space. As a result, joint fluid can be removed and injections performed without direct, large-needle injury to the articular cartilage. With the use of local anesthetic, this injection can help the clinician differentiate the etiology of knee pain. After pain has been eliminated as a confounding factor, the knee can be reexamined to assess structural integrity of the ligaments and menisci. For the reasons previously noted, the extended-leg lateral suprapatellar approach is the preferred technique to perform knee joint aspirations and injections.

| Indications | ICD-9 Code | ICD-10 Code |
|---|---|---|
| Knee pain | 719.46 | M25.569 |
| Knee sprain, unspecified site | 844.9 | S83.90 |
| Knee arthritis, unspecified | 716.96 | M13.96 |
| Knee osteoarthritis, primary | 715.16 | M17.10 |
| Knee osteoarthritis, posttraumatic | 716.16 | M12.569 |
| Knee osteoarthritis, secondary | 715.26 | M17.5 |

**Relevant Anatomy:** (Fig. 8.15)

## PATIENT POSITION

- Lying supine on the examination table with the knee extended, or slightly flexed and supported with folded towels or chucks pads as needed for patient comfort.
- Rotate the patient's head away from the side that is being injected. This minimizes anxiety and pain perception.

## LANDMARKS

1. With the patient lying supine on the examination table, the clinician stands lateral to the affected knee.
2. Locate the superior aspect of the patella.
3. Draw a line vertically 1 cm superior to the proximal margin of the patella (Fig. 8.16).
4. Next, draw a line horizontally along the posterior edge of the patella.
5. Identify the point where these two lines intersect.
6. At that site, press firmly on the skin with the retracted tip of a ballpoint pen. This indention represents the entry point for the needle.
7. After the landmarks are identified, the patient should not move the knee.

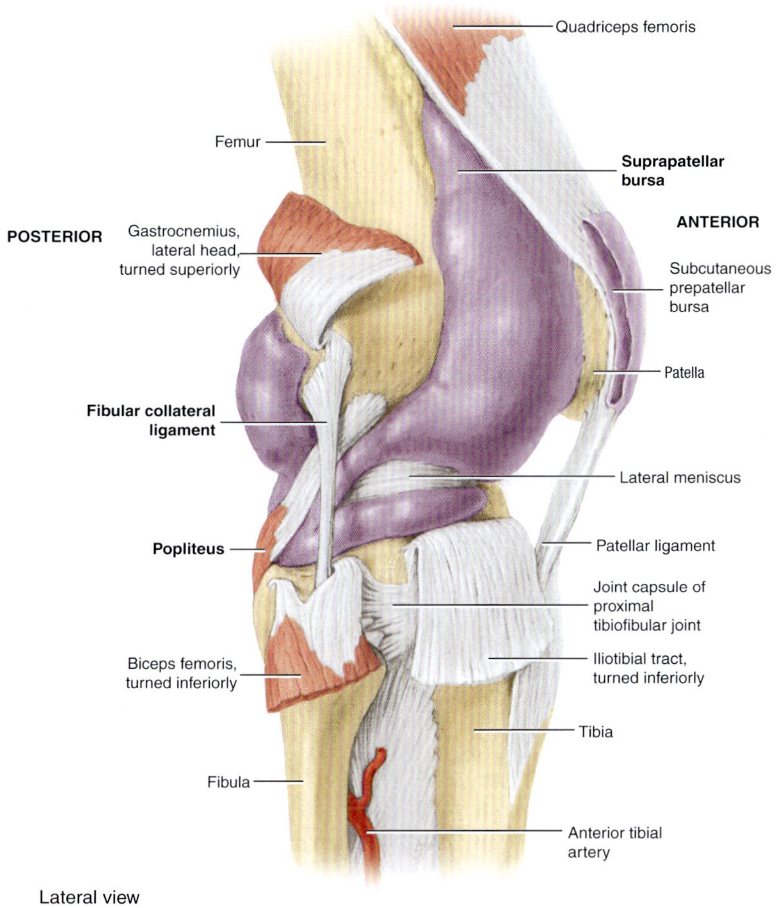


**FIGURE 8.15** ● Lateral aspect of the right knee showing the extent of the knee joint capsule (in purple). (Adapted from Tank PW, Gest TR. *Lippincott Williams & Wilkins Atlas of Anatomy*. Philadelphia, PA: Lippincott Williams & Wilkins, 2009.)

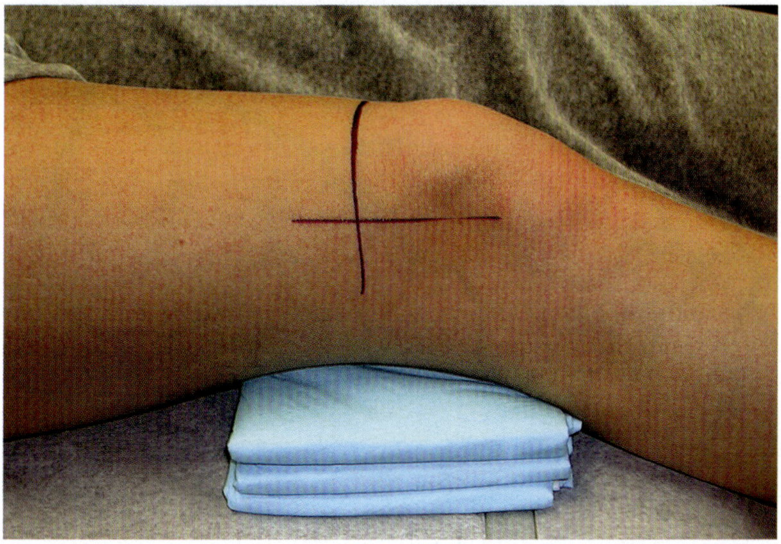

**FIGURE 8.16** ● Lateral aspect of the right knee with lines drawn.

## ANESTHESIA

- Local anesthesia of the skin using topical vapocoolant spray.
- (Optional) Local anesthesia and vasoconstriction of the skin and soft tissues may be augmented using an injection of up to 10 mL of 1% lidocaine with epinephrine (see "Pearls").

## EQUIPMENT

- (Optional) 10-mL syringe—for local tissue anesthesia
- 20- to 60-mL syringe—for aspiration
- 5-mL syringe—for injection of the anesthetic/corticosteroid mixture
- (Optional) 25-gauge, 1½ in. needle—for local tissue anesthesia
- 18-gauge, 1½ in. needle—for aspiration
- (Optional) 10 mL of 1% lidocaine with epinephrine—for local tissue anesthesia
- 3 mL of 1% lidocaine without epinephrine—to dilute the corticosteroid
- 1 mL of the corticosteroid solution (40 mg of triamcinolone acetonide)
- Viscosupplementation agent of choice—if indicated
- One alcohol prep pad
- Two povidone–iodine prep pads
- Sterile gauze pads
- Sterile adhesive bandage
- Nonsterile, clean chucks pad

## TECHNIQUE

1. (Optional) Use ultrasound to image the knee joint structures using an adjacent, but separate, acoustic window (Fig. 8.17). This allows separate imaging from the injection site so that there is no contamination from the ultrasound gel. Alternatively, the entire site may be prepped in an aseptic manner and sterile ultrasound gel utilized (Fig. 8.18).

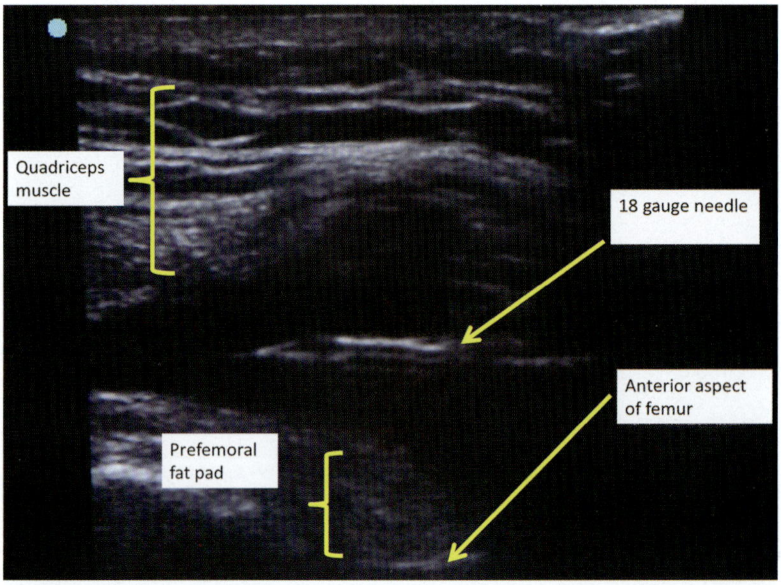


**FIGURE 8.17** Ultrasound imaging of knee joint.

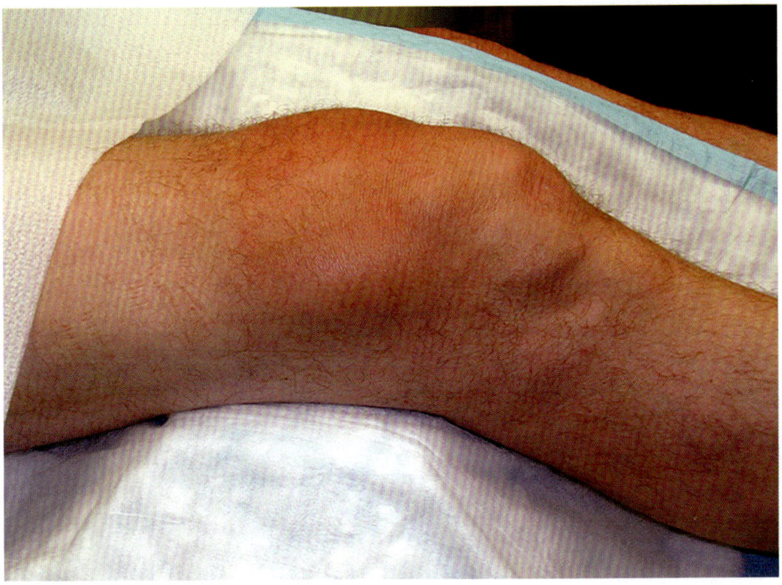

***FIGURE 8.18*** • Right knee joint—distended with intraarticular fluid. Note bulging of the joint capsule (suprapatellar bursa) proximal to the patella.

2. Create an aseptic insertion site by wiping with a single alcohol prep pad followed by two 10% povidone–iodine prep pads. Allow this site to completely dry by evaporation.
3. Achieve good local anesthesia by using topical vapocoolant spray.
4. (Optional) Using the no-touch technique, introduce the 25-gauge, 1½ in. needle for local anesthesia at the insertion site. Inject up to 10 mL of 1% lidocaine with epinephrine to provide adequate local anesthesia. Deposit the anesthetic under the skin, in the soft tissue at the joint capsule, and over the periosteum.
5. Position the 18-gauge, 1½ in. needle and syringe perpendicularly to the skin, parallel to the floor, at a right angle to the other two previously drawn skin lines and with the tip of the needle directed medially.
6. Using the aseptic, no-touch technique, quickly introduce that needle at the insertion site.
7. Advance the needle under the quadriceps tendon and toward the anterior surface of the distal femur until the needle tip is located in the joint capsule. Apply suction to the syringe while advancing the needle. The appearance of fluid in the syringe confirms that the joint capsule has been entered (Fig. 8.19). If fluid is aspirated, stop advancing the needle. The needle may contact the distal femur itself. Should that happen, withdraw the needle a few centimeters and advance the needle as needed to "walk" it over the femur and into the joint capsule.
8. Multiple syringes may be required in order to drain all of the synovial fluid if a large effusion is present.
9. If injection following aspiration is elected, remove the large syringe from the 18-gauge needle and then attach the 5-mL syringe filled with the anesthetic/steroid solution (Fig. 8.20) or a proprietary glass syringe prefilled with viscosupplement (Fig. 8.21).
10. Inject the anesthetic/steroid solution as a bolus into the knee joint capsule. The injected solution should flow smoothly into the joint space. If increased resistance

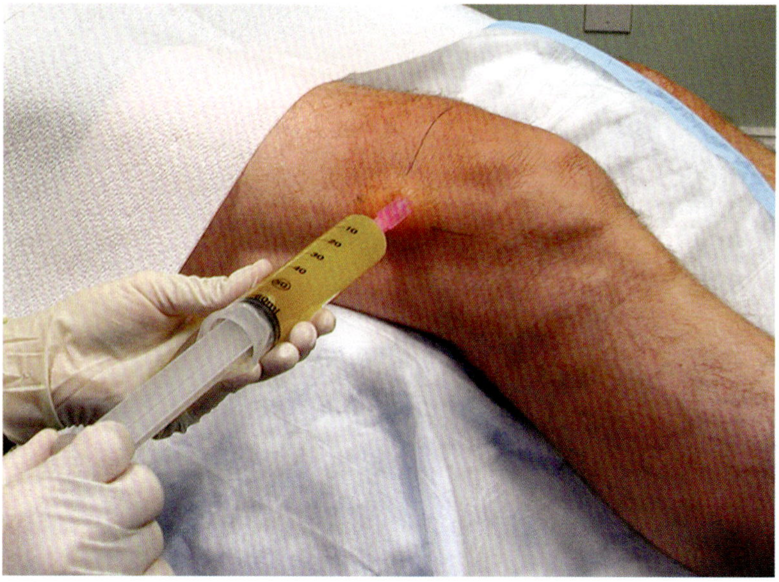

*FIGURE 8.19* ● Right knee aspiration of distended joint using the preferred lateral suprapatellar approach.

is encountered, advance or withdraw the needle slightly, and confirm aspiration of a small amount of joint fluid before attempting further injection (Fig. 8.20).

11. Following injection of the corticosteroid solution or viscosupplement, withdraw the needle.
12. Apply a sterile adhesive bandage.
13. Instruct the patient to move his or her knee through its full range of motion. This movement distributes the steroid solution throughout the knee joint.
14. Reexamine the knee in 5 min to confirm pain relief.

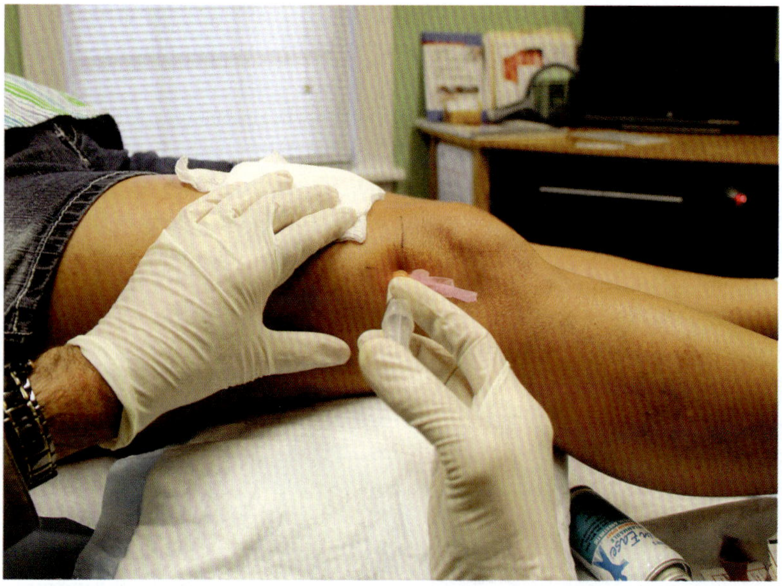

*FIGURE 8.20* ● Right knee corticosteroid injection.

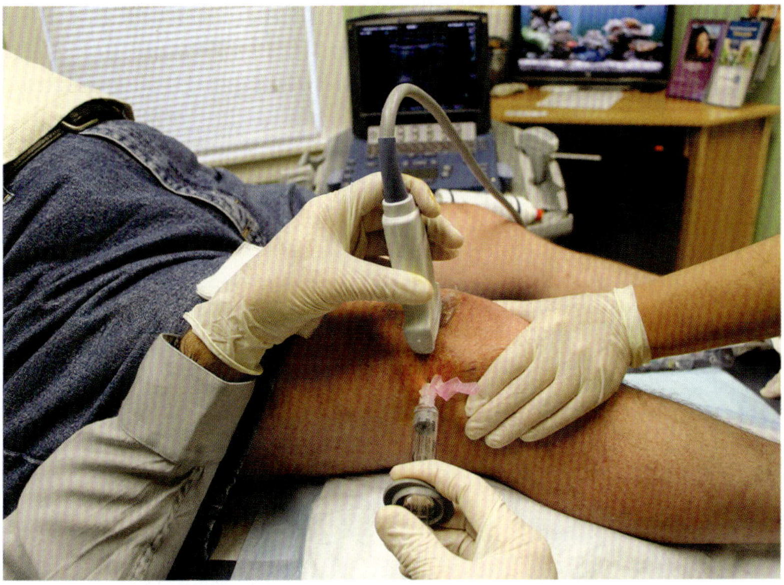

*FIGURE 8.21* • Right knee viscosupplementation injection - using ultrasound guidance.

## AFTERCARE

- Avoid more than light use of the affected knee over the next 2 weeks.
- Use other complementary treatment modalities including physical therapy as indicated.
- Consider follow-up examination in 2 weeks.

**CPT code:** 20610—Arthrocentesis, aspiration, and/or injection of major joint or bursa

## PEARLS

- Although both the lateral and medial approaches may be used, the preferred approach is from the lateral aspect. This approach affords the operator more room, avoids inadvertent kicking of the clinician by the patient with the uninvolved leg, and preserves patient modesty.
- Usually, this procedure can be conducted in a pain-free manner with the use of topical vapocoolant spray. However, an occasional patient may complain of pain when the 18-gauge needle is advanced into contact with the joint capsule. In this case, that needle should be withdrawn and a 1½ in., 25-gauge needle advanced in the same direction. A total of up to 10 mL of 1% lidocaine with epinephrine is deposited under the skin, in the soft tissue at the joint capsule, and over the periosteum. In almost all such cases where pain is reported, it is the author's experience to observe with ultrasound that the synovial membrane is thickened and presumably inflamed.
- If the clinician encounters the unusual situation of experiencing difficulty finding the joint capsule, then either of the following maneuvers can be attempted.
  - Firmly squeeze the anterodistal aspect of the patella and displace it posteriorly and proximally (the "cupping" maneuver) thereby shifting the joint fluid and filling the suprapatellar pouch.
  - Redirect the needle in a distal direction to target the undersurface of the patella. However, this technique may potentially result in injury to the patellar cartilage.

- Ultrasound-guided aspiration and injection are indicated when an effusion is not detected, or in a very obese patient. Ultrasound is also very useful in locating fluid in the knee joint to ensure the accuracy when injecting expensive viscosupplement products.

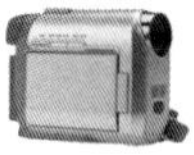

A video clip showing a knee injection can be found in the companion eBook.

# Knee Joint—Lateral Midpatellar Approach

The supine, extended-leg lateral midpatellar approach to the knee joint is relatively easy to perform and is well accepted by patients. As noted previously, injection through this portal has a high likelihood of success. Because of supine positioning, patients do not see the approaching needle and anxiety is diminished. This approach is considered a safe procedure since there are no major arteries or nerves in the immediate path of the needle. Since the needle tip may come into contact with the lateral aspect of the patellar cartilage, direct trauma may result, but this is usually lateral to the appositional joint surface and should not be clinically significant. With the use of local anesthetic, this injection can help the clinician differentiate the etiology of knee pain. After pain has been eliminated as a confounding factor, the knee can be reexamined to assess structural integrity of the ligaments and menisci.

| Indications | ICD-9 Code | ICD-10 Code |
|---|---|---|
| Knee pain | 719.46 | M25.569 |
| Knee sprain, unspecified site | 844.9 | S83.90 |
| Knee arthritis, unspecified | 716.96 | M13.96 |
| Knee osteoarthritis, primary | 715.16 | M17.10 |
| Knee osteoarthritis, posttraumatic | 716.16 | M12.569 |
| Knee osteoarthritis, secondary | 715.26 | M17.5 |

**Relevant Anatomy:** (see Fig. 8.15)

- See previous chapter

## PATIENT POSITION

- Lying supine on the examination table with the knee extended or slightly flexed and supported with folded towels or chucks pads as needed for patient comfort.
- Rotate the patient's head away from the side that is being injected. This minimizes anxiety and pain perception.

## LANDMARKS

1. With the patient lying supine on the examination table, the clinician stands lateral to the affected knee.
2. Locate the lateral aspect of the patella.
3. Have the patient relax the quadriceps muscles; then, apply pressure to the medial aspect of the patella in order to displace it laterally.
4. Identify the sulcus at the midpatella that develops between the lateral undersurface of the patella and the lateral femoral condyle (Fig. 8.22).

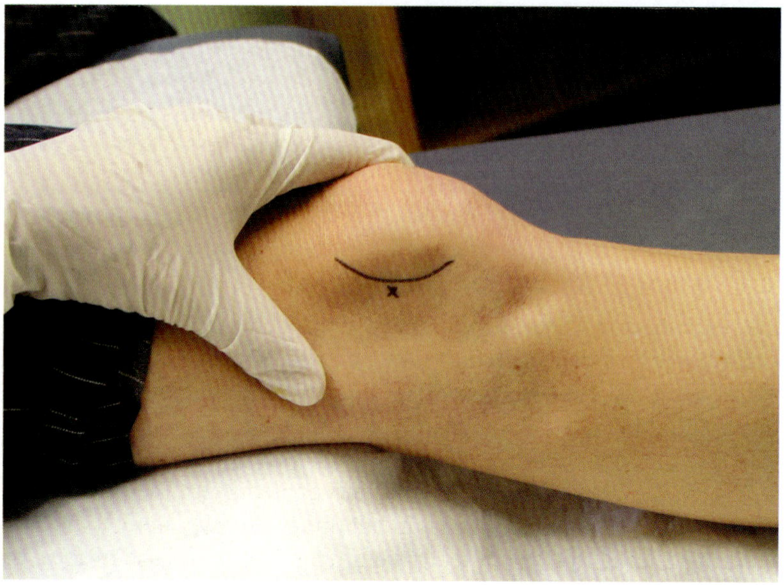

**FIGURE 8.22** ● Lateral aspect of the right knee with patella outlined and injection site drawn.

5. At that site, press firmly on the skin with the retracted tip of a ballpoint pen. This indention represents the entry point for the needle.
6. After this landmark is identified, the patient should not move the knee.

## ANESTHESIA

- Local anesthesia of the skin using topical vapocoolant spray.
- (Optional) Local anesthesia and vasoconstriction of the skin and soft tissues may be augmented using an injection of 2 to 3 mL of 1% lidocaine with epinephrine (see Pearls).

## EQUIPMENT

- (Optional) 5-mL syringe—for injected local tissue anesthesia
- 20- to 60-mL syringe—for aspiration
- 5-mL syringe—for injection of the anesthetic/corticosteroid mixture
- (Optional) 25-gauge, 1 in. needle—for local tissue anesthesia
- 18-gauge, 1½ in. needle—for aspiration
- (Optional) 2 to 3 mL of 1% lidocaine with epinephrine—for local tissue anesthesia
- 3 mL of 1% lidocaine without epinephrine—to dilute the corticosteroid
- 1 mL of the steroid solution (40 mg of triamcinolone acetonide)
- Viscosupplementation agent of choice—if indicated
- One alcohol prep pad
- Two povidone–iodine prep pads
- Sterile gauze pads
- Sterile adhesive bandage
- Nonsterile, clean chucks pad

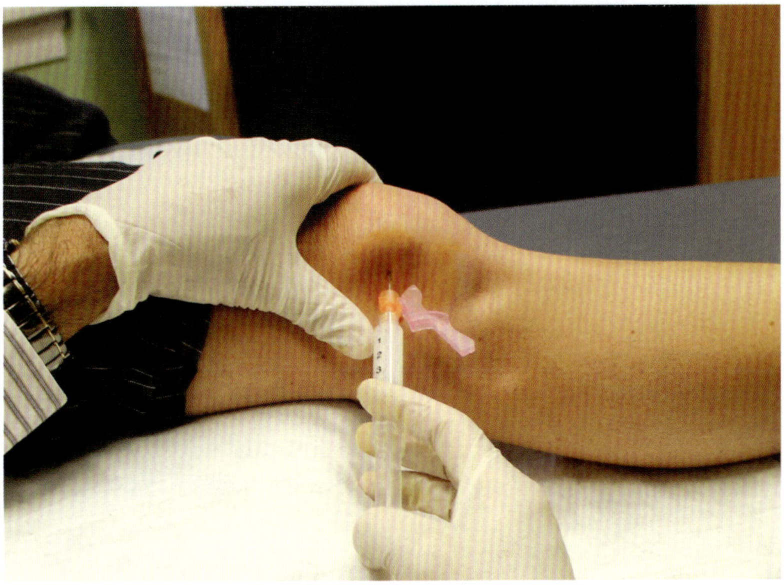

*FIGURE 8.23* • Right knee injection using the lateral midpatellar approach.

## TECHNIQUE

1. (Optional) Use ultrasound to image the knee joint structures using an adjacent, but separate, acoustic window. This allows separate imaging from the injection site so that there is no contamination from the ultrasound gel. Alternatively, the entire site may be prepped in an aseptic manner and sterile ultrasound gel utilized.
2. Create an aseptic insertion site by wiping with a single alcohol prep pad followed by two 10% povidone–iodine prep pads. Allow this site to completely dry by evaporation.
3. Achieve good local anesthesia by using topical vapocoolant spray.
4. (Optional) Using the no-touch technique, introduce the 25-gauge, 1 in. needle for local anesthesia at the insertion site. Inject 2 to 3 mL of 1% lidocaine with epinephrine to provide adequate local anesthesia. Deposit the anesthetic under the skin and in the soft tissue at the joint capsule.
5. Have the patient relax the quadriceps muscles; then, have an assistant apply pressure to the medial aspect of the patella in order to displace it laterally.
6. Position the 18-gauge, 1½ in. needle and syringe over the previously marked injection site in a medial direction and with the needle tip angled up underneath the patella and over the lateral femoral condyle.
7. Using the aseptic, no-touch technique, quickly introduce that needle at the insertion site.
8. Advance the needle medially underneath the patella and over the lateral femoral condyle until the needle tip is located in the joint capsule. Apply suction to the syringe while advancing the needle. The appearance of fluid in the syringe confirms that the joint capsule has been entered (Fig. 8.23). If fluid is aspirated, stop advancing the needle.
9. Multiple syringes may be required in order to drain all of the synovial fluid if a large effusion is present.
10. If injection following aspiration is elected, remove the large syringe from the 18-gauge needle and then attach the 5-mL syringe filled with the anesthetic/steroid solution or a proprietary glass syringe prefilled with viscosupplement.

11. Inject the anesthetic/steroid solution as a bolus into the knee joint capsule. The injected solution should flow smoothly into the joint space. If increased resistance is encountered, advance or withdraw the needle slightly, and confirm aspiration of a small amount of joint fluid before attempting further injection.
12. Following injection of the corticosteroid solution or viscosupplement, withdraw the needle.
13. Apply a sterile adhesive bandage.
14. Instruct the patient to move his or her knee through its full range of motion. This movement distributes the steroid solution throughout the knee joint.
15. Reexamine the knee in 5 min to confirm pain relief.

## AFTERCARE

- Avoid more than light use of the affected knee over the next 2 weeks.
- Use other complementary treatment modalities including physical therapy as indicated.
- Consider follow-up examination in 2 weeks.

**CPT code:** 20610—Arthrocentesis, aspiration, and/or injection of major joint or bursa

## PEARLS

- Although both the lateral and medial approaches may be used, the preferred approach is from the lateral aspect. This approach affords the operator more room, avoids inadvertent kicking of the clinician by the patient with the uninvolved leg, and preserves patient modesty.
- Usually, this procedure can be conducted in a pain-free manner with the use of topical vapocoolant spray. However, an occasional patient may complain of pain when the 18-gauge needle is advanced into contact with the joint capsule. In this case, that needle should be withdrawn and a 1 in., 25-gauge needle advanced in the same direction. A total of 2 to 3 mL of 1% lidocaine with epinephrine is deposited under the skin and in the soft tissue at the joint capsule.
- If the clinician encounters the unusual situation of experiencing difficulty finding the joint capsule, then either of the following maneuvers can be attempted.
  - Firmly squeeze the anterodistal aspect of the patella and displace it posteriorly and proximally (the "cupping" maneuver) thereby shifting the joint fluid and filling the suprapatellar pouch.
  - Abandon this approach and use the lateral suprapatellar portal. Alternatively, ultrasound imaging may be utilized.
- Ultrasound-guided aspiration and injection are indicated when an effusion is not detected or in a very obese patient. Ultrasound is also very useful in locating fluid in the knee joint to ensure the accuracy when injecting expensive viscosupplement products.

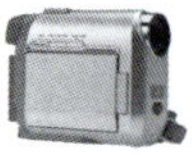

A video clip showing a knee injection can be found in the companion eBook.

# Knee Joint—Anteromedial and Anterolateral Approaches

Aspiration and injection of the knee joint are common procedures for primary care physicians. The infrapatellar anteromedial and anterolateral approaches to the knee joint are more difficult to perform than the extended-leg lateral approaches. They are also less accepted by patients since they are usually performed with patients sitting where they can see the approaching needle. There is increased anxiety with these procedures, and the patients are at increased risk of injury if they develop a vasovagal reaction and fall from the exam table. Alternatively, the patient may be placed supine with hip and knee flexion so the plantar aspect of the foot contacts the exam tabletop. Also, since these injections are intra-articular, the knee cartilage over the distal femur may suffer direct damage from gouging by the 18-gauge needle. For these reasons, and documented lower success rates as compared to the extended-leg approaches, the anteromedial and anterolateral techniques are considered secondary options.

| **Indications** | **ICD-9 Code** | **ICD-10 Code** |
|---|---|---|
| Knee pain | 719.46 | M25.569 |
| Knee sprain, unspecified site | 844.9 | S83.90 |
| Knee arthritis, unspecified | 716.96 | M13.96 |
| Knee osteoarthritis, primary | 715.16 | M17.10 |
| Knee osteoarthritis, posttraumatic | 716.16 | M12.569 |
| Knee osteoarthritis, secondary | 715.26 | M17.5 |

**Relevant Anatomy:** (see Fig. 8.15)

- See previous chapter

## PATIENT POSITION

- Lying supine on the examination table with the affected knee flexed at an angle of 90 degrees.
- Alternatively, the patient may be sitting on the examination table or a wheelchair with both knees flexed at 90 degrees.
- Rotate the patient's head away from the side that is being injected. This minimizes anxiety and pain perception.

## LANDMARKS

1. With the patient sitting up on the examination table or in a chair, the clinician sits on an exam stool in front of the affected knee.
2. With the patient lying supine on the examination table, the clinician stands medial or lateral to the affected knee.
3. Palpate the anterior aspect of the knee to locate the patellar tendon.

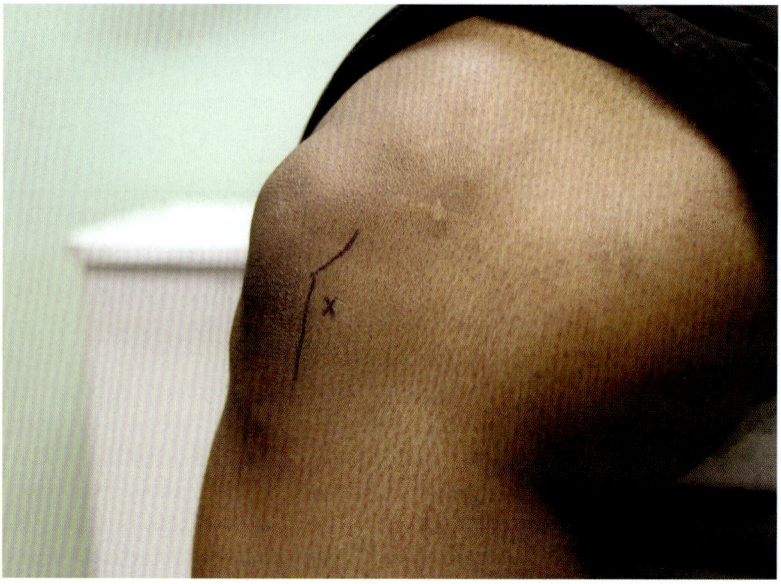

**FIGURE 8.24A** ● Anteromedial aspect of the right knee with injection sites drawn.

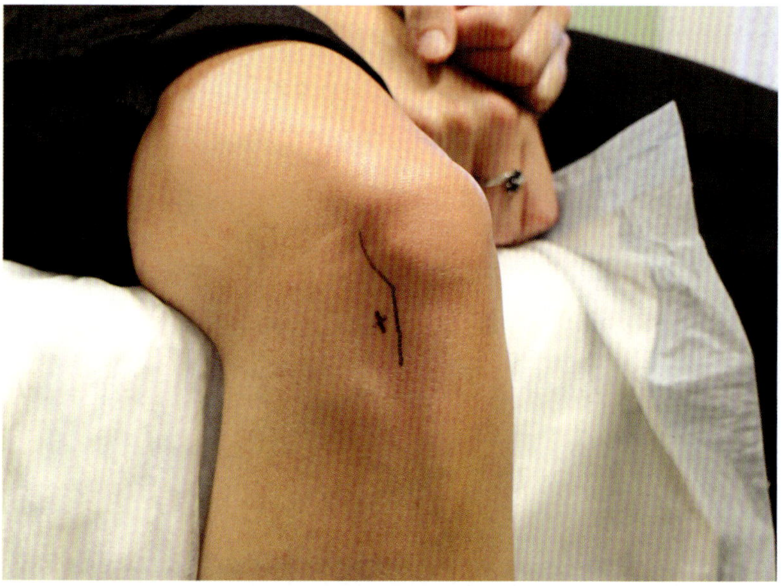

**FIGURE 8.24B** ● Anterolateral aspect of the right knee with injection sites drawn.

4. At the midpoint of the tendon, move about 1 cm medially or laterally. There is usually a depression at that spot. Mark it with ink.
5. At that site, press firmly on the skin with the retracted tip of a ballpoint pen. This indention represents the entry point for the needle.
6. After the landmarks are identified, the patient should not move the knee (Fig. 8.24A and B).

## ANESTHESIA

- Local anesthesia of the skin using topical vapocoolant spray.
- Local anesthesia and vasoconstriction of the skin and soft tissues may be augmented using an injection of up to 5 mL of 1% lidocaine with epinephrine (optional).

## EQUIPMENT

- (Optional) 5-mL syringe—for injected local tissue anesthesia
- 20- to 60-mL syringe—for aspiration
- 5-mL syringe—for injection of the anesthetic/corticosteroid mixture
- (Optional) 25-gauge, 1½ in. needle—for local tissue anesthesia
- 18-gauge, 1½ in. needle—for aspiration
- (Optional) Up to 5 mL of 1% lidocaine with epinephrine—for local tissue anesthesia
- 3 mL of 1% lidocaine without epinephrine—to dilute the corticosteroid
- 1 mL of the steroid solution (40 mg of triamcinolone acetonide)
- Viscosupplementation agent of choice—if indicated
- One alcohol prep pad
- Two povidone–iodine prep pads
- Sterile gauze pads
- Sterile adhesive bandage
- Nonsterile, clean chucks pad

## TECHNIQUE

1. (Optional) Use an ultrasound to image the knee joint using an adjacent, but separate, acoustic window. This allows imaging separate from the injection site so that there is no contamination from the ultrasound gel. Alternatively, the entire site may be prepped in an aseptic manner and sterile ultrasound gel utilized.
2. Create an aseptic insertion site by wiping with a single alcohol prep pad followed by two 10% povidone–iodine prep pads. Allow this site to completely dry by evaporation.
3. Achieve good local anesthesia by using topical vapocoolant spray.
4. (Optional) Using the no-touch technique, introduce the 25-gauge, 1½ in. needle for local anesthesia at the insertion site. Inject a total of up to 5 mL of 1% lidocaine with epinephrine to provide adequate local anesthesia. Deposit the anesthetic under the skin, in the soft tissues, and over the periosteum.
5. Position the 18-gauge, 1½ in. needle and syringe perpendicular to the skin with the tip of the needle directed at a 45-degree angle into the center of the knee.
6. Using the no-touch technique, introduce that needle at the insertion site (Fig. 8.25A and B).
7. Advance the needle toward the center of the knee until the needle tip is located in the joint capsule. Apply suction to the syringe while advancing the needle. The appearance of fluid in the syringe indicates that the joint capsule has been entered.
8. Multiple syringes may be required in order to drain all of the synovial fluid.
9. If injection following aspiration is elected, remove the large syringe from the 18-gauge needle and then attach the 10-mL syringe filled with the steroid solution or the proprietary syringe prefilled with viscosupplement.
10. Inject the steroid solution as a bolus into the knee joint capsule. The injected solution should flow smoothly into the joint space. If increased resistance is encountered, advance or withdraw the needle slightly before attempting further injection.
11. Following injection of the corticosteroid solution or viscosupplement, withdraw the needle.

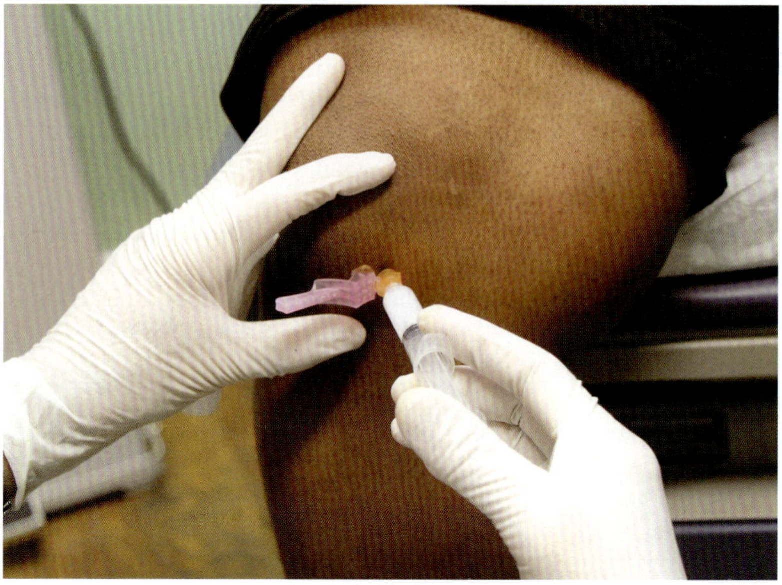

A

**FIGURE 8.25A** ● Right knee injection using the anteromedial approach.

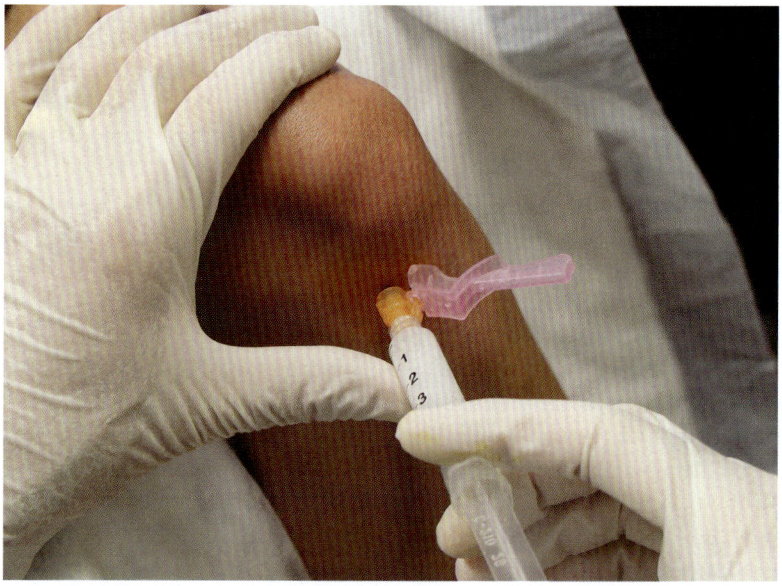

B

**FIGURE 8.25B** ● Right knee injection using the anterolateral approach.

12. Apply a sterile adhesive bandage.
13. Instruct the patient to move his or her knee through its full range of motion. This movement distributes the steroid solution throughout the knee joint.
14. Reexamine the knee in 5 min to confirm pain relief.

## AFTERCARE

- Avoid more than light use of the affected knee over the next 2 weeks.
- Use other complementary treatment modalities including physical therapy as indicated.
- Consider follow-up examination in 2 weeks.

**CPT code:** 20610—Arthrocentesis, aspiration, and/or injection of major joint or bursa

## PEARLS

- Because of potential direct needle injury to articular cartilage, the infrapatellar approach should only be used in circumstances where the suprapatellar approach cannot be performed. This may occur in patients with local cellulitis or soft tissue injury or in a patient confined to a wheelchair who cannot be easily moved onto an examination table.
- Ultrasound-assisted aspiration and injection are indicated in the situation where an effusion is not present or is a small "pocket" of fluid. Ultrasound is also very useful in locating fluid in the knee joint to ensure the accuracy of injecting expensive viscosupplementation products.

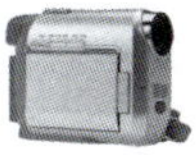

Video clips showing anteromedial and anterolateral knee injections can be found in the companion eBook.

# Prepatellar Bursitis

Prepatellar bursitis is a relatively common aspiration and injection site for primary care physicians. Successful aspiration is usually easy because the location of bursa is readily evident. The subcutaneous prepatellar bursa may become inflamed and accumulate fluid when subjected to repeated excessive pressure or friction. The fluid may consist of blood in acute trauma, thick proteinaceous mucoid fluid after repetitive injury, or purulence if infected. Corticosteroids should never be administered if an infectious bursitis is suspected.

A large-diameter needle is appropriate as this technique is used to aspirate large volume of fluid. Occasionally, the clinician may elect to inject a steroid solution if the fluid recollects—as long as an infection can be excluded. However, there are no studies found in the peer-reviewed medical literature that address any injection treatment.

| Indication | ICD-9 Code | ICD-10 Code |
|---|---|---|
| Prepatellar bursitis | 726.65 | M70.40 |

## Relevant Anatomy

- Relevant Anatomy: (Fig. 8.26)

## PATIENT POSITION

- Lying supine on the examination table with the affected knee extended or slightly flexed and supported with folded towels or chucks pads as needed for patient comfort.
- Rotate the patient's head away from the side that is being injected. This minimizes anxiety and pain perception.

## LANDMARKS

1. With the patient lying supine on the examination table, the clinician stands lateral to the affected knee.
2. The point of maximal fluctuance is identified.
3. At that site, press firmly on the skin with the retracted tip of a ballpoint pen. This indention represents the entry point for the needle.
4. After the landmarks are identified, the patient should not move the knee.

## ANESTHESIA

- Local anesthesia of the skin using topical vapocoolant spray

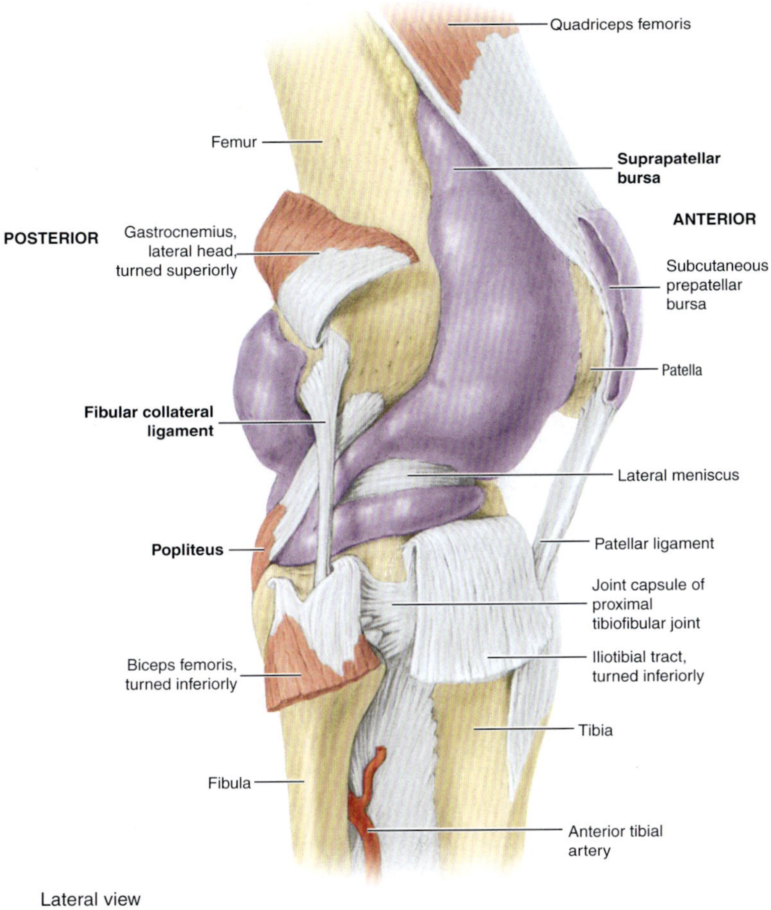


**FIGURE 8.26** • Lateral aspect of the right knee showing the extent of the knee joint capsule (in purple). (Adapted from Tank PW, Gest TR. *Lippincott Williams & Wilkins Atlas of Anatomy*. Philadelphia, PA: Lippincott Williams & Wilkins, 2009.)

## EQUIPMENT

- 20-mL syringe
- 3-mL syringe—for optional injection
- 18-gauge, 1½ in. needle
- 1 mL of 1% lidocaine without epinephrine—for optional injection
- 1 mL of the steroid solution (40 mg of triamcinolone acetonide)—for optional injection
- One alcohol prep pad
- Two povidone–iodine prep pads
- Sterile gauze pads
- Sterile adhesive bandage
- Nonsterile, clean chucks pad

## TECHNIQUE

1. Prep the insertion site with alcohol followed by the povidone–iodine pads.
2. Achieve good local anesthesia by using topical vapocoolant spray.
3. Position the 18-gauge needle and syringe with the tip of the needle directed toward the area of maximal fluid collection.
4. Using the no-touch technique, introduce the needle at the insertion site (Fig. 8.27).

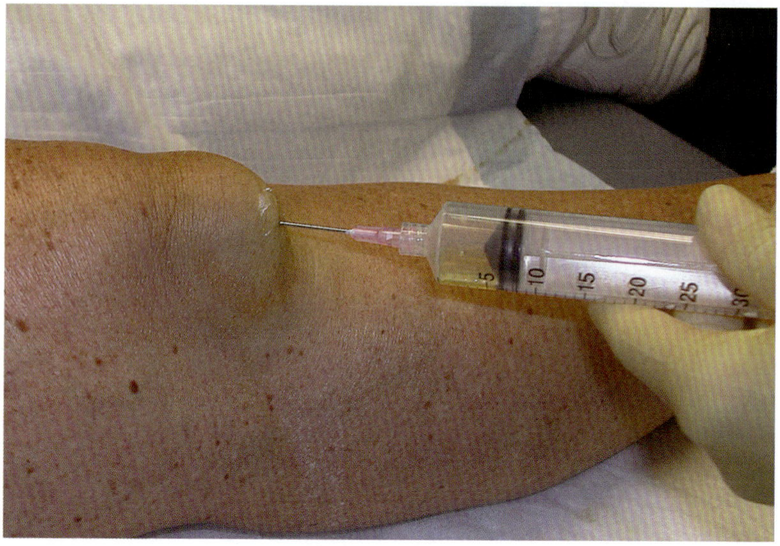

***FIGURE 8.27*** Prepatellar bursitis aspiration.

5. Advance the needle into the center of the bursa.
6. Aspiration should be easily accomplished. Use multiple syringes if the effusion is large.
7. (Optional) If injection following aspiration is elected, do not remove the needle. Grasp the hub of the 18-gauge needle, remove the large syringe, and then attach the 3-mL syringe filled with the steroid solution.
8. The injected solution should flow smoothly into the space. If increased resistance is encountered, advance or withdraw the needle slightly before attempting further injection.
9. Following complete aspiration, and possible injection of corticosteroid solution, withdraw the needle.
10. Apply a sterile adhesive bandage followed by a compressive elastic bandage.
11. Reexamine the knee in 5 min to confirm pain relief.

## AFTERCARE

- Avoid excessive use of the affected knee over the next 2 weeks.
- Consider the use of a knee compression wrap.
- NSAIDs, ice, and/or physical therapy as indicated.
- Consider follow-up examination in 2 weeks.

**CPT code:** 20605—Aspiration and/or injection of intermediate bursa

## PEARLS

- If the prepatellar bursitis is due to an infection or acute hemorrhagic event, do not follow aspiration with corticosteroid injection.
- Injection of corticosteroid solution is usually reserved for recurrent bursitis.

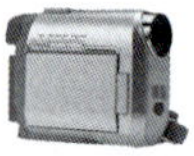

A video clip showing a prepatellar bursitis injection can be found in the companion eBook.

# Pes Anserine Syndrome

Injection of corticosteroids for the treatment of pes anserine syndrome is an unusual procedure for primary care physicians. The pes anserinus is the common insertion for the tendons of the sartorius, gracilis, and semitendinosus muscles. It is located over the medial aspect of the proximal tibia about 2 to 5 cm distal to the anteromedial joint margin of the knee. Since little is known regarding the structural defect responsible for this condition and it presents with features of bursitis, tendinitis, or both, this is simply referred to as pes anserine syndrome.[1] Pain and swelling may occur with overuse or excessive valgus stress on the knee. It is most commonly seen in overweight, middle-aged, and older women with knee osteoarthritis. Diabetes is a known risk factor as well. A small-diameter needle is appropriate as there will not be a fluid collection. Corticosteroids may be used to treat this condition, but this is controversial.[2–4]

| Indication | ICD-9 Code | ICD-10 Code |
|---|---|---|
| Pes anserine bursitis | 726.61 | M70.50 |

**Relevant Anatomy:** (Fig. 8.28)

## PATIENT POSITION

- Lying supine on the examination table with the affected knee extended or slightly flexed and supported with folded towels or chucks pads as needed for patient comfort.
- Rotate the patient's head away from the side that is being injected. This minimizes anxiety and pain perception.

## LANDMARKS

1. With the patient lying supine on the examination table, the clinician stands lateral to the affected knee.
2. The point of maximal tenderness over the proximal medial anterior tibia is identified.
3. At that site, press firmly on the skin with the retracted tip of a ballpoint pen. This indention represents the entry point for the needle.
4. After the landmarks are identified, the patient should not move the knee.

## ANESTHESIA

- Local anesthesia of the skin using topical vapocoolant spray

## EQUIPMENT

- 3-mL syringe
- 25-gauge, 1 in. needle

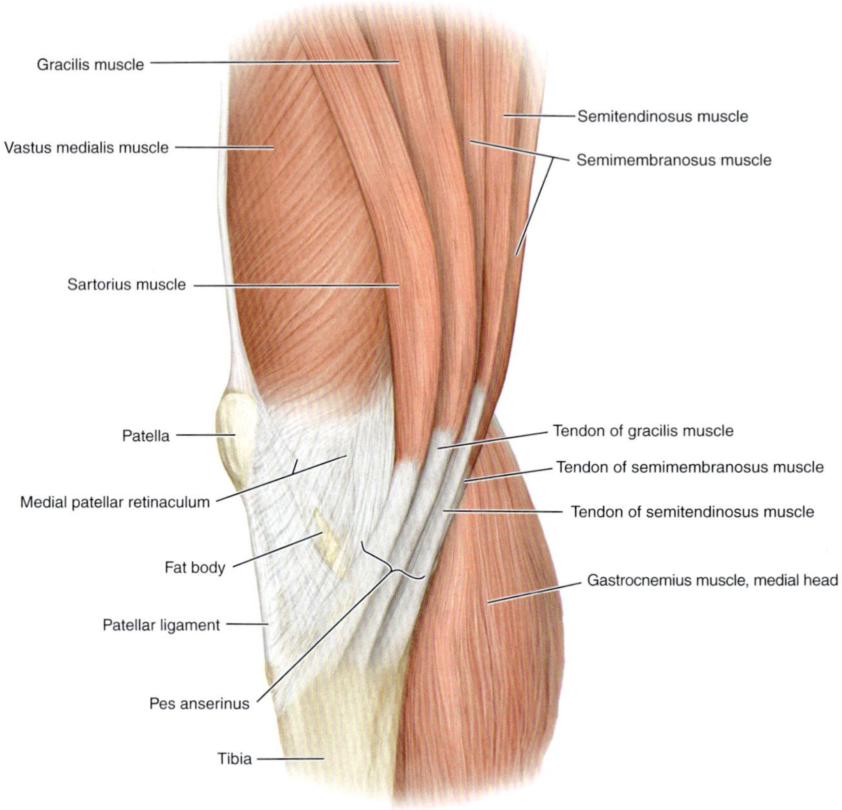


**FIGURE 8.28** Medial aspect of the right knee/leg. (Adapted from Tank PW, Gest TR *Lippincott Williams & Wilkins Atlas of Anatomy*. Philadelphia, PA: Lippincott Williams & Wilkins, 2009.)

- 1 mL of 1% lidocaine without epinephrine
- 0.5 to 1 mL of the steroid solution (20 to 40 mg of triamcinolone acetonide)
- One alcohol prep pad
- Two povidone–iodine prep pads
- Sterile gauze pads
- Sterile adhesive bandage
- Nonsterile, clean chucks pad

## TECHNIQUE

1. Prep the insertion site with alcohol followed by the povidone–iodine pads.
2. Achieve good local anesthesia by using topical vapocoolant spray.
3. Position the needle and syringe perpendicular to the skin with the tip of the needle directed toward the area of maximal tenderness at the insertion of the tendons.
4. Using the no-touch technique, introduce the needle at the insertion site (Fig. 8.29).
5. Advance the needle toward the bone of the proximal medial tibia. Back up the needle 1 to 2 mm.
6. Inject the steroid solution as a bolus into this area. The injected solution should flow smoothly into the space. If increased resistance is encountered, advance or withdraw the needle slightly before attempting further injection.
7. Following injection of the corticosteroid solution, withdraw the needle.
8. Apply a sterile adhesive bandage.

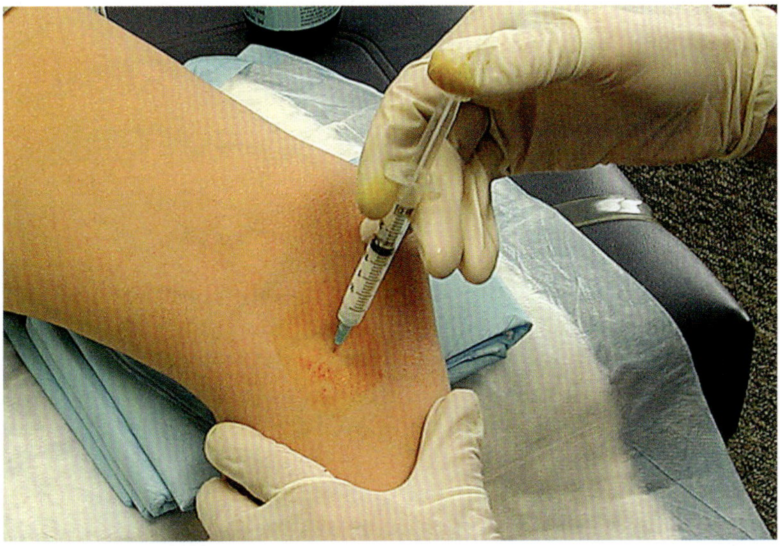

***FIGURE 8.29*** • Left knee pes anserine bursitis injection.

9. Instruct the patient to massage this area and move his or her knee through its full range of motion. This movement distributes the steroid solution throughout the pes anserine bursa and related tendons.
10. Reexamine the pes anserine bursa in 5 min to confirm pain relief.

## AFTERCARE

- Avoid excessive knee extension and adduction over the next 2 weeks.
- Consider the use of a compression wrap.
- NSAIDs, ice, heat, and/or physical therapy as indicated.
- Consider follow-up examination in 2 weeks.

**CPT code:** 20551—Injection of single tendon origin or insertion

## PEARLS

- The pes anserine bursa is superficial. As a result, this injection can be complicated by the development of skin atrophy and hypopigmentation. Avoid the development of a subdermal wheal while injecting the corticosteroid solution.
- Since this is an unusual diagnosis, also consider a medial meniscal tear, chondral fracture, or osteonecrosis of the tibia.

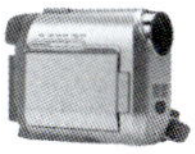

A video clip showing a pes anserine syndrome injection can be found in the companion eBook.

## REFERENCES

1. Helfenstein M Jr, Kuromoto J. Anserine syndrome. *Rev Bras Reumatol*. 2010;50(3):313–327.
2. Vega-Morales D, Esquivel-Valerio JA, Negrete-López R, et al. Safety and efficacy of methylprednisolone infiltration in anserine syndrome treatment. *Rheumatol Clin*. 2012;8(2):63–67.
3. Yoon HS, Kim SE, Suh YR, et al. Correlation between ultrasonographic findings and the response to corticosteroid injection in pes anserinus tendinobursitis syndrome in knee osteoarthritis patients. *J Korean Med Sci*. 2005;20(1):109–112.
4. Kang I, Han SW. Anserine bursitis in patients with osteoarthritis of the knee. *South Med J*. 2000;93(2):207–209.

# Iliotibial Band Friction Syndrome

Iliotibial band syndrome is a common overuse injury typically seen in runners, cyclists, and military recruits. Affected patients report lateral knee pain associated with repetitive motion activities. Several etiologies have been proposed for iliotibial band syndrome, including friction of the iliotibial band as it rubs against the lateral femoral epicondyle, compression of the fat and connective tissue deep to the iliotibial band, and chronic inflammation of the iliotibial band bursa.[1] Another factor is a greater strain throughout the support phase of running.[2] In the acute phase, treatment includes activity modification, ice, nonsteroidal anti-inflammatory medication, and corticosteroid injection in cases of severe pain or swelling.[3] However, there is a paucity of research available and only a single, small study to support the use of injected corticosteroids.[4] A small-diameter needle is appropriate as there will not be a fluid collection.

| Indication | ICD-9 Code | ICD-10 Code |
|---|---|---|
| Iliotibial band syndrome | 728.89 | M76.30 |

**Relevant Anatomy:** (Fig. 8.30)

## PATIENT POSITION

- Lying supine on the examination table with the affected knee extended or slightly flexed and supported with folded towels or chucks pads as needed for patient comfort.
- Rotate the patient's head away from the side that is being injected. This minimizes anxiety and pain perception.

## LANDMARKS

1. With the patient lying supine on the examination table, the clinician stands lateral to the affected knee.
2. The point of maximal tenderness over the lateral femoral condyle is identified.
3. At that site, press firmly on the skin with the retracted tip of a ballpoint pen. This indention represents the entry point for the needle.
4. After the landmarks are identified, the patient should not move the knee.

## ANESTHESIA

- Local anesthesia of the skin using topical vapocoolant spray.

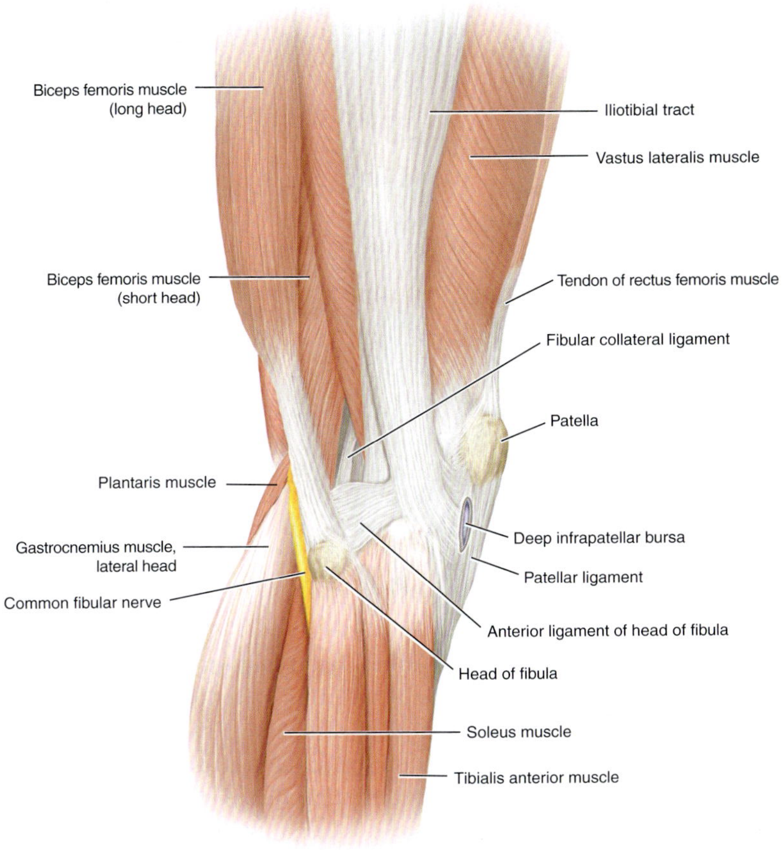


**FIGURE 8.30** • Lateral aspect of the right knee/leg. (Adapted from Tank PW, Gest TR. *Lippincott Williams & Wilkins Atlas of Anatomy*. Philadelphia, PA: Lippincott Williams & Wilkins, 2009.)

## EQUIPMENT

- 3-mL syringe
- 25-gauge, 1 in. needle
- 1 mL of 1% lidocaine without epinephrine
- 0.5 to 1 mL of the steroid solution (20 to 40 mg of triamcinolone acetonide)
- One alcohol prep pad
- Two povidone–iodine prep pads
- Sterile gauze pads
- Sterile adhesive bandage
- Nonsterile, clean chucks pad

## TECHNIQUE

1. Prep the insertion site with alcohol followed by the povidone–iodine pads.
2. Achieve good local anesthesia by using topical vapocoolant spray.
3. Position the needle and syringe perpendicular to the skin with the tip of the needle directed toward the area of maximal tenderness over the lateral femoral condyle.
4. Using the no-touch technique, introduce the needle at the insertion site (Fig. 8.31).

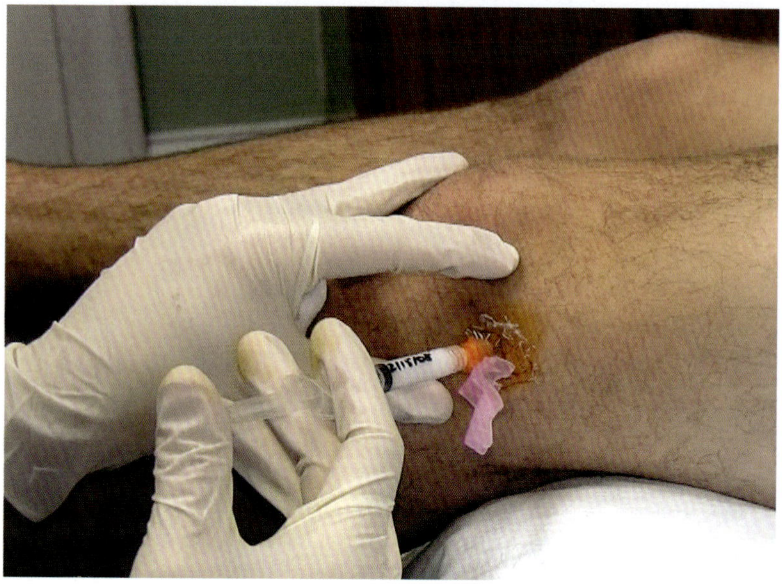

**FIGURE 8.31** ● Left leg iliotibial band injection.

5. Advance the needle through the iliotibial band and touch the bone of the lateral femoral condyle. Back up the needle 1 to 2 mm.
6. Inject the steroid solution as a bolus into this area. The injected solution should flow smoothly into the tissues. If increased resistance is encountered, advance or withdraw the needle slightly before attempting further injection.
7. Following injection of the corticosteroid solution, withdraw the needle.
8. Apply a sterile adhesive bandage.
9. Instruct the patient to massage this area and move his or her knee through its full range of motion. This movement distributes the steroid solution throughout the pes anserine bursa and related tendons.
10. Reexamine the lateral aspect of the knee in 5 min to confirm pain relief.

## AFTERCARE

- Relative rest with avoidance of the precipitating activity for at least 2 weeks.
- Iliotibial band stretching exercises.
- NSAIDs, ice, heat, and/or physical therapy as indicated.
- Consider follow-up examination in 2 weeks.

**CPT code:** 20551—Injection of single tendon origin or insertion

## PEARLS

- The iliotibial band can be superficial, especially in thin persons. As a result, this injection can be complicated by the development of skin atrophy and hypopigmentation. Avoid the development of a subdermal wheal while injecting the corticosteroid solution.

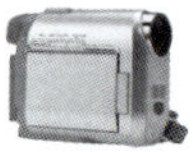

A video clip showing an iliotibial band friction syndrome injection can be found in the companion eBook.

## REFERENCES

1. Strauss EJ, Kim S, Calcei JG, et al. Iliotibial band syndrome: evaluation and management. *J Am Acad Orthop Surg*. 2011;19(12):728–736.
2. Hamill J, Miller R, Noehren B, et al. A prospective study of iliotibial band strain in runners. *Clin Biomech (Bristol, Avon)*. 2008;23(8):1018–1025.
3. Fredericson M, Weir A. Practical management of iliotibial band friction syndrome in runners. *Clin J Sport Med*. 2006;16(3):261–268.
4. Gunter P, Schwellnus MP. Local corticosteroid injection in iliotibial band friction syndrome in runners: a randomised controlled trial. *Br J Sports Med*. 2004;38(3):269–272.

# Tibialis Posterior Tendonitis

The tibialis posterior muscle originates from the interosseous membrane and the adjacent posterior surface of the tibia in the proximal third of the leg. It courses behind the medial malleolus, passes under the flexor retinaculum, and inserts into the tuberosity of the navicular bone. The muscle plantar flexes the ankle and inverts the foot. Tibialis posterior tendon dysfunction is an often unrecognized disabling cause of progressive flatfoot deformity and is the most frequently ruptured tendon in the rear foot. Tenosynovitis of the tibialis posterior tendon occurs as a result of altered mechanics of the foot, acute trauma, and chronic overuse or with inflammatory conditions such as rheumatoid arthritis. Patients present with pain, difficulty walking, and swelling along the medial malleolus and the arch of the foot. Conservative management includes the use of orthotics, stretching, as well as eccentric and concentric progressive resistive exercises.[1] Discrete injections of corticosteroids may be of some benefit to decrease pain and facilitate physical therapy, but there is little evidence-based support for this recommendation. Surgery is required in the case of tendon rupture.

| Indication | ICD-9 Code | ICD-10 Code |
|---|---|---|
| Tibialis posterior tenosynovitis | 726.72 | M76.829 |

**Relevant Anatomy:** (Fig. 8.32)

## PATIENT POSITION

- Supine on the examination table with the hip in full external rotation, knee slightly flexed, and the ankle in a neutral position.
- Alternatively, lying on the examination table on the affected side with the knee slightly flexed and the ankle in a neutral position.
- Rotate the patient's head away from the side that is being injected. This minimizes anxiety and pain perception.

## LANDMARKS

1. With the patient lying supine on the examination table, the clinician stands or sits medial to the affected ankle.
2. Palpate the medial malleolus of the tibia.
3. Locate the tibialis posterior tendon immediately behind and below the medial malleolus.
4. Determine the location of maximal tenderness along the tendon.
5. Identify a point along the tendon 1 cm distal to the point of maximal tenderness and mark it in ink.
6. At that site, press firmly on the skin with the retracted tip of a ballpoint pen. This indention represents the entry point for the needle.
7. After the landmarks are identified, the patient should not move the ankle.

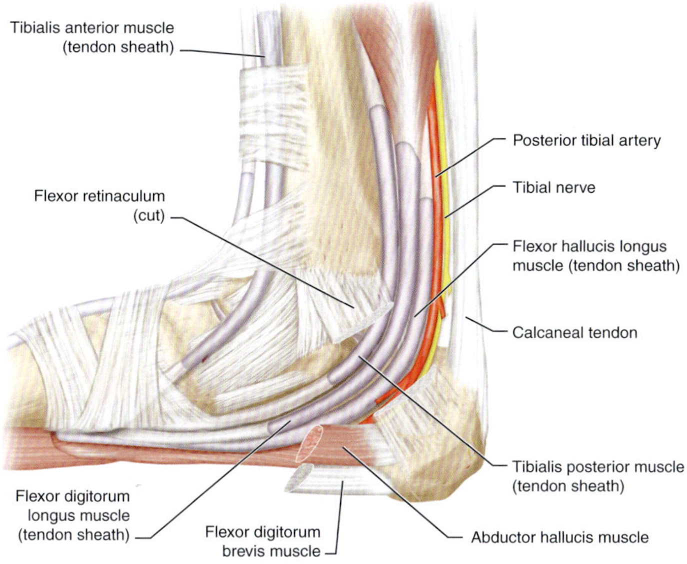


**FIGURE 8.32** • Medial aspect of the right foot. (From Tank PW, Gest TR. *Lippincott Williams & Wilkins Atlas of Anatomy*. Philadelphia, PA: Lippincott Williams & Wilkins, 2009.)

## ANESTHESIA

- Local anesthesia of the skin with topical vapocoolant spray

## EQUIPMENT

- 3-mL syringe
- 25-gauge, 5/8 in. needle
- 0.5 mL of 1% lidocaine without epinephrine
- 0.5 mL of the steroid solution (20 mg of triamcinolone acetonide)
- One alcohol prep pad
- Two povidone–iodine prep pads
- Sterile gauze pads
- Sterile adhesive bandage
- Nonsterile, clean chucks pad

## TECHNIQUE

1. Prep the insertion site with alcohol followed by the povidone–iodine pads.
2. Achieve good local anesthesia by using topical vapocoolant spray.
3. Position the needle and syringe with the needle tip directed proximally at a 30-degree angle to the surface of the skin.
4. Using the no-touch technique, introduce the needle at the insertion site (Fig. 8.33).
5. Advance the needle until it touches the tibialis posterior tendon. Back up the needle 1 to 2 mm.
6. Slowly inject the volume of the syringe around the tendon. The injected solution should flow smoothly into the synovial sheath. If increased resistance is encountered, advance or withdraw the needle slightly before attempting further injection.
7. Following injection of the corticosteroid solution, withdraw the needle.

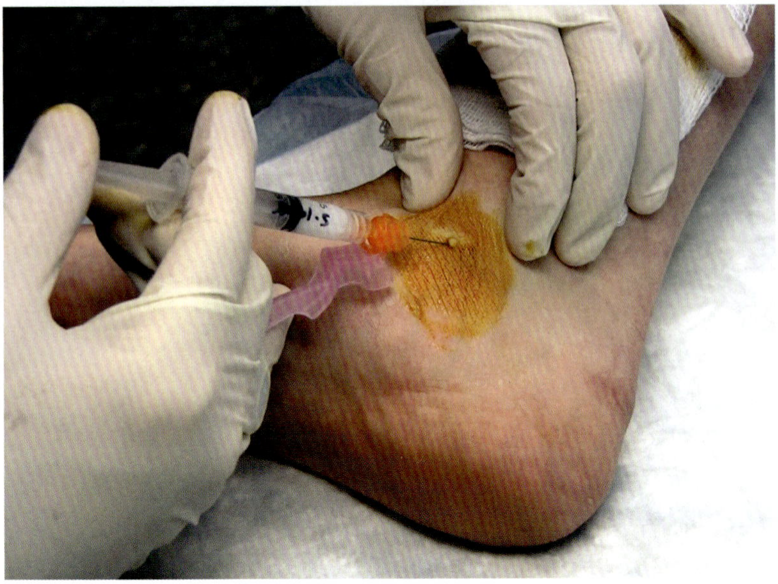


*FIGURE 8.33* Tibialis posterior tendonitis injection.

8. Instruct the patient to move his or her ankle through its full range of motion. This movement distributes the steroid solution throughout the tibialis posterior tendon sheath.
9. Reexamine the tendon in 5 min to confirm pain relief.

## AFTERCARE

- Avoid excessive use of the foot over the next 2 weeks.
- Begin a program of physical therapy.
- Use orthotics or "motion-control" running shoes if there is excessive foot pronation.
- NSAIDs, ice, and heat as indicated.
- Consider follow-up examination in 2 weeks.

**CPT code:** 20550—Injection of single tendon sheath

## PEARLS

- This injection can be superficial. Depositing corticosteroid in the subcutaneous tissues can result in the complication of skin atrophy and hypopigmentation. Avoid the development of a subdermal wheal while performing all injections of corticosteroid solutions.

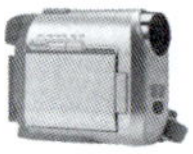

A video clip showing a tibialis posterior tendonitis injection can be found in the companion eBook.

## REFERENCE

1. Kulig K, Reischl SF, Pomrantz AB, et al. Nonsurgical management of posterior tibial tendon dysfunction with orthoses and resistive exercise: a randomized controlled trial. *Phys Ther*. 2009;89(1):26–37.

# Tarsal Tunnel Syndrome

Tarsal tunnel syndrome is a rare condition encountered in primary care. It represents an entrapment neuropathy of the posterior tibial nerve or its branches as it passes underneath the flexor retinaculum at the level of the medial malleolus. It may occur due to trauma from crush injury, stretch injury, fractures, dislocations, and severe ankle sprains. Other causes include overuse in athletes, valgus foot deformity, compression from bony prominences, and systemic conditions such as diabetes, hypothyroidism, rheumatoid arthritis, or amyloidosis. Typical symptoms include pain and paresthesias that radiate from the medial ankle. A positive Tinel sign may be elicited posterior to the medial malleolus. Electrodiagnostic tests frequently yield false-negative results.[1] Conservative treatment options include relative rest, physical therapy, orthotics, splints, and, perhaps, the injection of corticosteroids. However, there is no literature basis for the use of injections. Complete surgical decompression of the tarsal tunnel is required for patients with persistent symptoms.[2]

| Indication | ICD-9 Code | ICD-10 Code |
|---|---|---|
| Tarsal tunnel syndrome | 355.5 | G57.50 |

**Relevant Anatomy:** (Fig. 8.34)

## PATIENT POSITION

- Supine on the examination table with the hip in full external rotation, the knee slightly flexed, and the ankle in a neutral position.
- Alternatively, lying on the examination table on the affected side with the knee slightly flexed and the ankle in a neutral position.
- Rotate the patient's head away from the side that is being injected. This minimizes anxiety and pain perception.

## LANDMARKS

1. With the patient lying supine on the examination table, the clinician stands medial to the affected ankle.
2. Locate the medial malleolus of the tibia and then the insertion of the Achilles tendon into the calcaneus.
3. Midway between these two structures, palpate the posterior tibial artery.
4. The posterior tibial nerve is located about 0.5 cm posterior to the posterior tibial artery. Mark the nerve with ink.
5. At that site, press firmly on the skin with the retracted tip of a ballpoint pen. This indention represents the entry point for the needle.
6. After the landmarks are identified, the patient should not move the ankle.

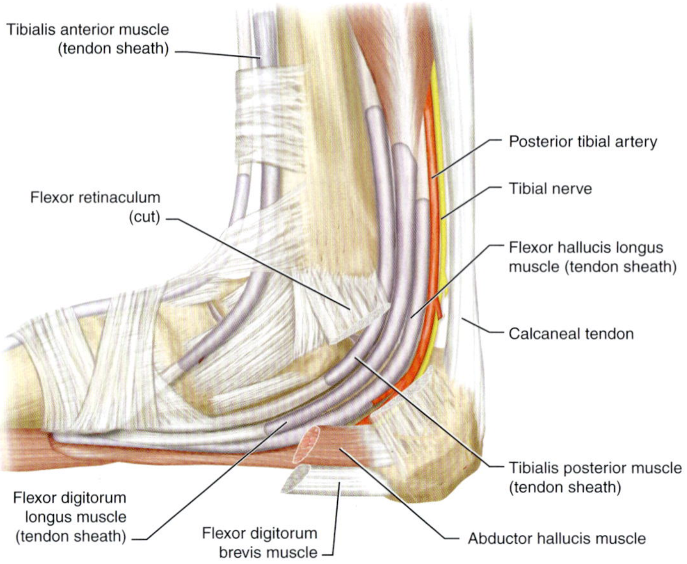


***FIGURE 8.34*** Medial aspect of the right foot. (From Tank PW, Gest TR. *Lippincott Williams & Wilkins Atlas of Anatomy*. Philadelphia, PA: Lippincott Williams & Wilkins, 2009.)

## ANESTHESIA

- Local anesthesia of the skin using a topical vapocoolant spray.

## EQUIPMENT

- 3-mL syringe
- 25-gauge, 5/8 in. needle
- 0.5 mL of 1% lidocaine without epinephrine
- 0.5 mL of the steroid solution (20 mg of triamcinolone acetonide)
- One alcohol prep pad
- Two povidone–iodine prep pads
- Sterile gauze pads
- Sterile adhesive bandage
- Nonsterile, clean chucks pad

## TECHNIQUE

1. Prep the insertion site with alcohol followed by the povidone–iodine pads.
2. Achieve good local anesthesia by using a topical vapocoolant spray.
3. Position the needle and syringe with the needle tip directed perpendicularly to the surface of the skin with the tip of the needle directed laterally toward the nerve.
4. Using the no-touch technique, introduce the needle at the insertion site (Fig. 8.35).
5. Advance the needle about 1 cm deep. If any pain, paresthesia, or numbness is encountered, back up the needle 1 to 2 mm.
6. Aspirate with the syringe to ensure that the needle tip is not in the posterior tibial artery or vein.
7. Slowly inject the volume of the syringe as a bolus around the posterior tibial nerve and into the tarsal tunnel. If increased resistance is encountered, advance or withdraw the needle slightly before attempting further injection.

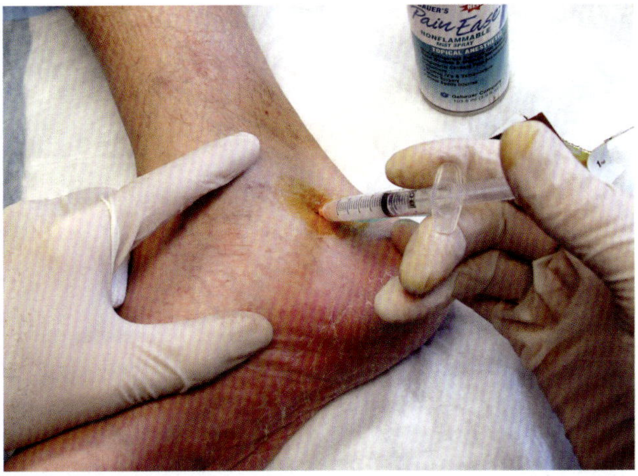


*FIGURE 8.35* ● Tarsal tunnel injection.

8. Following injection of the corticosteroid solution, withdraw the needle.
9. Apply a sterile adhesive bandage.
10. Instruct the patient to move his or her ankle through its full range of motion. This movement distributes the steroid solution along the nerve and throughout the tarsal tunnel.
11. Reexamine the foot in 5 min to confirm pain relief or the development of numbness in the distribution of the posterior tibial nerve from the local anesthetic.

## AFTERCARE

- Avoid excessive use of the foot over the next 2 weeks.
- Begin a program of physical therapy.
- Use orthotics or "motion-control" running shoes if there is excessive foot pronation.
- Consider splinting—especially at night.
- NSAIDs, ice, and heat as indicated.
- Consider follow-up examination in 2 weeks.

**CPT code:** 64450—Injection, nerve block, therapeutic, other peripheral nerve or branch

## PEARLS

- Warn the patient that the posterior tibial nerve may be contacted when using this approach. Ask him or her to calmly report any pain or electrical shock sensation without jerking his or her foot away.
- This injection can be superficial. Depositing corticosteroid in the subcutaneous tissues can result in the complication of skin atrophy and hypopigmentation. Avoid the development of a subdermal wheal while performing all injections of the corticosteroid solutions.

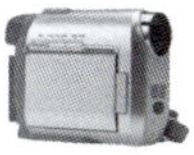

A video clip showing a tarsal tunnel syndrome injection can be found in the companion eBook.

## REFERENCES

1. Ahmad M, Tsang K, Mackenney PJ, et al. Tarsal tunnel syndrome: a literature review. *Foot Ankle Surg.* 2012;18(3):149–152.
2. Franson J, Baravarian B. Tarsal tunnel syndrome: a compression neuropathy involving four distinct tunnels. *Clin Podiatr Med Surg.* 2006;23(3):597–609.

# Ankle Joint—Anterolateral Approach

Injection of the ankle joint is a fairly uncommon procedure in primary care. Ankle joint pain may occur following a trauma or with osteoarthritis, gout, rheumatoid arthritis, or other inflammatory conditions. Conservative treatment of osteoarthritis includes the use of nonsteroidal anti-inflammatory drugs, orthotics, and ankle braces. A small study demonstrated benefit of corticosteroid injections.[1] A recent report demonstrates effectiveness of this particular approach, especially when combined with imaging placement.[2] There is increasing data on improvement in pain and function in patients treated with hyaluronic acid viscosupplements.[3,4] However, this treatment is not approved by the U.S. Food and Drug Administration at the time of publication. The gold standard for operative intervention in end-stage degenerative arthritis remains arthrodesis, but evidence for the superiority in functional outcomes of total ankle arthroplasty is increasing.[5] A small-diameter needle is appropriate as this technique is primarily used to inject steroid solution into the ankle joint. Occasionally, there will be a small amount of joint fluid to be aspirated.

| **Indications** | **ICD-9 Code** | **ICD-10 Code** |
|---|---|---|
| Ankle pain | 719.47 | M25.579 |
| Ankle sprain, unspecified site | 845.00 | S93.401 |
| Ankle arthritis, unspecified | 716.97 | M12.9 |
| Ankle osteoarthritis, primary | 715.17 | M19.079 |
| Ankle osteoarthritis, posttraumatic | 716.17 | M12.579 |
| Ankle osteoarthritis, secondary | 715.27 | M19.279 |

**Relevant Anatomy:** (Fig. 8.36)

## PATIENT POSITION

1. Supine on the examination table.
2. The knee on the affected side is placed in 90 degrees of flexion.
3. The ankle is slightly plantar flexed so that the plantar surface is in full contact with the chucks pad covering the exam table.
4. Rotate the patient's head away from the side that is being injected. This minimizes anxiety and pain perception.

## LANDMARKS

1. With the patient lying supine on the examination table, the clinician stands lateral to the affected ankle.
2. Locate the junction between the fibula, distal tibia, and talus over the anterolateral aspect of the ankle.

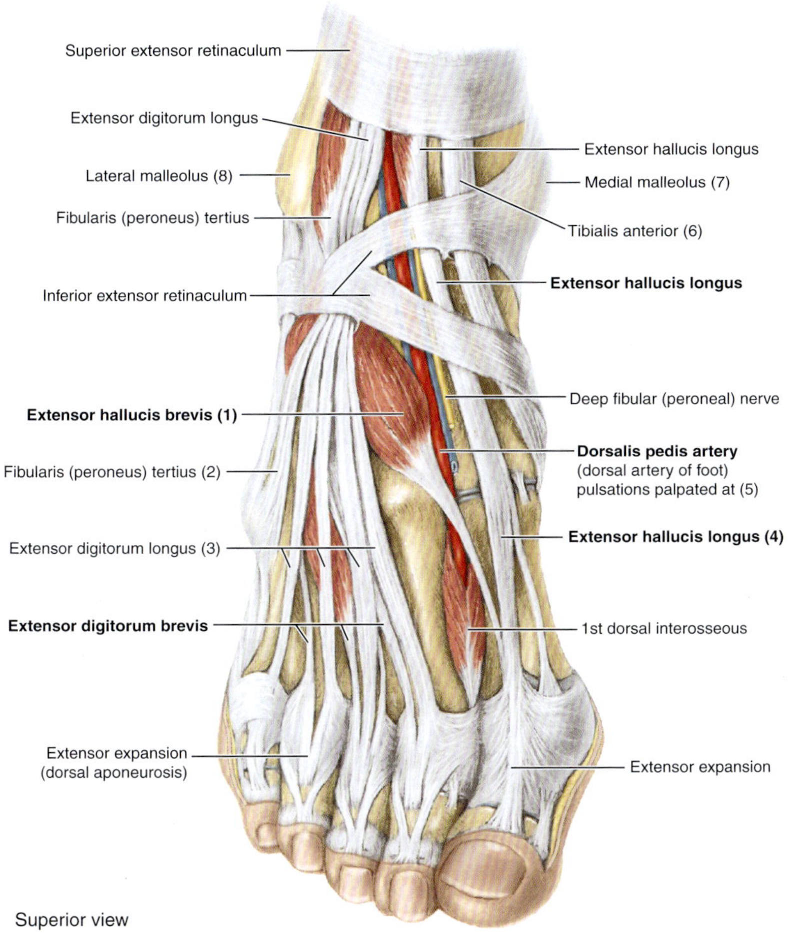


***FIGURE 8.36*** • Anterior aspect of the right ankle. (Adapted from Tank PW, Gest TR. *Lippincott Williams & Wilkins Atlas of Anatomy*. Philadelphia, PA: Lippincott Williams & Wilkins, 2009.)

3. Mark a point over this articulation. There is normally a depression in that area.
4. At that site, press firmly on the skin with the retracted tip of a ballpoint pen. This indention represents the entry point for the needle.
5. After the landmarks are identified, the patient should not move the ankle.

## ANESTHESIA

- Local anesthesia of the skin using topical vapocoolant spray

## EQUIPMENT

- 20-mL syringe—for optional aspiration
- 3-mL syringe—for injection
- 20-gauge, 1 in. needle—for optional aspiration
- 25-gauge, 1½ in. needle—if not aspirating fluid
- 1 mL of 1% lidocaine without epinephrine
- 1 mL of the steroid solution (40 mg of triamcinolone acetonide)
- One alcohol prep pad

- Two povidone–iodine prep pads
- Sterile gauze pads
- Sterile adhesive bandage
- Nonsterile, clean chucks pad

## TECHNIQUE

1. Prep the insertion site with alcohol followed by the povidone–iodine pads.
2. Achieve good local anesthesia by using topical vapocoolant spray.
3. Position the needle and syringe perpendicular to the skin with the tip of the needle directed toward the center of the ankle.
4. Using the no-touch technique, introduce the needle at the insertion site (Fig. 8.37).
5. Advance the needle into the ankle joint. This places the needle tip between the distal tibia and fibula in the ankle joint.
6. If aspirating, withdraw the fluid using a 20-gauge, 1½ in. needle with the 20-mL syringe.
7. If only injecting corticosteroid solution, use a 25-gauge, 1½ in. needle with the 3-mL syringe.
8. If injection following aspiration is elected, remove the large syringe from the 20-gauge needle and then attach the 3-mL syringe filled with the steroid solution.
9. Inject the steroid solution as a bolus into the ankle joint. The injected solution should flow smoothly into the space. If increased resistance is encountered, advance or withdraw the needle slightly before attempting further injection.
10. Following injection of the corticosteroid solution, withdraw the needle.
11. Apply a sterile adhesive bandage.
12. Instruct the patient to move his or her ankle through its full range of motion. This movement distributes the steroid solution throughout the ankle joint.
13. Reexamine the ankle in 5 min to confirm pain relief.

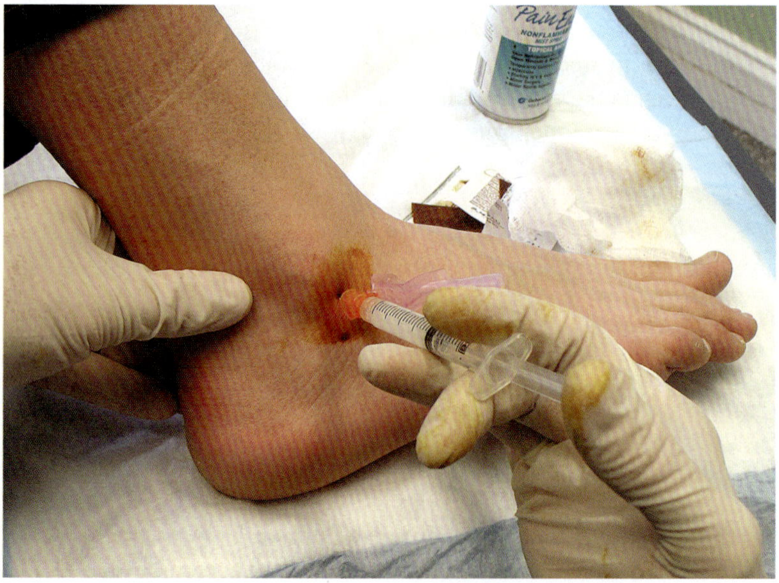

**FIGURE 8.37** Right anterolateral ankle joint injection.

## AFTERCARE

- Consider the use of an ankle brace.
- Avoid vigorous use of the ankle over the next 2 weeks.
- NSAIDs, ice, and/or physical therapy as indicated.
- Consider follow-up examination in 2 weeks.

**CPT code:** 20605—Arthrocentesis, aspiration, and/or injection of intermediate joint or bursa

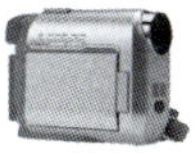

A video clip showing an ankle joint injection can be found in the companion eBook.

## REFERENCES

1. Ward ST, Williams PL, Purkayastha S. Intra-articular corticosteroid injections in the foot and ankle: a prospective 1-year follow-up investigation. *J Foot Ankle Surg*. 2008;47(2):138–144.
2. Fox MG, Wright PR, Alford B, et al. Lateral mortise approach for therapeutic ankle injection: an alternative to the anteromedial approach. *AJR Am J Roentgenol*. 2013;200(5):1096–1100.
3. Lucas Y, Hernandez J, Darcel V, et al. Viscosupplementation of the ankle: a prospective study with an average follow-up of 45.5 months. *Orthop Traumatol Surg Res*. 2013;99(5):593–599.
4. Chang KV, Hsiao MY, Chen WS, et al. Effectiveness of intra-articular hyaluronic acid for ankle osteoarthritis treatment: a systematic review and meta-analysis. *Arch Phys Med Rehabil*. 2013;94(5):951–960.
5. Grunfeld R, Aydogan U, Juliano P. Ankle arthritis: review of diagnosis and operative management. *Med Clin North Am*. 2014;98(2):267–289.

# Ankle Joint—Anteromedial Approach

Injection of the ankle joint is a fairly uncommon procedure in primary care. Ankle joint pain may occur following a trauma or with osteoarthritis, gout, rheumatoid arthritis, or other inflammatory conditions. Conservative treatment of osteoarthritis includes the use of nonsteroidal anti-inflammatory drugs, orthotics, and ankle braces. A small study demonstrated benefit of corticosteroid injections.[1] There is increasing data on improvement in pain and function in patients treated with hyaluronic acid viscosupplements.[2,3] However, this treatment is not approved by the U.S. Food and Drug Administration at the time of publication. The gold standard for operative intervention in end-stage degenerative arthritis remains arthrodesis, but evidence for the superiority in functional outcomes of total ankle arthroplasty is increasing.[4] A small-diameter needle is appropriate as this technique is primarily used to inject steroid solution into the ankle joint. Occasionally, there will be a small amount of joint fluid to be aspirated.

| Indications | ICD-9 Code | ICD-10 Code |
|---|---|---|
| Ankle pain | 719.47 | M25.579 |
| Ankle sprain, unspecified site | 845.00 | S93.401 |
| Ankle arthritis, unspecified | 716.97 | M12.9 |
| Ankle osteoarthritis, primary | 715.17 | M19.079 |
| Ankle osteoarthritis, posttraumatic | 716.17 | M12.579 |
| Ankle osteoarthritis, secondary | 715.27 | M19.279 |

**Relevant Anatomy:** (Fig. 8.38)

## PATIENT POSITION

- Supine on the examination table.
- The knee on the affected side is placed in 90 degrees of flexion.
- The ankle is slightly plantar flexed so that the plantar surface is in full contact with the chucks pad covering the exam table.
- Rotate the patient's head away from the side that is being injected. This minimizes anxiety and pain perception.

## LANDMARKS

1. With the patient lying supine on the examination table, the clinician stands medial to the affected ankle.
2. Locate the junction between the fibula, distal tibia, and talus over the anterolateral aspect of the ankle.
3. Identify the anterior tibialis tendon.

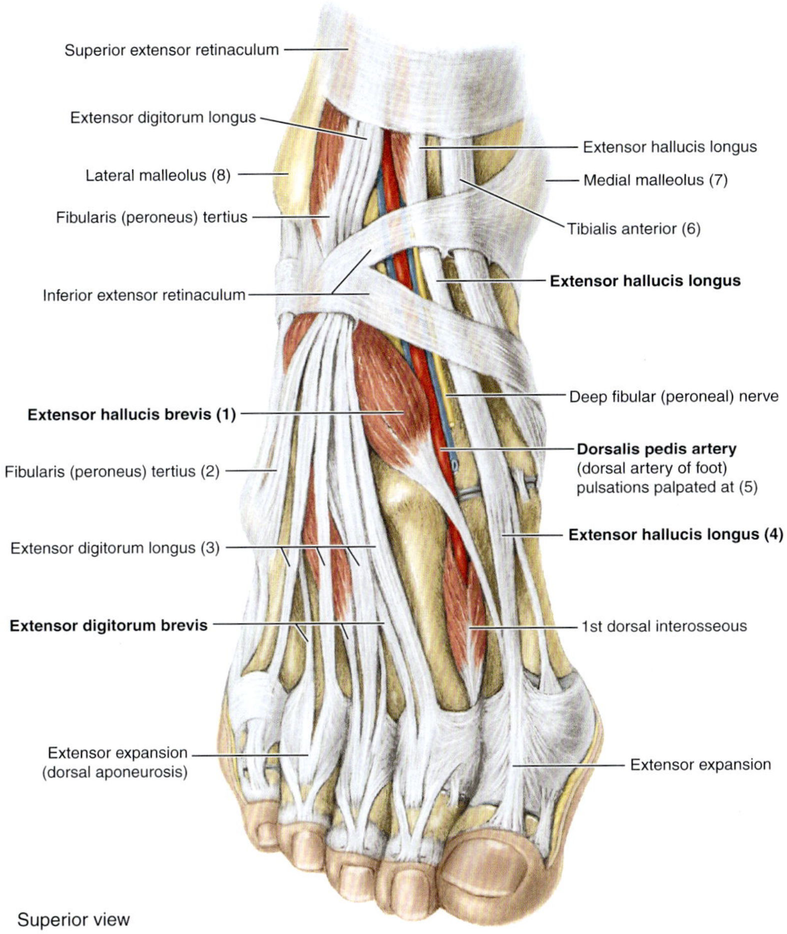


**FIGURE 8.38** ● Right anterior ankle. (Adapted from Tank PW, Gest TR. *Lippincott Williams & Wilkins Atlas of Anatomy*. Philadelphia, PA: Lippincott Williams & Wilkins, 2009.)

4. Mark a point over the ankle joint line that is 1 cm medial to the anterior tibialis tendon. There is normally a depression in that area.
5. At that site, press firmly on the skin with the retracted tip of a ballpoint pen. This indention represents the entry point for the needle.
6. After the landmarks are identified, the patient should not move the ankle.

## ANESTHESIA

- Local anesthesia of the skin using topical vapocoolant spray.

## EQUIPMENT

- 20-mL syringe—for optional aspiration
- 3-mL syringe—for injection
- 20-gauge, 1 in. needle—for optional aspiration
- 25-gauge, 1½ in. needle—if not aspirating fluid
- 1 mL of 1% lidocaine without epinephrine
- 1 mL of the steroid solution (40 mg of triamcinolone acetonide)

- One alcohol prep pad
- Two povidone–iodine prep pads
- Sterile gauze pads
- Sterile adhesive bandage
- Nonsterile, clean chucks pad

## TECHNIQUE

1. Prep the insertion site with alcohol followed by the povidone–iodine pads.
2. Achieve good local anesthesia by using topical vapocoolant spray.
3. Position the needle and syringe perpendicular to the skin with the tip of the needle directed toward the center of the ankle.
4. Using the no-touch technique, introduce the needle at the insertion site (Fig. 8.39).
5. Advance the needle into the ankle joint. This places the needle tip between the distal tibia and fibula in the ankle joint.
6. If aspirating, withdraw the fluid using a 20-gauge, 1½ in. needle with the 20-mL syringe.
7. If only injecting corticosteroid solution, use a 25-gauge, 1½ in. needle with the 3-mL syringe.
8. If injection following aspiration is elected, remove the large syringe from the 20-gauge needle and then attach the 3-mL syringe filled with the steroid solution.
9. Inject the steroid solution as a bolus into the ankle joint. The injected solution should flow smoothly into the space. If increased resistance is encountered, advance or withdraw the needle slightly before attempting further injection.
10. Following injection of the corticosteroid solution, withdraw the needle.
11. Apply a sterile adhesive bandage.
12. Instruct the patient to move his or her ankle through its full range of motion. This movement distributes the steroid solution throughout the ankle joint.
13. Reexamine the ankle in 5 min to confirm pain relief.

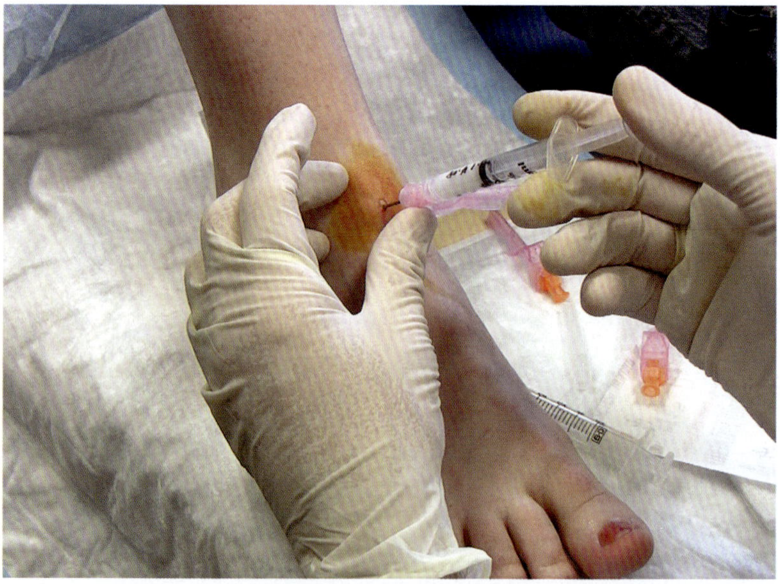

***FIGURE 8.39*** Right anteromedial ankle joint injection.

## AFTERCARE

- Consider the use of an ankle brace.
- Avoid vigorous use of the affected ankle over the next 2 weeks.
- NSAIDs, ice, and/or physical therapy as indicated.
- Consider follow-up examination in 2 weeks.

**CPT code:** 20605 – Arthrocentesis, aspiration, and/or injection of intermediate joint or bursa

## PEARLS

- Insert the needle medially to the anterior tibialis tendon in order to avoid injury to the anterior tibial artery, anterior tibial vein, and peroneal nerve.

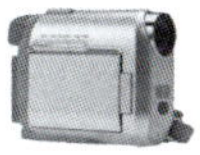

A video clip showing an ankle joint injection can be found in the companion eBook.

## REFERENCES


1. Ward ST, Williams PL, Purkayastha S. Intra-articular corticosteroid injections in the foot and ankle: a prospective 1-year follow-up investigation. *J Foot Ankle Surg*. 2008;47(2):138–144.
2. Lucas Y, Hernandez J, Darcel V, et al. Viscosupplementation of the ankle: a prospective study with an average follow-up of 45.5 months. *Orthop Traumatol Surg Res*. 2013;99(5):593–599.
3. Chang KV, Hsiao MY, Chen WS, et al. Effectiveness of intra-articular hyaluronic acid for ankle osteoarthritis treatment: a systematic review and meta-analysis. *Arch Phys Med Rehabil*. 2013;94(5):951–960.
4. Grunfeld R, Aydogan U, Juliano P. Ankle arthritis: review of diagnosis and operative management. *Med Clin North Am*. 2014;98(2):267–289.

# Fibularis Brevis Tendonitis

Injection of corticosteroids for the treatment of tendonitis of the fibularis brevis (formerly known as the peroneus brevis) tendon is a fairly uncommon procedure for primary care physicians. The fibularis longus and brevis tendons are often injured with inversion ankle sprains. This can cause chronic subluxation of the tendons. Overuse from repeated forceful plantar flexion and resisted foot eversion may also occur. Corticosteroid injections are provided, but without research support for this practice.

| Indication | ICD-9 Code | ICD-10 Code |
|---|---|---|
| Peroneus brevis tendonitis | 726.79 | M76.70 |

**Relevant Anatomy:** (Fig. 8.40)

## PATIENT POSITION

- Supine on the examination table.
- The ankle and the knee on the affected side are supported by placing rolled towels underneath them.
- The ankle is in a neutral position.
- Rotate the patient's head away from the side that is being injected. This minimizes anxiety and pain perception.

## LANDMARKS

1. With the patient lying supine on the examination table, the clinician stands lateral to the affected foot.
2. While the foot is held in a position of active eversion, identify tenderness at and immediately proximal to the head of the fifth metatarsal bone.
3. Palpate the fibularis brevis tendon along its course from posterior and distal to the lateral malleolus to its insertion into the head of the fifth metatarsal bone.
4. Locate the area of maximal tenderness.
5. At that site, press firmly with the retracted tip of a ballpoint pen. This indention represents the entry point for the needle.
6. After the landmarks are identified, the patient should not move the ankle.

## ANESTHESIA

- Local anesthesia of the skin using a topical vapocoolant spray.

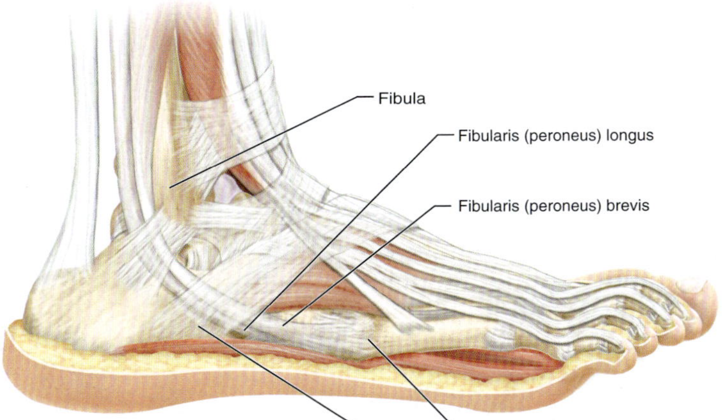


***FIGURE 8.40*** ● Lateral aspect of the right foot. (From Tank PW, Gest TR. *Lippincott Williams & Wilkins Atlas of Anatomy*. Philadelphia, PA: Lippincott Williams & Wilkins, 2009.)

## EQUIPMENT

- 3-mL syringe
- 25-gauge, 5/8 in. needle
- 0.5 mL of 1% lidocaine without epinephrine
- 0.5 mL of the steroid solution (20 mg of triamcinolone acetonide)
- One alcohol prep pad
- Two povidone–iodine prep pads
- Sterile gauze pads
- Sterile adhesive bandage
- Nonsterile, clean chucks pad

## TECHNIQUE

1. Prep the insertion site with alcohol followed by the povidone–iodine pads.
2. Achieve good local anesthesia by using a topical vapocoolant spray.
3. If treating tendonitis at the insertion of the fibularis brevis on the fifth metacarpal:
   a. Position the needle and syringe at an angle of 30 degrees to the skin with the needle tip directed distally.
   b. Using the no-touch technique, introduce the needle at the insertion site.
   c. Advance the needle slowly until the needle tip touches the tendon/bone junction. Back up the needle 1 to 2 mm.
   d. Inject the steroid solution slowly as a bolus around the insertion of the fibularis brevis tendon into the head of the fifth metatarsal. The injected solution should flow smoothly into the space. If increased resistance is encountered, advance or withdraw the needle slightly before attempting further injection.
4. If treating tendonitis along the course of the fibularis brevis tendon proximal to its insertion:
   a. Position the needle and syringe at an angle of 30 degrees to the skin with the needle tip directed proximally.
   b. Using the no-touch technique, introduce the needle at the insertion site (Fig. 8.41).

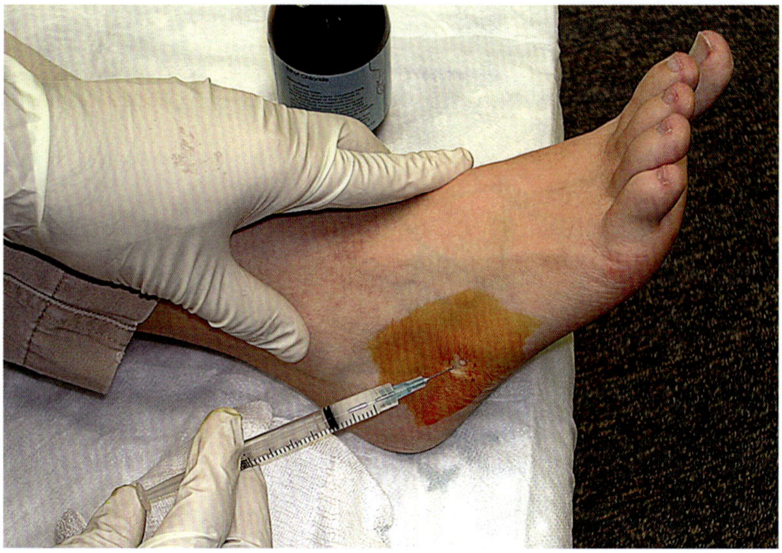

**FIGURE 8.41** ● Injection of the right fibularis brevis tendon insertion.

c. Advance the needle slowly until the needle tip touches the tendon. Back up the needle 1 to 2 mm.
d. Inject the steroid solution slowly as a bolus around the fibularis brevis tendon. A small bulge in the shape of a sausage may develop in the tendon sheath. The injected solution should flow smoothly into the tenosynovial space. If increased resistance is encountered, advance or withdraw the needle slightly before attempting further injection.

5. Following injection of the corticosteroid solution, withdraw the needle.
6. Apply a sterile adhesive bandage.
7. Instruct the patient to move his or her ankle through its full range of inversion and eversion. This movement distributes the steroid solution throughout the fibularis brevis tenosynovial sheath.
8. Reexamine the foot in 5 min to confirm pain relief.

## AFTERCARE

- Ensure no excessive plantar flexion over the next 2 weeks by the use of an ankle–foot orthotic or walking cast.
- NSAIDs, ice, heat, and/or physical therapy as indicated.
- Consider follow-up examination in 2 weeks.

**CPT code:** 20550—Injection of single tendon sheath

## PEARLS

- The fibularis brevis tendon is superficial. As a result, this injection can be complicated by the development of skin atrophy and hypopigmentation. Avoid the development of a subdermal wheal while injecting the corticosteroid solution.

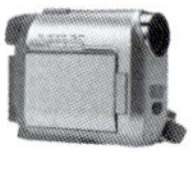

A video clip showing a fibularis brevis tendon injection can be found in the companion eBook.

# Plantar Fasciitis

Injection of corticosteroids for the treatment of plantar fasciitis is a common procedure for primary care physicians. Plantar fasciitis is a repetitive motion injury with inflammation in the origin of the plantar aponeurosis at the medial tubercle of the calcaneus. It is usually caused by an excessive pronation of the foot—especially in persons with pes planus. The pain with this condition is worst when bearing weight after a period of rest. Conservative treatment modalities include rest, orthotics, stretching, therapeutic exercise, tension night splints, anti-inflammatory medications, and injections. Corticosteroids have been a mainstay of treatment and demonstrate at least short-term symptomatic improvement.[1,2] Efficacy increases with ultrasound guidance.[3,4] Other injection treatment options may include platelet-rich plasma[5,6] and botulinum toxin.[7,8] Surgical procedures are considered if conservative management fails.

| Indication | ICD-9 Code | ICD-10 Code |
|---|---|---|
| Plantar fasciitis | 728.71 | M72.2 |

**Relevant Anatomy:** (Fig. 8.42)

## PATIENT POSITION

- Supine on the examination table with the hip in full external rotation, the knee slightly flexed, and the ankle in a neutral position.
- Alternatively, lying on the examination table on the affected side with the knee slightly flexed and the ankle in a neutral position.
- Rotate the patient's head away from the side that is being injected. This minimizes anxiety and pain perception.

## LANDMARKS

1. With the patient lying supine on the examination table, the clinician stands medial to the affected foot.
2. Identify the point of maximal tenderness over the plantar aspect of the foot. This is usually just medial of midline over the medial tubercle of the calcaneus.
3. Draw a vertical line down the posterior border of the tibia.
4. Draw a horizontal line one fingerbreadth above the plantar surface.
5. Mark the point where these two lines intersect over the medial aspect of the foot.
6. At that site, press firmly on the skin with the retracted tip of a ballpoint pen. This indention represents the entry point for the needle.
7. After the landmarks are identified, the patient should not move the foot or ankle.

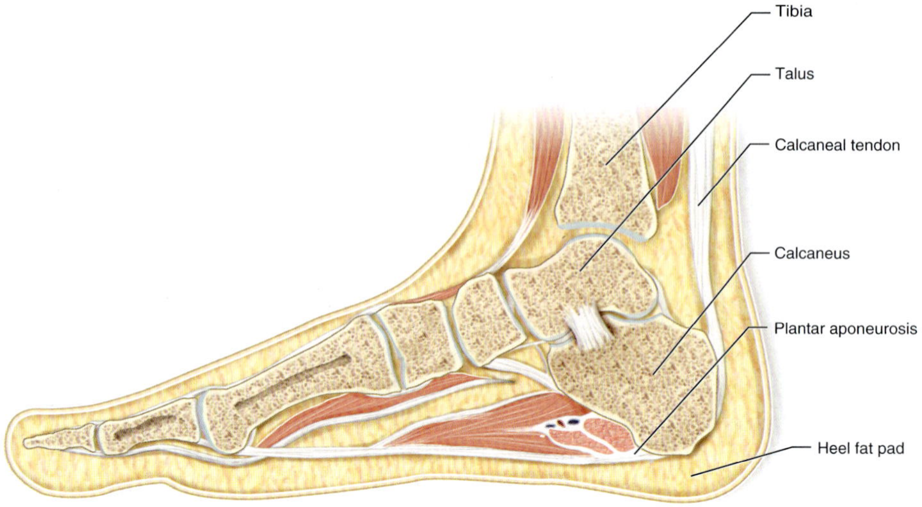


**FIGURE 8.42** ● Medial right foot—sagittal section. (From Tank PW, Gest TR. *Lippincott Williams & Wilkins Atlas of Anatomy*. Philadelphia, PA: Lippincott Williams & Wilkins, 2009.)

## ANESTHESIA

- Local anesthesia of the skin using a topical vapocoolant spray.

## EQUIPMENT

- 3-mL syringe
- 25-gauge, 1½ in. needle
- 1 mL of 1% lidocaine without epinephrine
- 1 mL of the steroid solution (40 mg of triamcinolone acetonide)
- One alcohol prep pad
- Two povidone–iodine prep pads
- Sterile gauze pads
- Sterile adhesive bandage
- Nonsterile, clean chucks pad

## TECHNIQUE

1. Prep the insertion site with alcohol followed by the povidone–iodine pads.
2. Achieve good local anesthesia by using topical vapocoolant spray.
3. Position the needle and syringe perpendicular to the skin and the intersection of the two landmark lines with the tip of the needle directed laterally.
4. Using the no-touch technique, introduce the needle at the insertion site (Fig. 8.43).
5. Advance the needle toward the medial tubercle of the calcaneus until the needle tip is located at the origin of the plantar fascia.
6. Inject the steroid solution as a bolus at the origin of the plantar fascia. The injected solution should flow smoothly into the space. If increased resistance is encountered, advance or withdraw the needle slightly before attempting further injection.
7. Following injection of the corticosteroid solution, withdraw the needle.
8. Apply a sterile adhesive bandage.
9. Instruct the patient to massage the area and then take several steps. This movement distributes the steroid solution along the plantar fascia.
10. Reexamine the foot in 5 min to confirm pain relief.

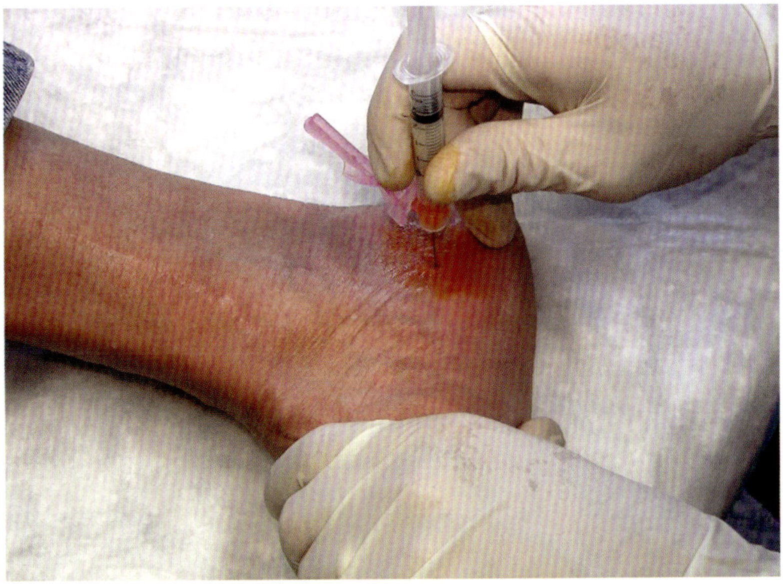

*FIGURE 8.43* • Right foot plantar fasciitis injection.

## AFTERCARE

- NSAIDs, ice, heat, and/or physical therapy as indicated.
- Instruct the patient to perform heel cord stretching exercises four times a day.
- Wear proper shoes or orthotics as indicated.
- Consider the use of a tension night splint.
- Consider follow-up examination in 2 weeks.

**CPT code:** 20550—Injection of aponeurosis

## PEARLS

- The plantar fascia injection may be quite painful. This is especially true if the injection is performed through the plantar surface of the foot. The medial approach described above minimizes the pain of this procedure. Vapocoolant spray should always be used.
- Notice the thickness of the plantar fat pad in the anatomic drawing. The injection should be placed superior to the fat pad in order to prevent fat atrophy in this critical area.

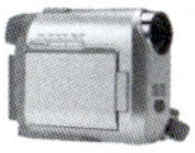

A video clip showing a plantar fasciitis injection can be found in the companion eBook.

## REFERENCES

1. Ball EM, McKeeman HM, Patterson C, et al. Steroid injection for inferior heel pain: a randomised controlled trial. *Ann Rheum Dis*. 2013;72(6):996–1002.
2. Kim C, Cashdollar MR, Mendicino RW, et al. Incidence of plantar fascia ruptures following corticosteroid injection. *Foot Ankle Spec*. 2010;3(6):335–337.
3. Chen CM, Chen JS, Tsai WC, et al. Effectiveness of device-assisted ultrasound-guided steroid injection for treating plantar fasciitis. *Am J Phys Med Rehabil*. 2013;92(7):597–605.

4. McMillan AM, Landorf KB, Gilheany MF, et al. Ultrasound guided corticosteroid injection for plantar fasciitis: randomised controlled trial. *BMJ*. 2012;344:e3260.
5. Martinelli N, Marinozzi A, Carnì S, et al. Platelet-rich plasma injections for chronic plantar fasciitis. *Int Orthop*. 2013;37(5):839–842.
6. Ragab EM, Othman AM. Platelets rich plasma for treatment of chronic plantar fasciitis. *Arch Orthop Trauma Surg*. 2012;132(8):1065–1070.
7. Díaz-Llopis IV, Gómez-Gallego D, Mondéjar-Gómez FJ, et al. Botulinum toxin type A in chronic plantar fasciitis: clinical effects 1 year after injection. *Clin Rehabil*. 2013;27(8):681–685.
8. Elizondo-Rodriguez J, Araujo-Lopez Y, Moreno-Gonzalez JA, et al. A comparison of botulinum toxin a and intralesional steroids for the treatment of plantar fasciitis: a randomized, double-blinded study. *Foot Ankle Int*. 2013;34(1):8–14.

# First Metatarsophalangeal Joint

The first metatarsophalangeal (MTP) joint of the foot is a relatively common aspiration and injection site for primary care physicians. This joint is the most commonly involved joint with gout and is frequently affected by osteoarthritis. Sivera et al.[1] have described the use of a 29-gauge needle to successfully aspirate this joint. Injected corticosteroids are also useful in patients with mild grades of hallux rigidus.[2]

| Indications | ICD-9 Code | ICD-10 Code |
|---|---|---|
| Pain of first MTP joint | 719.47 | M25.579 |
| Acute gouty arthritis, unspecified, toe | 274.0 | M10.079 |
| First MTP joint arthritis, unspecified | 716.97 | M12.9 |
| First MTP joint osteoarthritis, primary | 715.17 | M19.079 |
| First MTP joint osteoarthritis, posttraumatic | 716.17 | M19.179 |
| First MTP joint osteoarthritis, secondary | 715.27 | M19.279 |

**Relevant Anatomy:** (Fig. 8.44)

## PATIENT POSITION

- Supine on the examination table.
- The knee on the affected side is placed in 90 degrees of flexion.
- The ankle is slightly plantar flexed so that the plantar surface is in full contact with the chucks pad covering the exam table.
- Rotate the patient's head away from the side that is being injected. This minimizes anxiety and pain perception.

## LANDMARKS

1. With the patient lying supine on the examination table, the clinician stands medial to the affected foot.
2. Locate the first MTP joint with simultaneous palpation and flexion/extension of the great toe proximal phalanx. The patient will report tenderness in this joint, and there may be associated erythema and swelling.
3. The injection point is directly over the first MTP joint.
4. At that site, press firmly on the skin with the retracted tip of a ballpoint pen. This indention represents the entry point for the needle.
5. After the landmarks are identified, the patient should not move the foot or toe.

## ANESTHESIA

- Local anesthesia of the skin using topical vapocoolant spray

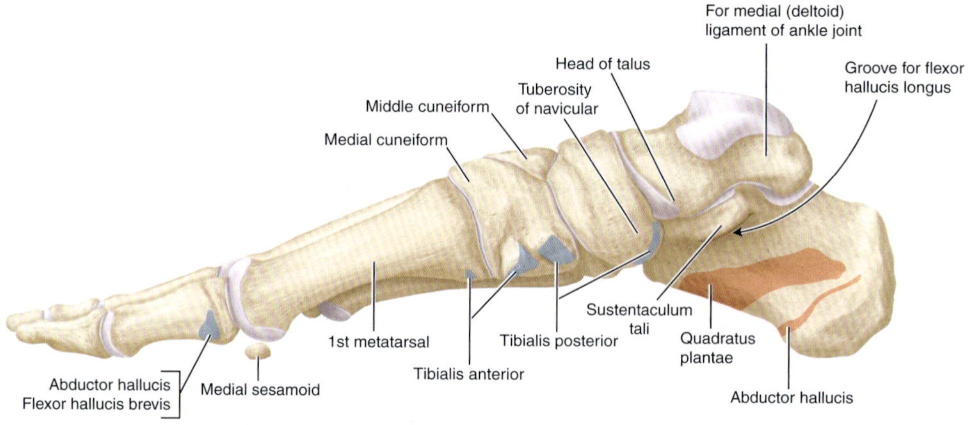


*FIGURE 8.44* Medial aspect of the right foot—bony anatomy. (Adapted from Tank PW, Gest TR. *Lippincott Williams & Wilkins Atlas of Anatomy*. Philadelphia, PA: Lippincott Williams & Wilkins, 2009.)

## EQUIPMENT

- 3-mL syringe
- 3-mL syringe—for optional aspiration
- 25-gauge, 1/2 in. needle
- 0.25 to 0.5 mL of 1% lidocaine without epinephrine
- 0.25 to 0.5 mL of the steroid solution (10 to 20 mg of triamcinolone acetonide)
- One alcohol prep pad
- Two povidone–iodine prep pads
- Sterile gauze pads
- Sterile adhesive bandage
- Nonsterile, clean chucks pad

## TECHNIQUE

1. Prep the insertion site with alcohol followed by the povidone–iodine pads.
2. Achieve good local anesthesia by using topical vapocoolant spray.
3. Position the needle and syringe perpendicular to the skin with the tip of the needle directed into the center of the joint.
4. Using the no-touch technique, introduce the needle at the insertion site (Fig. 8.45).
5. Advance the needle until the tip is located in the joint capsule. If the needle contacts bone or cartilage, back up the needle 1 to 2 mm.
6. If aspirating, withdraw fluid using the 25-gauge, 1/2 in. needle with a 3-mL syringe.
7. If injection following aspiration is elected, remove the 3-mL syringe from the 25-gauge needle and then attach the 3-mL syringe filled with the steroid solution.
8. If only injecting corticosteroid solution, use a 25-gauge, 1/2 in. needle with the 3-mL syringe.
9. Inject the steroid solution as a bolus into the joint capsule. The injected solution should flow smoothly into the space. If increased resistance is encountered, advance or withdraw the needle slightly before attempting further injection.
10. Following injection of the corticosteroid solution, withdraw the needle.
11. Apply a sterile adhesive bandage.

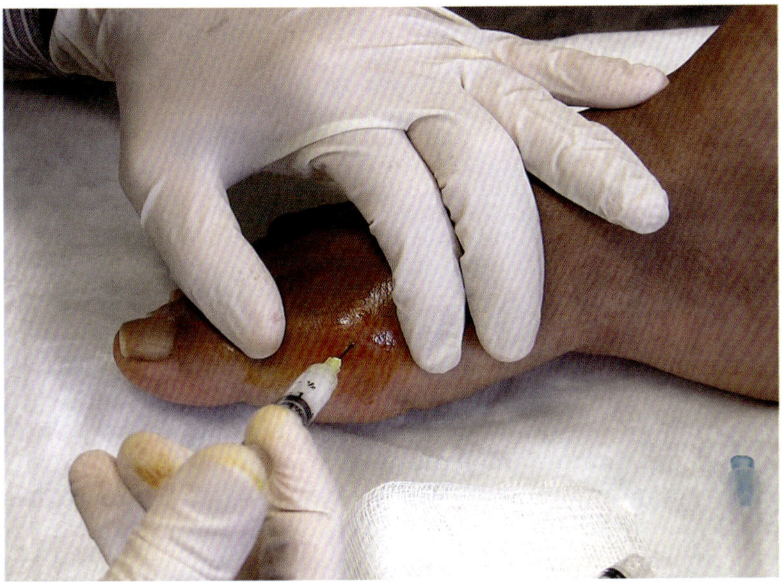

*FIGURE 8.45* • Right first MTP joint injection.

12. Instruct the patient to move his or her toe through its full range of motion. This movement distributes the steroid solution throughout the joint capsule.
13. Reexamine the first MTP joint in 5 min to confirm pain relief.

## AFTERCARE

- Avoid excessive movement of the first MTP joint over the next 2 weeks.
- NSAIDs, ice, and/or physical therapy as indicated.
- Consider the use of an ankle–foot orthotic or wooden-soled shoe.
- Consider follow-up examination in 2 weeks.

**CPT code:** 20600—Injection of small joint

## PEARLS

- Applying traction to the great toe in a distal direction may help open up the joint to accommodate the needle.

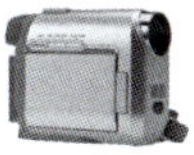

A video clip showing a first MTP joint injection can be found in the companion eBook.

## REFERENCES


1. Sivera F, Aragon R, Pascual E. First metatarsophalangeal joint aspiration using a 29-gauge needle. *Ann Rheum Dis*. 2008;67(2):273–275.
2. Solan MC, Calder JD, Bendall SP. Manipulation and injection for hallux rigidus: Is it worthwhile? *J Bone Joint Surg Br*. 2001;83:706–708.

# Morton Interdigital Neuroma

Compression of the interdigital nerves in the foot can result in a painful condition referred to as a Morton neuroma. This is a fairly common condition seen by primary care physicians. The condition is a repetitive compressive injury causing inflammation, perineural fibrosis, and enlargement of the interdigital nerve. Further compression of the neuroma causes symptoms of lancinating pain and dysesthesias with weight bearing—especially when wearing shoes with a narrow toe box. Usually, the neuroma lies between the second and third or the third and fourth metatarsal heads. Conservative treatment strategies include shoe-wear modifications, custom-made orthotics, and corticosteroid injections. Corticosteroid injections have shown to be effective interventions in the short to medium term.[1,2] They are less effective in the treatment of neuromas larger than 5 mm.[3] Sclerosant treatment with injections of alcohol shows short-term but not permanent resolution of symptoms for most patients and can be associated with considerable morbidity.[4] Patients who do not respond may require operative intervention with nerve decompression or neurectomy.

| Indication | ICD-9 Code | ICD-10 Code |
|---|---|---|
| Morton neuroma | 355.6 | G57.60 |

**Relevant Anatomy:** (Fig. 8.46)

## PATIENT POSITION

- Supine on the examination table.
- The knee on the affected side is placed in 90 degrees of flexion.
- The ankle is slightly plantar flexed so that the plantar surface is in full contact with the chucks pad covering the exam table.
- Rotate the patient's head away from the side that is being injected. This minimizes anxiety and pain perception.

## LANDMARKS

- With the patient lying supine on the examination table, the clinician stands or sits distal to the affected foot.
- Locate the site of maximal tenderness. This is found between the heads of the metatarsals. The most common site is between the second and third metatarsals.
- The injection point is on the dorsal aspect of the distal foot directly over the area of maximal tenderness. A tender nodule may be palpated occasionally at this site.
- At that site, press firmly on the skin with the retracted tip of a ballpoint pen. This indention represents the entry point for the needle.
- After the landmarks are identified, the patient should not move the foot.

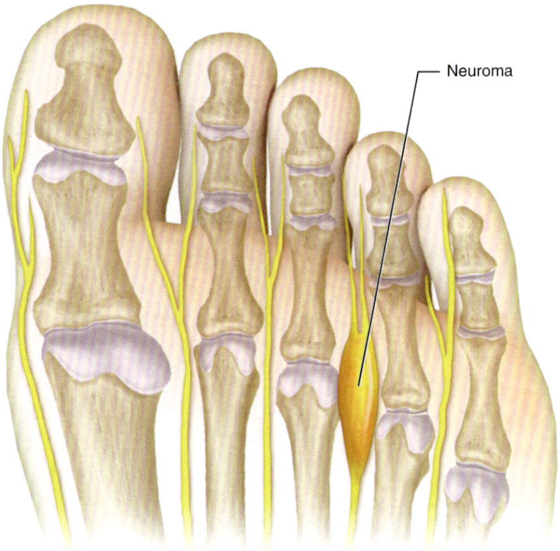


***FIGURE 8.46*** • Dorsal aspect of the right foot. (Adapted from Tank PW, Gest TR. *Lippincott Williams & Wilkins Atlas of Anatomy*. Philadelphia, PA: Lippincott Williams & Wilkins, 2009.)

## ANESTHESIA

- Local anesthesia of the skin using topical vapocoolant spray.

## EQUIPMENT

- 3-mL syringe
- 25-gauge, 1 in. needle
- 0.5 mL of 1% lidocaine without epinephrine
- 0.5 mL of the steroid solution (20 mg of triamcinolone acetonide)
- One alcohol prep pad
- Two povidone–iodine prep pads
- Sterile gauze pads
- Sterile adhesive bandage
- Nonsterile, clean chucks pad

## TECHNIQUE

1. Prep the insertion site with alcohol followed by the povidone–iodine pads.
2. Achieve good local anesthesia by using topical vapocoolant spray.
3. Position the needle and syringe perpendicular to the skin with the tip of the needle directed inferiorly between the affected metatarsal heads.
4. Using the no-touch technique, introduce the needle at the insertion site (Fig. 8.47).
5. Advance the needle until the needle tip is located between the metatarsal heads.
6. Inject the steroid solution as a bolus around the neuroma. The injected solution should flow smoothly into the space. If increased resistance is encountered, advance or withdraw the needle slightly before attempting further injection.
7. Following injection of the corticosteroid solution, withdraw the needle.
8. Apply a sterile adhesive bandage.
9. Instruct the patient to massage the area of injection. This movement distributes the steroid solution around the neuroma.
10. Reexamine the foot in 5 min to confirm pain relief.

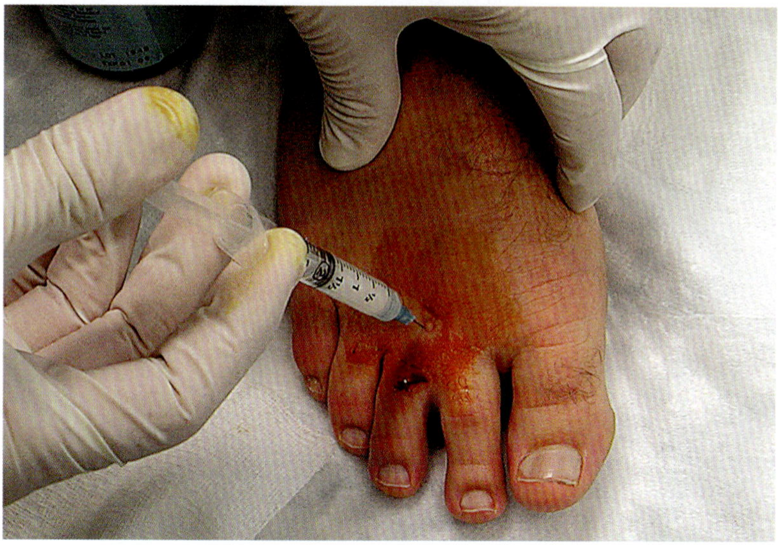

*FIGURE 8.47* ● Morton neuroma injection.

## AFTERCARE

- Avoid wearing shoes with a narrow toe box.
- NSAIDs, ice, and/or physical therapy as indicated.
- Consider metatarsal pads or custom orthotics.
- Consider follow-up examination in 2 weeks.

**CPT code:** 64455—Injection(s), anesthetic agent, and/or steroid, plantar common digital nerve(s) (e.g., Morton neuroma)

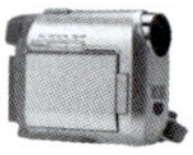

A video clip showing a Morton neuroma injection can be found in the companion eBook.

## REFERENCES

1. Markovic M, Crichton K, Read JW, et al. Effectiveness of ultrasound-guided corticosteroid injection in the treatment of Morton's neuroma. *Foot Ankle Int*. 2008;29(5):483–487.
2. Hassouna H, Singh D, Taylor H, et al. Ultrasound guided steroid injection in the treatment of interdigital neuralgia. *Acta Orthop Belg*. 2007;73(2):224–229.
3. Makki D, Haddad BZ, Mahmood Z, et al. Efficacy of corticosteroid injection versus size of plantar interdigital neuroma. *Foot Ankle Int*. 2012;33(9):722–726.
4. Gurdezi S, White T, Ramesh P. Alcohol injection for Morton's neuroma: a five-year follow-up. *Foot Ankle Int*. 2013;34(8):1064–1067.

APPENDIX 1

# Consent for Needle Aspiration and/or Injection

Date: ___________

I hereby authorize ______________________________________________

(Provider's name)

to perform upon ______________________________________________

(Patient's name)

the following procedure(s): ______________________________________________

______________________________________________

______________________________________________

The procedure(s) consists of: ______________________________________________

______________________________________________

______________________________________________

______________________________________________

(Describe in lay language)

Possible risks associated with the performance of a needle injection/aspiration may include but are not limited to:
Bleeding, Infection, Local pain, Fainting, Allergic reaction, or ________________

Possible risks with the use of injected corticosteroids may include but are not limited to:

**Feeling flushed**
**Tendon rupture**
**Abnormal skin color**
**Impaired immune response**
**Irregular menstrual periods**
**Flare-up of joint inflammation**
**Abnormal thinning of the skin**
**Worsening blood sugars in diabetes**
**Disturbance of hormone balance**

The nature of this procedure, methods of diagnosis/treatment, and possible alternatives have been explained to me by __________ or his/her associate. I am aware that there are certain risks associated with this procedure and that the practice of medicine and surgery is not an exact science. I acknowledge that no guarantees have been made to me concerning the results of the procedure or its interpretation.

I certify that I understand the contents of this form:

______________________________________________

Signature of patient or authorized representative

______________________________________________

Witness

IF THE PATIENT IS UNABLE TO CONSENT OR IS A MINOR, COMPLETE THE FOLLOWING:

The patient is a minor, ___ years of age, or is unable to consent because ______________

______________________________________________ (strike or define).

The undersigned hereby consents to the performance of the above described diagnostic/therapeutic procedure on the above patient as well as any tests, which are deemed necessary.

______________________________

Signature of authorized representative

APPENDIX 2

# Aspiration and Injection Aftercare Handout

You have just had a procedure done by: ______________________________

Your diagnosis is: ______________________________

The procedure involved placing a needle into the tissues to:

_____ withdraw fluid from the ______________________________

_____ inject "cortisone" into the ______________________________

_____ other ______________________________

**Please Follow These Instructions:**

**Recurring Pain:**
Injections are usually done using a local anesthetic such as lidocaine and cortisone. The anesthetic effect of the lidocaine usually lasts for about an hour and then wears off. At that time, your pain will return. Improvement in pain from the cortisone injection usually takes 24 to 48 h. So, expect the pain to return after an hour and hopefully go away in 1 to 2 days.

**Rest the Area:**
Be careful with the affected area/joint. Usually, the injected medicine causes the area to feel numb. Because you may not feel pain, it is very easy to cause further injury to the area. Do not use the area for anything more than mild essential movements for the next 2 weeks.

**Watch for Infection:**
Although every precaution has been taken to prevent infection, be alert for the following signs—fever above 100°F, increased warmth in the area, redness at the injection site, redness moving up the arm or leg, and swelling of the area. If *any* of these symptoms develop, call this office immediately at (INSERT PHONE NUMBER).

**Follow the Directions of Any Checked Boxes:**

- ❑ Apply ice to the area every 4 h for 20 min at a time for _____ day(s).
- ❑ Apply a heating pad to the area every 4 h for 20 min at a time for _____ day(s).
- ❑ Apply an elastic compression wrap to the area for _____ day(s).

- ❑ Perform stretching exercises as instructed.
- ❑ Wear a splint to the area for ____ day(s).
- ❑ Physical therapy referral.
- ❑ Take the following medicines in addition to your usual medications:

______________________________________________

______________________________________________

______________________________________________

**Return to this office** in ___ day(s)/week(s) for further evaluation and management of your condition.

APPENDIX 3

# Medical Record Documentation

*The following template is an example of documentation that may be used for a knee aspiration and injection procedure. Setting this up as a text template in an electronic medical record allows the practitioner the greatest documentation flexibility to deal with the inevitable variations encountered during the procedure.*

Patient name: ________________ Date: ________

**Procedure—Knee Aspiration and Injection**
Prior to performance of the knee aspiration and injection, a discussion of this procedure and alternative treatments was conducted with the patient. Possible complications were discussed, and all questions were answered.

**Lateral Suprapatellar Approach**
After informed consent was obtained, the patient was placed in a supine position on the examination table. A point at the intersection of a line drawn vertically 1 cm above the proximal margin of the patella and a line drawn horizontally along the posterior margin of the patella was identified and marked with the retracted tip of a ballpoint pen. The lateral aspect of the knee was aseptically prepped with alcohol and 10% povidone–iodine pads. Pain Ease mist topical vapocoolant spray was used to achieve good local anesthesia.

Following the no-touch technique, a 1½ in., 25-gauge needle was inserted and directed medially. 10 mL of 1% lidocaine with epinephrine was used to adequately anesthetize the skin and deep tissues including the knee joint capsule and periosteum over the anterior aspect of the distal femur. Next, a 1½ in., 18-gauge needle was directed medially into the knee joint capsule without any pain. ____ mL of ____ fluid was removed. Finally, a mixture of 3 mL of 1% lidocaine without epinephrine and 1 mL of triamcinolone acetonide (40 mg) was injected easily into the knee joint through the same 18-gauge needle.

The needle was withdrawn. No bleeding was encountered. The injection site was covered with a sterile Band-Aid.

The patient tolerated the procedure well without complications.
The patient reported complete relief of pain within 5 min.

________________________
Signature of medical provider

# Index

Note: Page numbers followed by 't' indicate tables and those in italic denote figures.

## E



## F



## G

**L**

## M



## N



## O



## P

## T



## U



## V



## W